Core Proces
Psychodynamic

Advancing Eff

Core Processes in Brief Psychodynamic Psychotherapy
Advancing Effective Practice

Edited by

Denise P. Charman
Victoria University

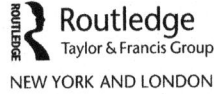
Taylor & Francis Group
NEW YORK AND LONDON

First published 2004 by Lawrence Erlbaum Associates, Inc.

This edition published 2015 by Routledge
711 Third Avenue, New York, NY 10017, USA
2 Park Square, Milton Park, Abingdon, Oxon, OX14 4RN

Routledge is an imprint of the Taylor & Francis Group, an informa business

Copyright © 2004 by Lawrence Erlbaum Associates, Inc.
All rights reserved. No part of the book may be reproduced in Any form, by photostat, microform, retrieval system, or any other means, without the prior written permission of the publisher.

ISBN 13 : 978-0-8058-4068-1 (pbk)

Cover design by Sean Trane Sciarrone

Library of Congress Cataloging-in-Publication Data

Core Processes in Brief Psychodynamic Psychotherapy: Advancing Effective Practice / Edited by Denise P. Charman.
    p. cm.
  ISBN 0-8058-4067-2 (cloth : alk. paper) – ISBN 0-8058-4068-0 (pbk. : alk paper)
    1. Brief psychotherapy. 2. Psychodynamic psychotherapy. 3. Evidence-based medicine.
  I. Charman, Denise, 1948-

RC480.55.C676 2003
616.89'14—dc21

2003040838

List of Contributors

Phillip Apostol, Center for Psychotherapy Research, Department of Psychiatry, University of Pennsylvania Health System, PA
Elizabeth G. Arnold, Private Practice, New York, NY
Ted P. Asay, Private Practice, Dallas, TX
Dawn Bennett, Clinical Psychology Service, St. Ives House, Blackburn, England
Denise P. Charman, Department of Psychology, Victoria University, Melbourne, Victoria, Australia
Paul Crits-Christoph, Center for Psychotherapy Research, University of Pennsylvania Medical Center, Philadelphia, PA
Michael Duffy, Counseling Psychology Program, Department of Educational Psychology, Texas A&M University, College Station, TX
Tracy D. Eells, Department of Psychiatry and Behavioral Sciences, University of Louisville, Louisville, KY
Barry A. Farber, Teachers College, Columbia University, New York, NY
Jackie Fosbury, The Diabetes & Endocrinology Day Centre, St Thomas' Hospital, London, England
Jesse D. Geller, Private Practice, New Haven, CT
Charles J. Gelso, Department of Psychology, University of Maryland, College Park, MD
Mary Beth Connolly Gibbons, Center for Psychotherapy Research, Department of Psychiatry, University of Pennsylvania Health System, Philadelphia, PA
Anne C. Graham, Department of Psychology, Victoria University, Melbourne, Victoria, Australia
Robert D. Hunt, Department of Psychology, Brigham Young University, Provo, UT
Anthony S. Joyce, Department of Psychiatry, University of Alberta, Edmonton, Alberta, Canada
Amelia H. Kaplan, Private Practice, Highland Park, NJ
Michael J. Lambert, Department of Psychology, Brigham Young University, Provo, UT
Robert Langs, Mount Sinai School of Medicine, New York, NY
Kenneth G. Lombart, Department of Psychological and Brain Sciences, University of Louisville, Louisville, KY

Mary McCallum, Private practice, Edmonton, Alberta, Canada

Stanley B. Messer, Graduate School of Applied and Professional Psychology, Rutgers, The State University of New Jersey, Piscataway, NJ

J. Christopher Muran, Brief Psychotherapy Research Program, Beth Israel Medical Center, New York, NY

Susan Allstetter Neufeldt, Counseling/Clinical/School Psychology Program, Graduate School of Education, University of California at Santa Barbara, Santa Barbara CA

John Ogrodniczuk, Psychiatry Department, University of British Columbia, Vancouver, BC, Canada

Glenys Parry, Community Health Sheffield NHS Trust, and University of Sheffield School of Health & Related Research, Sheffield, England

William Piper, Psychiatry Department, University of British Columbia, Vancouver, BC, Canada

Bonnie A. Rudolph, Department of Psychology and Sociology, Texas A&M International University, Laredo, TX

Jeremy D. Safran, Graduate Faculty of Political and Social Science, New School University, New York, NY

Lisa Wallner Samstag, Department of Psychology, Long Island University, Brooklyn, NY

David A. Vermeersch, Department of Psychology, Loma Linda University, Loma Linda, CA

Elizabeth R. Welfel, Counselor Education Programme, Cleveland State University, Cleveland, OH

Contents

List of Contributors	v
Preface	xi

PART I: INITIATING AND ASSESSING SUITABILITY FOR BRIEF PSYCHODYNAMIC PSYCHOTHERAPY

1. Effective Psychotherapy and Effective Psychotherapists 3
   Denise P. Charman

2. Optimizing Outcome Through Prediction and Measurement of Psychological Functioning 23
   Michael J. Lambert, Robert D. Hunt, and David A. Vermeersch

3. The First Interview 47
   Bonnie A. Rudolph

4. Assessing Patient Capacities for Therapy: Psychological-Mindedness and Quality of Object Relations 69
   Anthony S. Joyce and Mary McCallum

PART II: DETERMINING AND MAINTAINING A FOCUS

5. Outcomes and Factors Related to Efficacy of Brief Psychodynamic Therapy 103
   Stanley B. Messer and Amelia H. Kaplan

6. Case Formulation: Determining the Focus in Brief Dynamic Psychotherapy 119
   Tracy D. Eells and Kenneth G. Lombart

7. Constructing Interpretations and Assessing Their Accuracy 145
   Mary Beth Connolly Gibbons, Paul Crits-Christoph, and Phillip Apostol

8. The Evidence: Transference Interpretations and Patient Outcomes— 165
   A Comparison of "Types" of Patients
   John Ogrodniczuk and William Piper

PART III: KEEPING AN EYE ON THE RELATIONSHIP

9. Defining and Identifying Alliance Ruptures 187
   Lisa Wallner Samstag, J. Christopher Muran, and Jeremy D. Safran

10. The Power of Ground Rules 215
    Robert Langs

11. Countertransference and Its Management in Brief Dynamic Therapy 231
    Charles J. Gelso

12. Maintaining the Therapeutic Alliance: Resolving Alliance-Threatening Interactions Related to the Transference 251
    Dawn Bennett and Glenys Parry

PART IV: ENDING AND EVALUATING

13. Ending Therapy: Processes and Outcomes 275
    Denise P. Charman and Anne C. Graham

14. Termination, Posttermination, and Internalization of Therapy and the Therapist: Internal Representation and Psychotherapy Outcome 289
    Elizabeth G. Arnold, Barry A. Farber, and Jesse D. Geller

15. Measuring Clinically Significant Change 309
    Michael J. Lambert and Ted P. Asay

PART V: SPECIAL ISSUES

16. Critical Factors in Supervision: The Patient, the Therapist, and the Supervisor
    Susan Allstetter Neufeldt — 325

17. The Ethical Challenges of Brief Therapy
    Elizabeth Reynolds Welfel — 343

18. Curative Factors in Work With Older Adults
    Michael Duffy — 361

APPENDIX The Case Study: The Therapy, the Patient, and the Therapist
    Jackie Fosbury — 383

Author Index — 401
Subject Index — 415

Preface

All psychotherapy educators aspire to teach evidence-based psychotherapy. They encounter problems, not the least of which is reaching agreement about the meaning of the phrase "evidence based" (Slade & Priebe, 2001). Other problems result from the fact that to advocate one particular evidenced-based treatment over others is to ignore the reality that treatments need to be tailored to the population one is treating. The university where I teach is located in a socially and economically deprived outer metropolitan area. Our clinic patients are mainly from lower socioeconomic circumstances, often from chaotic, disorganized families and with histories of abuse and deprivation. Our clinical trainees rarely get the option of working on prescribed homogeneous disorders or with circumscribed problem behaviors.

This patient group is similar to the one that I worked with in the field prior to becoming an academic. Early in my career I had been known as a neurpsychologist and even as a behavioral psychologist. However, when I accepted a position as a child and family clinical psychologist in a community health service, I quickly found that the skills I had acquired were not sufficient and sought a theoretical framework that could adequately encompass the intergenerational and systemic issues within which I could describe the maladaptive patterns in relating that I observed in many of my patients. To improve my effectiveness, I sought further training in psychodynamic psychotherapy and family therapy, both of which provide systemic and developmental perspectives and means for conceptualizing the complex in a wide range of patients and presenting problems.

When I joined the Department of Psychology at Victoria University, the then Head of Department, Associate Professor Ross Williams, seemingly moving against the tide promoting only evidenced-based cognitive-behavioral therapies, had a vision of instruction in psychodynamic psychotherapy. I was given the task of teaching it, among other things, and was determined to do so from an evidence base. I found that this task was difficult because although the evidence appeared to be there, it was not easily accessible to staff or students. The books that were readily available included ones devoted to specific treatments for specific disorders requiring students to purchase too many texts; conceptual bases for psychotherapies too far removed from actual practice skills; manuals for practitioners written by practitioners with little evidence that their clinical wisdom was in fact wise; descriptions of different dynamic therapies that were difficult for students to translate into practice and evaluate for effectiveness; specific curative factors providing too much detail and not enough integration with practice; and techniques of psychotherapy outside any theoretical framework. These books did not satisfy my criteria for a good textbook: They were not based on a task analysis, not evidence based, or not theoretically integrated.

For teaching purposes, I had to cobble together my reports of research into a book of readings for easy access by students. This book of readings eventually developed into *Core Processes in Brief Psychodynamic Psychotherapy: Advancing Effective Practice*. This book is designed to meet the needs of those teaching, learning, and practicing psychodynamic therapy and who know that it is evidence based but find it hard to argue the case to those who are adamant that it is not. I hope as a result of this book, one of the outcomes will be that the argument for one form of therapy (as against another) will be more evenhanded.

Core Processes in Brief Psychodynamic Psychotherapy: Advancing Effective Practice emphasizes therapy as process rather than product (Charman, 2003). Yet the question remains about which "processes"? Because many students enter graduate programs with little or no psychodynamic psychotherapy experience, my view is that training needs to take a task analysis approach. In this approach, the task of therapy is divided into its various, usually sequential components or significant events, each event analyzed, taught separately, and then put together as an entire sequence. A task analysis approach is consistent with the delineation of "curative factors," that is, significant clinical events that are crucial for therapeutic change to be effective (Luborsky, Barber, & Beutler, 1993). These factors have been extensively researched.

In the context of psychodynamic psychotherapy, the tasks for the therapist are behavioral, cognitive, and affective. For example, a task analysis identifies these steps:

- Knowing what constitutes effectiveness as a therapist (cognitive).
- Conducting the first interview (behavioral).
- Forming a therapeutic relationship (cognitive-affective).
- Choosing between types of brief dynamic psychotherapies (cognitive).
- Maintaining the frame of therapy (behavioral-cognitive).

The encompassing curative factors include the following (Luborsky et al., 1993):

- Psychological health of the patient.
- Capacity of the patient for interpersonal relationships.
- The therapeutic alliance.
- Reliability and validity of dynamic formulations.
- Capacity to internalize representations of the therapist and the therapy.
- Characteristics of accurate interpretations.

By taking a task analytic approach grounded on the curative factors, *Core Processes in Brief Psychodynamic Psychotherapy* achieves a well-defined structure.

Part I focuses on the issues related to beginning brief psychodynamic psychotherapy. The first chapter summarizes concerns about establishing psychotherapy as evidence based and draws out some of the implications for training. The remaining chapters consider criteria by which patients are selected for (or excluded from) therapy. In practice, therapists rarely have the discretion to exclude suffering patients who come to them. They do, however, have the discretion to choose the type of therapy they will offer to a particular patient. The importance of prediction and measurement as a basis for informing clinical decision making, especially at intake is discussed. Skills for the first interview and evidence for them are presented. One of the therapists' tasks both during and after this first interview is to make judgments about the type of therapy to be offered. These judgments in psychodynamic work are based, in part, on the patient's psychological mindedness and quality of object relations, which play key roles in therapists' judgments about the appropriate type of therapy.

Part II discusses the focus of the work to be done in therapy. The need for a focus is first highlighted, and the variety of ways of defining a focus based on patient narratives is then reviewed. In brief work especially, the focus directs the nature of therapists' interventions. Two remaining chapters deal with constructing interpretations, assessing their accuracy, and providing evidence that accurate interpretations are related to patient outcomes.

Part III offers a more detailed examination of the relationship between therapist and patient. This part emphasizes the need for rapid establishment of a working alliance and for maintenance and monitoring of the relationship in the middle phases. Although it is now well documented that establishing an early positive alliance is related to positive outcomes (Horvath & Greenberg, 1994), for many patients and therapists the nature of the alliance can fluctuate. Indeed, some theorists say that there must be ruptures to precipitate change as and when they are successfully resolved. There are multiple ways of conceptualizing ruptures: for example, identifying misunderstandings considering therapists' actions that deviate from secure-frame therapy, or reenacting the patient's (or even the therapist's) repetitive maladaptive patterns. Chapters provide guidelines for recognizing these ruptures and restoring an effective working relationship. An important consideration is the therapist's capacity for self-reflection, that is, for monitoring countertransference and its impact on the therapy.

Part IV covers issues that are usually problematic as therapy ends. In brief therapy, of course, the end must be kept in mind from the beginning. Nevertheless, many aspects of termination in general and the last session in particular require careful consideration, as the termination experience appears to be related to patient satisfaction and outcome (Gelso & Woodhouse, 2002). Some longer term follow-up evaluations of brief psychodynamic psychotherapy have demonstrated a "sleeper effect" whereby patients continue to improve after therapy. This effect would appear to be related to the process of internalization, which needs encouragement to develop in patients. During, and especially at the end of therapy another question for therapists is whether their patients have achieved clinically significant change. One chapter provides guidelines for therapists seeking to monitor their own effectiveness.

Part V discusses issues in supervision and ethical concerns that matter deeply to educators, students, and practitioners alike. As practitioners often work with adult patients across the age range and much of the available process research focuses on young and middle-aged adults, a chapter on working with older adults has also been included in this part.

The authors are eminent psychotherapy researchers and practitioners and I am delighted that they agreed to contribute. They were recruited because of their allegiance to, or empircal work relevant to, relational models. Relational models are based on the assumption that psychological problems arise in the context of interpersonal relationships—they are the result of conflicting wishes in relation to others and need not be related to intrinsic instinctual drives such as sexual impulses or aggressive drives. I consider that the weight of evidence is in favor of therapies that emphasize interpersonal aspects of functioning.

Each author was asked to provide a "master lecture" on the designated topic, illustrated as he or she chose with case material. Because authors take a consistently relational approach, the findings are, as it were, precollated and readily accessible for the purposes of theory building. I hope that this book will facilitate the possible development of a metatheory of what makes different types of therapies, dynamic and nondynamic effective.

The authors were provided with one particular case study—that of the patient, "June." This case is described in the Appendix, which also incorporates an edited transcript of the third session, the one most often selected for psychodynamic psychotherapy research. Of course there are risks including such detail about a particular case, and these risks have been highlighted by Spence (2001). Over the years, I have read many transcripts in the course of supervision and research and listened to oral presentations by students and experienced therapists. Each one can give rise to conflicting clinical views. This may be the experience of the readers of this book and this case study. As the literature suggests, we can only look to the patient to give us feedback about our effectiveness. In the case of June, the last two sessions in particular demonstrate that the therapy was effective. Certainly the follow-up about June's level of functioning appears to support this conclusion. I encourage readers to seek and find their own responses to June's therapy and compare and contrast them with those described in this book.

I hope that this book will give pleasure to all who value psychodynamic approaches. I hope also that it will show that psychodynamic approaches and the scientist-professional model are compatible. There is a body of evidence about basic therapeutic processes, a deeper understanding of which will enhance clinical effectiveness.

ACKNOWLEDGMENTS

I thank all my patients (and clients) who have taught me so much about psychotherapy, including the multiple problems and pitfalls. I also thank my students and colleagues in the Department of Psychology where I developed my ideas for course curricula that culminated in this book. I thank Professor John Weinman in the Health Psychology Unit at United Dental and Medical Schools (as it then was) at Guy's Hospital in London who recommended me to Dr. Anthony Ryle and the Cognitive Analytic Therapy (CAT) Training Program. From there I found Jackie Fosbury who was conducting CAT with diabetes patients thereby combining both my major interests. Jackie and "June,"one of Jackie's patients, agreed to have their sessions audiotaped. I heartily thank them both. Barbara Tilden, one of my Honours in Psychology students, took on the task of mastering the English accent and transcribing the CAT therapy sessions. I thank my family, including my mother who came to live with me during the preparation of this book and helped with the myriad of little jobs to be done in editing such a book. The contributors to this book require special acknowledgment. Without them it would not have happened, but I also acknowledge their work more broadly, for their contributions to psychodynamic psychotherapy research, practice, and teaching. Last, I thank this book's publishers, Lawrence Erlbaum, Susan Milmoe, and Sondra Guideman in particular.

REFERENCES

Charman, D. (2003). Paradigms in current psychotherapy research: A critique and the case for evidence-based psychodynamic psychotherapy research. *Australian Psychologist*, *38*(1), 39-45.

Gelso, C. J., & Woodhouse, S. S. (2002). The termination of psychotherapy: What research tells us about the process of ending treatment. In G. S. Tryon (Ed.), *Counseling based on process research* (pp. 344-369). Boston: Allyn & Bacon.

Horvath, A. O., & Greenberg, L S. (Eds.). (1994). *The working alliance: Theory, research and practice*. New York: Wiley.

Luborsky, L., Barber, J. P., & Beutler, L. (1993). Introduction to special section: A briefing on curative factors in dynamic psychotherapy. *Journal of Consulting and Clinical Psychology*, *61*, 539-541.

Slade, M., & Priebe, S. (2001). Are randomized controlled trials the only gold that glitters? *British Journal of Psychiatry*, *179*, 286-287.

Spence, D. P. (2001). Dangers of anecdotal reports. *Journal of Clinical Psychology*, *57*(1), 37-41.

PART

I

INITIATING AND ASSESSING SUITABILITY FOR BRIEF PSYCHODYNAMIC PSYCHOTHERAPY

CHAPTER

1

Effective Psychotherapy and Effective Psychotherapists

Denise P. Charman
Victoria University

Psychotherapy is one of the most extensively researched treatments for mental disorders. When compared to no treatment or psychopharmacology, patient reports and comparative studies have demonstrated that psychotherapy is, in general, effective, efficient, and lasting (Asay & Lambert, 1999; Seligman, 1995). Researchers have also compared psychotherapy treatments hoping to find the most efficacious ones—a laudable undertaking. However, this undertaking has resulted in disenchantment on the part of many practitioners who feel keenly the gulf between research and practice (Talley, Strupp, & Butler, 1994). It is a paradox that efforts to demonstrate the beneficial effects of psychotherapy have led researchers to develop models and methodologies that are far removed from psychotherapy processes and practices.

The most stringent research is referred to as *efficacy research*, with the randomized controlled trial as the gold standard. Its methodology involves the comparison of manualized treatments administered by therapists who reach a criterion in competence and demonstrate satisfactory manual adherence. Treatments are delivered for a prescribed number of sessions to patients with clearly defined disorders who have been randomly allocated to treatment groups. Efficacy researchers have assumed that patients are not active in influencing outcomes, an assumption not well based (Tallman & Bohart, 1997) and now being discarded in drug trials (Bradley, 1997). Moreover, therapy in the field is not of fixed duration, is typically self-correcting rather than manualized, involves active rather than passive patients, and focuses on functioning not symptoms (Seligman, 1998).

It is not just practitioners who feel disenchantment. Researchers also appear to be frustrated because despite intense efforts, efficacy research comparing psychotherapy treatments has demonstrated that they appear to be equivalent (Stiles, Shapiro, & Elliott, 1986). Some researchers find this incredible. They believe that if efficacy research methodologies were more finely tuned, the superiority of one treatment (perhaps the one to which they have an allegiance) over another would inevitably be demonstrated and their beliefs justified (e.g., King, 1998).

Unfortunately, the response of researchers to their disenchantment, a call for even greater methodological rigor, increases practitioner disenchantment. I have referred to this as a call to "polish the gold standard" (Charman, 2003). Treatments are to be even more precisely prescribed and monitored and definitions of disorder are to be more stringent (Lampropoulos, 2000). Disorders are defined by the *Diagnostic and Statistical Manual of Mental Disorders* (4th ed.) or *International Classification of Diseases* (American Psychiatric Association, 1995), even though diagnostic categories do not capture the differences in patient dynamics within the same disorder and are generally unhelpful to psychotherapists.

Given this situation of mutual disenchantment, it is important to note that efficacy research and "efficacy-for-disorder" research (Charman, in press) have produced a number of important outcomes. For example, they have defined clearly and demonstrated as efficacious a number of empirically supported treatments (Lampropoulos, 2000; Nathan & Gorman, 1998; Roth & Fonagy, 1997) and treatment components (Beutler & Harwood, 2001) that therapists can incorporate into their psychotherapy practices. An array of treatment manuals has been produced along with measures of manual adherence and treatment competence and purity (Luborsky & Barber, 1993), which are excellent devices for training purposes.

Disenchantment with efficacy studies has led to the development of a variant approach referred to as *effectiveness research*, which focuses on the feasibility and clinical utility of psychotherapy treatments in the real world (Seligman, 1995). Support for effectiveness research can be seen in the advocacy for the Public Health Model by the National Institute for Mental Health (NIMH) (Niederehe, Street, & Lebowitz, 1999). This advocacy is heartening to practitioners, although they may still feel that even this model is more of the same, especially because there are moves to find a gold standard effectiveness methodology (e.g., Marginson et al., 2000).

Effectiveness research is packaged in an individualized form as the "patient-focused approach" advocated by Howard and his colleagues (e.g., Howard, Moras, Brill, Martinovich, & Lutz, 1996). This approach provides practitioners with a method to monitor the progress of their own patients by collecting data from each patient, which are mapped as an individualized patient recovery curve. Any patient curve can then be statistically compared with normed curves to determine if clinically meaningful change has occurred. It is essentially a case-based quality assurance system (Beutler, 2001) that addresses the question, "Is this patient's condition responding to the treatment that is being applied?" (Howard et al., 1996, p. 1060). The approach can signal when a patient is not improving sufficiently, enabling the therapist to adjust treatment. However, if practitioners find that they are less effective than desired, the patient-focused approach does not, as yet anyway, provide insight as to how they might adjust their treatment, as it does not monitor within-session events and is not related to psychotherapy theory.

TREATMENT RESEARCH IDENTIFIES EFFICACIOUS AND EFFECTIVE THERAPISTS

The relation between treatment research and real-world psychotherapy is not as dichotomized as the previous section implies. In the course of efficacy studies, researchers have identified efficacious therapists. Their findings prompt a revision of the research question away from which therapy is more efficacious to which therapist is. For example, researchers in the NIMH's Treatment of Depression Collaborative Research Program (TDRCP) generated therapeutic efficacy scores for all TDRCP therapists and reanalyzed their data (Blatt, Sanislow, Zuroff, & Pilkonis, 1996). The most efficacious therapists had patients improve significantly more, had less variability in patient outcomes, and had stronger alliances as perceived by patients. Alliance is considered a common factor across therapies. Efficacious therapists were not significantly different from less efficacious therapists on demographics or level of clinical experience.

Significantly, the two most efficacious therapists (from the placebo and imipramine treatments plus clinical management; Blatt et al., 1996) were providing treatments consistent with their preferred mode of working. This is what happens in the real world of psychotherapy: Psychotherapists opt to train in therapies of their own choosing and generally train for effectiveness in their preferred field. This finding highlights an important shortcoming in research methodologies. Therapists in research studies are not randomly allocated to treatment groups (only patients) and are often recruited to deliver a particular treatment via a process of self-selection, treatment preferences, and predisposing personal characteristics. The predilections of the therapist toward the therapy has been referred to as "therapy allegiance" by Wampold (2001), who suggested that this is another common factor across therapies.

Peer Identification of Effective Therapists

Recruitment processes for research therapists have often obliged peers or supervisors to nominate "good" therapists. Yet, it has been a consistent finding that when such good therapists were compared, their patient outcomes have shown great variability (e.g., Goldfried, Raue, & Castonguay, 1998; Masterton, Tolpin, & Sifneos, 1991). However, despite the apparent invalidity of their ratings of effectiveness, peer and supervisor ratings continue to be valued. Therefore, it is important to understand the bases for these ratings.

A pilot study consisting of a telephone survey ($n = 15$) of psychotherapists listed in the business telephone book sheds some light. Eighty percent of therapist respondents were psychodynamic in orientation and had at least six years experience. Respondents were asked, "In your opinion, what makes for a good psychotherapist?" The adjectives that respondents gave were categorized into dimensions, which were then ordered according to the number of respondents providing adjectives related to that dimension. The three most salient dimensions were, in order, personal qualities, interpersonal qualities, and training (equal to interpersonal qualities).

Respondents in the telephone survey described personal qualities using words and phrases such as "mindfulness," "not having an agenda," "concern for others," "intelligent," "not a rigid personality structure," "sense of self," "intuitive," "self-aware," "thoughtful," "knows own issues," "able to take care of self," "heart is able to be open," "patience," "creative," and "able to separate." These descriptive words convey a sense of *self-relatedness*. Therapist self-relatedness is the "interactive self-experience" with "self-awareness, self-control, self-esteem, and so forth, being manifested clinically in varying degrees of openness versus defensiveness" (Orlinsky, 1994, p. 105). No respondent used descriptors relating to suffering and survival, although earlier in human history and in some indigenous communities today suffering and survival have been significant life experience qualifications for shamans (Ellenberger, 1983). Indeed, psychotherapists, especially those who choose a psychodynamic orientation have been found likely to come from dysfunctional families (Halgin & Murphy, 1991).

Interpersonal qualities were indicated by respondents' use of words and phrases such as "listening," "responding," "having empathy," "an accepting presence," "being authentic," "genuine," "in tune," "trust in the inherent qualities of the other," and "available to the patient." *Interpersonal aspects* "reflect joint contributions to the global quality and atmosphere of the emergent dyadic/group process ... characterized in particular by varying levels of therapeutic teamwork" (Orlinsky, 1994, p. 105). The therapist respondents in the telephone survey did not use descriptive words available within their theoretical (psychodynamic) framework such as containment nor did they take into account the need to tailor technique according to the type of patient. For example, for a patient with paranoia, warmth, caring, and empathy may exacerbate the paranoia (Mohr, 1995).

Thus, the telephone survey confirmed that peers rely on assessment of personal and interpersonal qualities to assess effectiveness. The results were remarkably consistent in this small sample; therefore, a larger number of respondents may not alter the findings. However, on scrutiny, these nominated qualities are idealized and limited, for example by not being based on their personal experience as survivors or as having the ability to modify technique based on patient characteristics. Therefore, to the extent that peer ratings of therapist effectiveness are based on global judgments of personal and interpersonal qualities, it is little wonder that many studies have had mixed results in relating peer ratings to patient outcomes. Indeed, effectiveness as assessed by ratings by supervisors and peers have been found to be not consistent among each other (Najavits & Strupp, 1994), not reach significance (Luborsky, McLellan, Diguer, Woody, & Seligman, 1997), and not to be reliable (Lambert & Okiishi, 1997).

The ways in which personal and interpersonal qualities are related or unrelated to effectiveness have been addressed in a limited number of empirical studies. One of the earliest studies was conducted by Ricks (1974). It was a follow-up study of distressed male adolescents who had been seen by either Therapist A or Therapist B. When the adult clinical status of the patients was examined, both therapists were found to have been effective with less distressed patients. However, with very distressed patients Ricks found differential effectiveness related to personal and interpersonal qualities of the therapists. Therapist A, the "supershrink," had invested more time, made use of resources outside of therapy, was firm and direct with parents of the boys, encouraged moves to autonomy, implemented problem solving, was more consistent, and had strong alliances (Najavits & Strupp, 1994). That is, the supershrink had effective interpersonal qualities. On the other hand, Therapist B, the "subshrink," had invested less time, withdrew from the boys, was frightened of pathology, seemed to become depressed with difficult cases, and was hopeless about outcomes (Najavits & Strupp, 1994). In short, the subshrink had poor personal qualities. It appears that high and low therapist effectiveness may have different predictors, with poor therapist personal qualities associated with poor patient outcomes and good therapist interpersonal qualities with good patient outcomes.

The most effective therapists in the Najavits and Strupp (1994) study were distinguished from least effective therapists in that they had positive qualities of warmth, affirmation, understanding, helping, and protecting. The most effective therapists had few actively negative qualities and were more self-critical. Less effective therapists in the Najavits and Strupp study were more actively hostile (Najavits & Strupp, 1994), had hostile introjects, or were high on scales of dissaffiliativeness (Hilliard, Henry, & Strupp, 2000). That is, less effective therapists had controlling and hostile views of themselves, which were related to engaging in more patient interactions that were more hostile, were less prone to grant friendly autonomy, and gave mixed messages that were simultaneously affiliative and hostile (Henry, Schacht, & Strupp, 1990; Strupp, 1993).

Thus, the therapist's (not just the patient's) capacity to relate is very important for patient outcome (Hilliard et al., 2000; Luborksy, Barber, & Crits-Christoph, 1999). Hostility in the therapist denies patients the opportunity to attain the hopefulness that therapy will be helpful (Snyder, Michael, & Cheavers, 1999) and achieve remoralization (Howard, Orlinsky, & Lueger, 1994). The two maxims of "do no harm" and "instill hope" have been given vital new tighter meanings based on research findings.

Lafferty, Beutler, and Crago (1989) found that the least effective psychotherapists (of 30 trainees) had less empathy and valued comfort, stimulation, and intellectual goals more than effective therapists did. These personal qualities, however, can make for success as a student and as an academic. There lies a conundrum in the identification of effective therapists by academic psychotherapists.

The previously mentioned studies support the call by Stein and Lambert (1995) for graduate programs to emphasize personal qualities of trainees in selection. This is especially important because Hilliard et al. (2000) found that extensive training in psychodynamic psychotherapy was not adequate in correcting the impact of therapists' own interpersonal histories on their psychotherapeutic work. Such findings confirm Strupp's (1976) early call for psychodynamic psychotherapy research and psychotherapy training research to be interdependent. There are research opportunities here on the relation between selection, effectiveness, and personal and interpersonal qualities, especially with the development of circumplex models, for example Structural Analysis of Sequential Behavior (Benjamin, 1996), Millon Personality Model (Muran, Samstag, Jilton, Batchelder, & Winston, 1997), and Inventory of Interpersonal Problems (Horowitz, Rosenberg, & Bartholomew, 1993). An alternative to good selection process is to mandate personal psychotherapy as a component of training. However, this alternative does not seem ethical at this time because positive psychotherapy outcomes cannot be guaranteed (Mohr, 1995).

Effectiveness Defined as Patient Outcomes

Because peer and supervisor reports are not reliable and valid assessments of therapist effectiveness, effectiveness needs to be defined in alternative ways. It is likely that these alternatives will be based on work samples

(Luborsky et al., 1997) and criteria for assessing work samples based on patient outcomes (e.g., Lueger et al., 2001).

Interestingly, changes in patient status as an outcome of psychotherapy are not usually measured by changes in diagnosis. Patient outcome is a complex, multidimensional construct that has been operationally defined in multifarious ways. Examples include measures of symptomology, interpersonal functioning, social role performance, and specific treatment targets such as cognitions, behavior, affect, or physiological arousal (Docherty & Streeter, 1993). Patient outcomes assessed at the end of therapy with multiple measures have consistently revealed inconsistent results across those measures even in the same study, with some measures showing improvement and others not. This creates a confusing picture (Elkin, 1994; Hilliard et al., 2000).

This confusion may be due to the lack of an apparent theoretical rationale for the selection of outcome measures. Howard and his colleagues (Howard, Moras, Brill, Martinovich, & Lutz, 1996; Howard, Orlinsky, & Lueger, 1994) in their phase model have provided a theoretical rationale. This model has not yet been widely adopted. However, it does indicate that the nature of any expected beneficial outcome would be related to the phase of treatment that the patient has completed. Sequential improvement in outcomes would be expected, first in subjective well-being such as fulfilled expectations or increased hope (remoralization), then symptom reduction (remediation), and finally recovery of life functioning (rehabilitation; Orlinsky, 1994). This model implies that phase-related outcome measures should be assessed throughout treatment and clinically meaningful change monitored according to the expected phase-related changes. It is unknown if this order of recovery always applies. Sometimes the patient may show improvement in functioning before subjective well-being.

The confusing picture is also related to outcome measures varying according to vantage point: that is, whether it is the patient, observer, or therapist doing the rating. However, from alliance studies patient self-reports appear to be the best predictors of patient outcomes (Horvath & Greenberg, 1994). After all, it is the patient who needs to experience the outcome.

Confusion abounds for other reasons, which are related to the timing of the measurement of therapy outcomes. End-of-therapy assessment may indicate that some therapies seem unproductive, but these therapies may have latent effects (demonstrated at follow-up). Moreover, immediate effects of other therapies may later dissipate (Docherty & Streeter, 1993). Therefore, it is important in research to have follow-up assessment of therapy outcomes. However, this type of follow-up has usually been considered by psychotherapists as contrary to psychotherapy best practice because it intrudes on the patient.

Effectiveness Defined as Patient Dropout

Another alternative conceptualization of therapist effectiveness is patient dropout rate in which the number of sessions attended is contrasted with the number of sessions planned. If less sessions are attended, the therapist is considered not to have maintained the patient in needed treatment. However, it is equally as likely that patients have dropped out for positive reasons as for negative reasons. Patients may have had their initially low expectations fulfilled and their symptoms improved (Warner et al., 2001). They may have "fled into health" (Malan, 1993). Howard et al. (1996) showed that by the eighth session, approximately 50% of patients had shown measurable improvement. Similarly, in a meta-analysis of the value of psychotherapy, Smith, Glass, and Miller (1980) showed that positive impacts occurred in the first 6 to 8 sessions. Moreover, from a health economics perspective, fewer sessions is surely a sign of effectiveness! The figure of 6 to 8 sessions is not magical because as Lambert, Hansen, and Finch (2001) reported, their more distressed samples took 10, 13, or more sessions to show a 50% recovery rate. Thus, to be effective with more distressed patients, therapists do need to be able to maintain their patients in therapy for more sessions.

Of course, patients do drop out for negative reasons and the proportions of patients who drop out can depend on the effectiveness of the therapist. If we accept Howard's (Howard et al., 1994) figures, then by the eighth session, 50% of patients have improved, but 50% of those who have stayed that long have not improved. Of course, the staying patients may or may not have deteriorated (Beutler, 2001) and not deteriorating can be a beneficial outcome. If the patient has not improved, the treating therapist may be ineffective, but curiously the patient has remained in therapy. Thus, for any given therapist, the patients who continue in treatment and indeed who remain in research studies long enough to complete outcome measures may be quite different from those who have left prematurely (Stein & Lambert, 1995).

Therefore, if we assess therapist effectiveness by dropout rate, we really need to understand the reasons patients give at the time of dropping out and we need to assess whether gains have been made or not. That is, dropout rate by itself is an ambiguous sign and should not be used as a sole outcome measure.

Variability in Effectiveness

In studies using patient outcomes as measures of therapist effectiveness, research therapists have shown variability in their outcomes. Variability has ranged from improvement for most if not all patients to less than chance. For example, Luborsky et al. (1997) found that for 22 therapists, the range of percentage improvement was from "slightly negative" to "slightly more than 80% improvement" (p. 60). Orlinsky and Howard (1980) studied 23 therapists and found that 25% ($n = 6$) were effective in that 70% of their patients improved and less than 10% deteriorated. The least effective therapists had beneficial results with less than 50% (44%) of patients. The less effective therapists also had at least 10% negative effects, which may actually be a conservative figure based on the review by Mohr (1995).

There is a broad range of reasons that may account for variability in effectiveness. For example, effectiveness may vary according to type of patient (Zuroff et al., 2000), type of disorder (Luborsky et al., 1997), pretreatment functioning (Lambert et al., 2001), gender (Barkham et al., 2001), whether the therapist is working in his or her preferred orientation (Elkin, 1994), and level of experience (Stein & Lambert, 1995). Effectiveness may also depend on the type of workplace where, of course, therapists are selected for employment according to employment criteria. Stein and Lambert (1995) noted in their review a study that found no outcome differences in therapists of different levels of training in university counseling centers, but differences were found in community mental health services in which less trained therapists had much higher premature dropout rates. Lambert et al. (2001) noted that treatment sites had significantly different survival curves depicting patient outcome changes over time. These findings imply that psychotherapy trainers may need to anticipate patient and situational factors that their trainees will have to deal with postgraduation and adjust their curricula accordingly.

EFFECTIVENESS AND TRAINING

Training and effectiveness have always been associated in practitioners' minds; however, early research reviews showed little correspondence (Smith, Glass, & Miller, 1980). This bleak conclusion has been popularized (e.g., S. Miller, personal communication, July 3, 2000). Stein and Lambert (1995) proffered one explanation for findings of equivalence. They argued that less trained therapists have a higher dropout rate, which can distort research producing findings of equivalent effectiveness, as the proportion of patients who complete therapy with good outcomes is less for less trained therapists than the proportion for more trained therapists. Even if the bleak conclusion was true, because of pressures for legal, financial, and therapeutic accountability, learning only as part of an apprenticeship or with a mentor or supervisor is no longer satisfactory, even though it is an important component of ensuring one's effectiveness (Halgin & Murphy, 1991).

However, the conclusion that there is no relation between training and effectiveness is not true. Researchers know from experience and research that there is an association between training and effectiveness. Training is essential to methodically transmit the knowledge and skills required for practicing. Training is especially important in brief work because psychotherapists need to be able to think and act in short time frames for the benefit of their patients. Stein and Lambert (1995) in their extensive review of the research, concluded, "it is clear that a modest but fairly consistent treatment effect size is associated with training level for a number of measures of patient improvement" (p. 192). The relation between training and effectiveness is depicted in Table 1.1.

Less trained, lay, or nonprofessional therapists are effective in behavior therapy and counseling (Stein & Lambert, 1995). They have more difficulty with time intensive and complex forms of therapy. Therapists with more training are more effective with patients across the age range, with bigger caseloads and do better with brief treatments and in psychodynamic work. They also do better in marital work.

Less effective therapists are limited in the range of patients they can deal with (Orlinsky & Howard, 1980). The range does not appear to be determined by disorder or life problem but rather by the quantity of distress

TABLE 1.1
A Model of Effectiveness and Training and Patient Type

Effectiveness	High Training Levels[a]	Low Training Levels
High	Patients with complex presentations, serious and difficult problems	Restricted range of patients, problems and personality styles[b]
	Psychotic patients who receive non-behavioral therapies[d]	Target problems[c]
	Over-control problems[e]	Younger age groups[b]
	All age groups	Simple counseling
	Long-term work (>15 sessions)	Specific behavior therapy
	Psychodynamic therapy	
	Brief treatments	
	Marital therapy	
Low	Therapists able to develop strong alliances but show poor outcome[g,h]	Patients similar to therapists[f]
	Therapists with admired personal and interpersonal qualities but may not adjust their mode of working to match the patient	Less distressed patients
	Less distressed patients	

[a]Training is associated with greater life experience and more psychotherapy experience. [b]Stein and Lambert (1995). [c]Shapiro, Firth-Cozens, and Stiles (1989). [d]Smith, Glass, and Miller (1980). [e]Outcome and level of training are not related for under-control problems such as aggression and impulsivity (Stein & Lambert, 1995). [f]Orlinsky and Howard (1980). [g]Najavits and Strupp (1994). [h]Horvath, Gaston, and Luborsky (1993).

and complexity of the presentation in the patient (Luborsky et al., 1997). Research has shown that less effective therapists can be effective when their patients are less distressed (Elkin, 1994; Ricks, 1974). This relation between effectiveness and training confirms the practice of adopting a triage model of allocating patients to trainees according to their perceived capacity to manage patient distress.

One of the observations of less effective therapists is that they may be able to form positive alliances, but alliance can fail to predict positive outcomes (Horvath, Gaston, & Luborsky, 1993). For example, in one research study (Najavits & Strupp, 1994), the therapist who obtained the highest alliance score was one of the less effective therapists, having at least two patients leave treatment early and at least one negative outcome case. Najavits and Strupp explained this by noting that on occasion less effective therapists may compensate by developing a style that is superficially therapeutic. Another feature noted in less effective therapists is that they have been found to rate patients as more involved and themselves as more supportive than did therapists who were more effective. This less critical stance in relation to themselves is consistent with Mohr's (1995) observation that therapists can overestimate their own effectiveness.

Thus, the challenge to higher education training institutions is to select personally and interpersonally talented graduates who can adjust their own processes in response to the patient that they have and who can learn to be highly effective with patients who are more distressed or who have complex presentations. In a comparison of cognitive-behavioral therapy and psychodynamic-interpersonal therapy, the results support equivalence between treatments; however, cognitive-behavioral therapy appeared to be better able to effect change in clients with well-assimilated problems (Hardy, Shapiro, Stiles, & Barkham, 1998). For all clients, therapy was more effective when the individual needs of the clients were responded to flexibly. As both treatments in the Sheffield Psychotherapy Research Projects were delivered by the same therapists, crossover effects were likely in that "PI [psychodynamic-interpersonal] procedures aimed at maintaining the therapeutic alliance and dealing with affect may be 'borrowed' by CB [cognitive-behavioral] therapies as part of the collaborative approach" (Hardy et al., 1998, p. 188). For example, we know that patients with low quality of object relations require supportive therapies, but even then outcomes are not guaranteed (Piper et al., 1999). Clearly, therapy research and training research need to combine to develop effective ways and means of working with patients with low quality of object relations to produce effective outcomes. This is especially important because many more such patients are presenting to public mental health clinics and are characteristic of today's clinical population.

Training and Manuals

The preponderance of manuals now available would seem to indicate that they become the basis of training in graduate programs. Manuals are appealing because they are readily available, targeted at specific populations, and designed to ensure cohesiveness of treatment approach. The Vanderbilt II studies (Strupp, 1993) found that manuals helped trainees acquire prescribed techniques, reduced their variability in effectiveness, and resulted in improvement to their interviewing styles. However, training may not show immediate outcomes in terms of effectiveness with patients. The issues here parallel those for determining effectiveness of therapy by examining patient outcomes. Therapists have been shown to have decreased performance immediately after training (Najavits & Strupp, 1994), although one might expect a latency effect such that trainees would continue to improve as they internalize and consolidate their knowledge and skills.

Unfortunately, manuals do not guarantee effectiveness (Elkin, 1994). This has been shown in efficacy studies in which all research therapists undertook significant training as part of their preparation for the randomized controlled trials (Blatt et al., 1996; Crits-Christoph et al., 1991). In the event they still demonstrated differential effectiveness, which was not the result of level of manual adherence or treatment competence. The downside of manual use is that therapists can adhere too little in their actual practice or can adhere too much and lose their flexibility. Greater adherence has also been related to therapist hostility (Strupp, 1993). In addition, training from manuals, even when that training emphasized ongoing therapeutic transactions, is not adequate in correcting the impact of therapists' own interpersonal histories on their psychotherapeutic work (Hilliard et al., 2000).

There are other nonspecific factors impinging on effectiveness over and above the competent use of a manual. The question is because most available manuals presume that trainees are already trained in the fundamentals of psychotherapy (Butler & Strupp, 1993), how are the fundamentals and the nonspecific factors to be taught to ensure effectiveness with patients?

SEEKING AN EVIDENCE BASE FOR PSYCHOTHERAPY PRACTICE

Psychotherapy is defined as "an interpersonal *process* [italics added] designed to bring about modifications of feelings, cognitions, attitudes and behavior which have proved troublesome to the person seeking help from a trained professional" (Strupp, 1976, p. 3). An alternative definition is that psychotherapy is "a planned, emotionally charged confiding *interaction* [italics added] between a trained, socially sanctioned healer and a sufferer" (Frank, 1982, as cited in Halgin & Murphy, 1995, p. 437). Both of these definitions emphasize the interaction or process dimensions of psychotherapy. Therefore, it is logical to teach psychotherapy as a process. This can be consistent with the mantra to teach evidence-based therapies because there is a large body of process research that provides an evidence base.

Process research has differed from the previously discussed models of research. It generally has special methodological features because it "addresses questions pertaining to the mechanisms of change of therapy and what transpires between therapist and patient and the impact of intervening events on the moment-to-moment or interim changes during treatment" (Kazdin, 1991, p. 297). It identifies critical and active ingredients (Hayes, Castonguay, & Goldfried, 1996), which are then related to patient outcomes both within the session and at the end of therapy.

There has been debate about what constitutes good process research. One argument is about the conceptual basis with some advocating a nontheoretical stance or discovery-oriented approach to develop theory that is pantheoretical (Hill, 1990). Others argue that it should not be driven by what can appear to be arbitrary personal interests (Garfield, 1990; Hayes et al., 1996; Stiles & Shapiro, 1994) or by superficial eclecticism (Orlinsky & Russell, 1990). Why ignore the discovery-oriented results of the past 100 years or more? It has been argued elsewhere in psychology that research should be based in theory. Similarly, process research should be based in theory (Hayes et al., 1996; Luborsky et al., 1999).

Theory-driven process research is already available within psychodynamic psychotherapy research. Psychodynamic psychotherapy is uniquely placed with a long tradition of understanding and working with complex and difficult patients. Its aim is to "focus on achieving understanding of *intentionality* (motivation) from the point of view of the patient" (Luborksy et al., 1999, p. 281). Moreover, most therapists practice psychodynamic psychotherapy with residents in general psychiatry training programs, mostly (67%) conducting brief and short-term psychodynamic psychotherapy (Tasman, 1993).

Psychodynamic Psychotherapy Empiricism and Research

It has to be acknowledged that psychodynamic and psychoanalytic empiricism and research have a proud but not flawless tradition. Empiricism in psychodynamic psychotherapy is centered on clinical data with a reliance on the use of case reports and case studies. These reports and case studies are often imbued with clinical intuition and clinical beliefs, one of which is that talented and trained practitioners can recognize psychic phenomena, for example, Klein's (1975) paranoid-schizoid position and the depressive position. However, as Wallerstein (1993) stated, skilled practitioners can construct differing but equally plausible and compelling formulations and have no way of testing the alternatives; when testing has been attempted, expert practitioners have not agreed on core conflicts (Malan, 1993).

These problems of lack of reliability and questionable validity in clinical empiricism are not necessarily unremediable. One of the first psychotherapists to put psychoanalysis on a consistently empirical footing was Robert Langs who tightly operationalized his clinical judgment and developed means for validating interventions moment by moment (Langs, 1988). Validation comes from examining how the patient responds to each therapist intervention. This method is contrasted with the practice of therapists silently validating their proposed intervention by weighing the evidence for and against it before they have intervened (Dorpat, 1994). Thus, empiricism can be more rigorous by examining in-session events and patient in-session responses (outcomes). Indeed, empiricism based on case studies methodology has become more rigorous in recent years and more formalized as a credible research methodology, with advice being offered to clinicians from writers such as Spence (1993) and Fonagy and Moran (1993). There are also journals devoted to case study research, a range of qualitative methodologies and computerized methods of analysis of interview transcripts and narratives.

As for psychodynamic research (as distinct from psychodynamic empiricism), there has been some defensiveness about psychodynamic psychotherapy's underresearched status (e.g., Barber & Crits-Christoph, 1995), even though it is considered "probably efficacious" as an empirically validated treatment (Roth and Fonagy, 1997). However, Roth and Fonagy noted that the absence of evidence for efficacy is not evidence of ineffectiveness. In one way, this seems to be an appeal for evenhandedness in the debate. Psychodynamic psychotherapy researchers generally have had little faith in randomized controlled trials to determine the truth about efficaciousness of treatments. Yet they have often been urged to demonstrate the efficacy of their therapy using these very methods (Bohart, 2000). The resolution of the tensions will be based around a review of the nature of evidence. The myth that psychodynamic psychotherapy is not evidence based is belied in the finding that 18 out of 40 psychotherapy research programs have been devoted to dynamically oriented psychotherapy research (Beutler & Crago, 1991). Even if the myth was true, most psychodynamic psychotherapy practitioners and researchers have not appeared to be troubled by this state of affairs. In fact, most psychodynamic practitioners and researchers have appeared to sidestep the entire debate about evidence-based treatments. Having waited this long, their stance seems to have merit, as there appears to be renewed interest in theory-driven process empiricism and research.

Psychodynamic Psychotherapy Process Research

There is a myriad of theoretical positions under the rubric of psychodynamic psychotherapy, but overall they can be roughly categorized into two models. The first is the drive/structural model, which is definitely an intrapsychic model with an emphasis on the mental life within the individual patient. It views the mind as dynamic with inherent drives and "body-based, constitutionally wired fantasies" (Mitchell, 2000, p. x). This model has recently been associated with Malan, Davanloo, and Sifneos (see Messer & Warren, 1995). The second is object relations or the relational model with a focus on the nature of human relatedness and emotional bonds with significant others—objects. Mental life involves the internal mental representations of objects or aspects of objects and not real persons. Relational therapies also emphasize the establishment of safety and the preservation of the self before any attempt to analyze more complex themes. A third model is based on interpersonal theory of actual relationships or actual transactions between people and is associated with Sullivan (1953). In recent times, interpersonal and relational models have become interwoven (Mitchell, 2000). Both models require reliable and valid methods of depicting the relevant patient psychodynamics for use in research and clinical application. The importance of doing so and the related clinical and research issues are considered in this book by referring to the interpersonal or relational model in particular.

One method of operationally defining relationship patterns is the Core Conflictual Relationship Theme method (CCRT; Luborsky & Crits-Christoph, 1998). In this method, interview transcripts are examined to identify relationship episodes. Episode themes are then decoded to identify the patient's inherent wishes (W), their perceived responses of the other (RO; person in the episode) and responses of the self to the other (RS). Luborsky and Crits-Christoph (1998) classified ROs and RSs as either being positive or negative. A negative response is defined as one where the patient perceives interference with satisfaction of their wishes has occurred or is expected to occur. A positive response is one in which there is no actual or expected interference with the satisfaction of wishes or there is a sense of mastery in being able to deal with personal wishes. CCRT has been shown to be reliable and valid (Barber & Crits-Christoph, 1993), even though studies have been based on relatively small sample sizes. However, each patient in each sample has generated about four complete relationship episodes per session transcript.

These interactional patterns have been evident in patient narratives about their therapists. That is, the CCRT method has been applied to formulate the interactional relationship between therapist and patient—that is, the patient transference (Fried, Crit-Christoph, & Luborsky, 1998). Moreover, the relationship patterns evident with the therapist were similar to those described by the patient with other people. This adds support to an assumption within object relations that relationships are patterns of interaction that are repetitive and are reenacted in therapy relationships.

As yet, it remains unclear how these narrative-derived CCRTs about the therapist are related to the therapeutic alliance as measured by patient self-report. Research has consistently shown that alliance is significant and accounts for more variance in patient outcome than treatment (Asay & Lambert, 1999). The quality of the alliance between patient and therapist, especially the patient's perspective of that alliance, has been shown to be related to patient outcome (Horvath & Greenberg, 1994). However, measures of alliance as standardized paper-and-pencil indexes are generally unable to depict the idiosyncratic interactional patterns that unfold between patient and therapist. The measures do not inform clinicians about what to expect to be manifested in the relationship or how to recognize ruptures in the alliance. This is an area in which methods to depict the interactional patterns can complement and help interpret measures of the alliance.

Another key feature of relational therapy is the assessment of the patient's capacity for object relations. This capacity has been evaluated in clinical settings by determining if the patient has had at least one continuous supporting relationship and the nature of that relationship. Piper and his colleagues (Piper et al., 1999; Piper & Duncan, 1999) demonstrated that this capacity can be reliably and validly measured and found that it is related to patient outcome. A further key feature of relational therapy is to consider the capacity of the therapist to respond to the patient, that is, to monitor the therapist's own quality of object relations. Therapists' own characteristic interactional patterns require some understanding, as these can affect their capacity to form positive alliances with patients and the accuracy of their perceptions of these alliances. For example, research has shown that therapists' poor ratings of alliance early in therapy are related to poor patient outcomes. However, the reasons for this finding remain obscure, although therapists' views of process (alliance is one example) have been found to be significantly related to their personal history (Hilliard et al., 2000).

Clearly more needs to be understood about the origins of poor alliance and its relation to interactional patterns between patient and therapist. Developments in research based on relational models of psychodynamic psychotherapy offer great potential in elucidating the relevant dynamics.

In summary, psychotherapy researchers need to return to an appreciation of psychotherapy as a set of processes involving two people. Theory-driven research and teaching facilitate a coherent approach to studying and learning them. Relational therapy has been shown to be effective and its processes have been subjected to much empirical scrutiny. Whatever one's theoretical allegiance, an understanding of the psychodynamics of interactions can contribute to effectiveness, especially in relation to the alliance.

REFERENCES

American Psychiatric Association. (1995). *Diagnostic and statistical manual of mental disorders: DSM-IV: International version with ICD-10 codes* (4th ed.). Washington, DC: Author.
Asay, T., & Lambert, M. (1999). The empirical case for the common factors. In B. L. Duncan, M. A. Hubble, & S. D. Miller (Eds.), *The heart & soul of change: What works in therapy* (pp. 23–55). Washington, DC: American Psychological Association.
Barber, J. P., & Crits-Christoph, P. (1995). *Dynamic therapies for psychiatric disorders (Axis I)*. New York: Basic Books.
Barkham, M., Marginson, F., Leach, C., Lucock, M., Mellor-Clark, J., Evans, C., Benson, L., Connell, J., Audin, K., & McGrath, G. (2001). Service profiling and outcomes benchmarking using the CORE-OM: Toward practice-based evidence in the psychological therapies. *Journal of Consulting and Clinical Psychology, 69,* 184–196.
Benjamin, L. S. (1996). Introduction to the special section on Structural Analysis of Social Behavior. *Journal of Consulting and Clinical Psychology, 64,* 1203–1212.
Beutler, L. E. (2001). Comparisons among quality assurance systems: From outcome assessment to clinical utility. *Journal of Consulting and Clinical Psychology, 69,* 197–204.
Beutler, L. E., & Crago, M. (Eds.). (1991). *Psychotherapy research: An international review of programmatic studies.* Washington, DC: American Psychological Association.
Beutler, L. E., & Harwood, T. M. (2001). Antiscientific attitudes: What happens when scientists are unscientific? *Journal of Clinical Psychology, 57,* 43–51.
Blatt, S. J., Sanislow, C. A., Zuroff, D. C., & Pilkonis, P. A. (1996). Characteristics of effective therapists: Further analyses of data from the National Institute of Mental Health treatment of depression collaborative research program. *Journal of Consulting and Clinical Psychology, 64,* 1276–1284.
Bohart, A. C. (2000). Paradigm clash: Empirically supported treatments versus empirically supported empirical practice. *Psychotherapy Research, 10,* 488–493.
Bradley, C. (1997). Psychological issues in clinical trial design. *The Irish Journal of Psychology, 18,* 67–87.
Butler, S. F., & Strupp, H. H. (1993). Effects of training experienced dynamic therapists to use a psychotherapy manual. In N. E. Miller, L. Luborsky, J. P. Barber, & J. P. Docherty (Eds.), *Psychodynamic treatment research: A handbook for clinical practice* (pp. 191–210). New York: Basic Books.
Charman, D. P. (2003). Paradigms in current psychotherapy research: A critique and the case for evidence-based psychodynamic psychotherapy. *Australian Psychologist, 38*(1), 39–45.
Crits-Christoph, P., Baranackie, K., Kurcias, J. S., & Beck, A. T. (1991). Meta-analysis of therapist effects in psychotherapy outcome studies. *Psychotherapy Research, 1*(2), 81–91.
Docherty, J. P., & Streeter, M. J. (1993). Progress and limitations in psychotherapy research: A focus on depression. *Journal of Psychotherapy Practice and Research, 2,* 100–118.
Dorpat, T. (1994). Foreword. In R. Langs (Ed.), *Doing supervision and being supervised* (pp. vii–xii). London: Karnac Books.
Elkin, I. (1994). The NIMH Treatment depression collaborative research program: Where we began and where we are. In A. E. Bergin & S. L. Garfield (Eds.), *Handbook of psychotherapy and behavior change* (4th ed., pp. 114–139). New York: Wiley.

Ellenberger, H. F. (1983). *The discovery of the unconscious: The history and evolution of dynamic psychiatry.* New York: Basic Books.
Fonagy, P., & Moran, G. (1993). Selecting single case research designs for practitioners. In N. E. Miller, L. Luborsky, J. P. Barber, & J. P. Docherty (Eds.), *Psychodynamic treatment research: A handbook for clinical practice* (pp. 62–95). New York: Basic Books.
Fried, D., Crits-Christoph, P., & Luborsky, L. (1998). The parallel of the CCRT for the therapists with the CCRT for other people. In L. Luborsky & P. Crits-Christoph (Eds.), *Understanding transference: The core conflictual relationship theme method* (2nd ed., pp. 165–174). Washington, DC: American Psychological Association.
Garfield, S. L. (1990). Issues and methods in psychotherapy process research. *Journal of Consulting and Clinical Psychology, 58,* 273–280.
Goldfried, M. R., Raue, P. J., & Castonguay, L. G. (1998). The therapeutic focus in significant sessions of master therapists: A comparison of cognitive-behavioral and psychodynamic-interpersonal interventions. *Journal of Consulting and Clinical Psychology, 66,* 803–810.
Halgin, R. P., & Murphy, R. A. (1995). Issues in the training of psychotherapists. In B. M. Bongar & L. E. Beutler (Eds.), *Comprehensive textbook of psychotherapy: Theory and practice* (Vol. 1, pp. 434–455). London: Oxford University Press.
Hardy, G. E., Shapiro, D. A., Stiles, W. B., & Barkham, M. (1998). When and why does cognitive-behavioral treatment appear more effective than psychodynamic-interpersonal treatment? Discussion of the findings from the Second Sheffield Psychotherapy Project. *Journal of Mental Health, 7*(2), 179–190.
Hayes, A. M., Castonguay, L. G., & Goldfried, M. R. (1996). The study of change in psychotherapy: A reexamination of the process-outcome correlation paradigm. Comment on Stiles and Shapiro (1994). *Journal of Consulting and Clinical Psychology, 64,* 909–914.
Henry, W. P., Schacht, T. E., & Strupp, H. H. (1990). Patient and therapist introject, interpersonal process, and differential psychotherapy outcome. *Journal of Consulting and Clinical Psychology, 58,* 768–774.
Hill, C. E. (1990). Exploratory in-session process research in individual psychotherapy: A review. *Journal of Consulting and Clinical Psychology, 58,* 288–294.
Hilliard, R. B., Henry, W. P., & Strupp, H. H. (2000). An interpersonal model of psychotherapy: Linking patient and therapist developmental history, therapeutic process, and types of outcomes. *Journal of Consulting and Clinical Psychology, 68,* 125–133.
Horowitz, L. M., Rosenberg, S. E., & Bartholomew, K. (1993). Interpersonal problems, attachment styles, and outcomes in brief dynamic psychotherapy. *Journal of Consulting & Clinical Psychology, 61,* 549–560.
Horvath, A. O., Gaston, L., & Luborsky, L. (1993). The therapeutic alliance and its measures. In N. E. Miller, L. Luborsky, J. P. Barber, & J. P. Docherty (Eds.), *Psychodynamic treatment research: A handbook for clinical practice* (pp. 247–273). New York: Basic Books.
Horvath, A. O., & Greenberg, L. S. (Eds.). (1994). *The working alliance: Theory, research, and practice.* New York: Wiley.
Howard, K. I., Moras, K., Brill, P. L., Martinovich, Z., & Lutz, W. (1996). Evaluation of psychotherapy: Efficacy, effectiveness, and patient progress. *American Psychologist, 51,* 1059–1064.
Howard, K. I., Orlinsky, D. E., & Lueger, R. J. (1994). Clinically relevant outcome research in individual psychotherapy. *British Journal of Psychiatry, 165,* 4–8.
Kazdin, A. E. (1991). Treatment research: The investigation and evaluation of psychotherapy. In M. Hersen, A. E. Kazdin, & A. S. Bellack (Eds.), *The clinical psychology handbook* (2nd ed., pp. 292–312). New York: Pergamon.
King, R. (1998). Evidence-based practice: Where is the evidence? The case of cognitive behaviour therapy and depression. *Australian Psychologist, 33,* 83–88.
Klein, M. (1975). *Envy and gratitude and other works 1946–1963.* London: Virago.
Lafferty, P., Beutler, L. E., & Crago, M. (1989). Differences between more and less effective psychotherapists: A study of select therapist variables. *Journal of Consulting and Clinical Psychology, 57*(1), 76–80.

Lambert, M. J., Hansen, N. B., & Finch, A. E. (2001). Patient-focused research: Using patient outcome data to enhance treatment effects. *Journal of Consulting and Clinical Psychology, 69,* 159–172.
Lampropoulos, G. K. (2000). A reexamination of the empirically supported treatments critiques. *Psychotherapy Research, 10,* 474–487.
Langs, R. (1988). *A primer of psychotherapy.* New York: Gardner Press.
Luborsky, L., & Barber, J. P. (1993). Benefits of adherence to psychotherapy manuals, and where to get them. In N. E. Miller, L. Luborsky, J. P. Barber, & J. P. Docherty (Eds.), *Psychodynamic treatment research: A handbook for clinical practice* (pp. 211–226). New York: Basic Books.
Luborksy, L., Barber, J. P., & Crits-Christoph, P. (1999). Theory-based research for understanding the process of dynamic psychotherapy. *Journal of Consulting and Clinical Psychology, 58,* 281–287.
Luborsky, L., & Crits-Christoph, P. (Eds.). (1998). *Understanding transference: The Core Conflictual Relationship Theme Method* (2nd ed.). Washington, DC: American Psychological Association.
Luborsky, L., McLellan, A. T., Diguer, L., Woody, G., & Seligman, D. A. (1997). The psychotherapist matters: Comparison of outcomes across twenty-two therapist and seven patient samples. *Clinical Psychology: Science and Practice, 4,* 53–65.
Lueger, R. J., Howard, K. I., Martinovich, Z., Lutz, W., Anderson, E. E., & Grissom, G. (2001). Assessing treatment progress of individual patients using expected treatment response models. *Journal of Consulting and Clinical Psychology, 69,* 150–158.
Malan, D. H. (1993). *Individual psychotherapy and the science of psychodynamics.* Oxford, England: Butterworth-Heinemann.
Marginson, F. R., Barkham, M., Evans, C., McGrath, G., Clark, J. M., Audin, K., & Connell, J. (2000). Measurement and psychotherapy: Evidence-based practice and practice-based evidence. *British Journal of Psychiatry, 177,* 123–130.
Masterton, J. F., Tolpin, M., & Sifneos, P. E. (1991). *Comparing psychoanalytic psychotherapies.* New York: Brunner/Mazel.
Messer, S. B., & Warren, C. S. (1995). *Models of brief psychodynamic therapy: A comparative approach.* New York: Guilford.
Mitchell, S. A. (2000). *Relationality: From attachment to intersubjectivity.* Hillsdale, NJ: The Analytic Press.
Mohr, D. C. (1995). Negative outcome in psychotherapy: A critical review. *Clinical Psychology: Science and Practice, 2,* 1–27.
Muran, J. C., Samstag, L. W., Jilton, R., Batchelder, S., & Winston, A. (1997). Development of a suboutcome strategy to measure interpersonal process in psychotherapy from an observer perspective. *Journal of Clinical Psychology, 53,* 405–420.
Najavits, L. M., & Strupp, H. H. (1994). Differences in the effectiveness of psychodynamic therapists: A process-outcome study. *Psychotherapy, 31,* 114–123.
Nathan, P. E., & Gorman, J. M. (Eds.). (1998). *A guide to treatments that work.* New York: Oxford University Press.
Niederehe, G., Street, L. L., & Lebowitz, B. D. (1999). NIMH support for psychotherapy research: Opportunities and questions. *Prevention and Treatment,* Vol. 2, Article 0003a, posted March 21. http://journals.apa.org/prevention/volume2/pre0020003a.html
Orlinsky, D. (1994). Research based knowledge as the emergent foundation for clinical practice in psychotherapy. In P. F. Talley, H. H. Strupp, & S. F. Butler (Eds.), *Psychotherapy research and practice: Bridging the gap* (pp. 99–123). New York: Basic Books.
Orlinsky, D. E., & Howard, K. I. (1980). Gender and psychotherapy outcome. In A. M. Brodsky & R. T. Hare-Mustin (Eds.), *Women and psychotherapy* (pp. 3–34). New York: Guilford.
Orlinsky, D. E., & Russell, R. L. (1990). Tradition and change in psychotherapy research: Note on the fourth generation. In R. L. Russell (Ed.), *Reassessing psychotherapy research* (pp. 185–214). New York: Guilford.
Piper, W. E., & Duncan, S. C. (1999). Object relations theory and short-term dynamic psychotherapy: Findings from the Quality of Object Relations Scale. *Clinical Psychology Review, 19*(6), 669–685.

Piper, W. E., Joyce, A. S., Rosie, J. S., Ogrodniczuk, J. S., McCallum, M., O'Kelly, J. G., & Steinberg, P. I. (1999). Prediction of dropping out in time-limited, interpretive individual psychotherapy. *Psychotherapy, 36*, 267–273.

Ricks, D. F. (1974). Supershrink: Methods of a therapist judged successful on the basis of adult outcome of adolescent patients. In D. Ricks, A. Thomas, & M. Roff (Eds.), *Life history research in psychopathology* (Vol. III, pp. 275–297). Minneapolis: University of Minnesota Press.

Roth, A., & Fonagy, P. (1997). *What works for whom? A critical review of psychotherapy research.* New York: Guilford.

Seligman, M. E. P. (1995). The effectiveness of psychotherapy: The consumer reports study. *American Psychologist, 50*, 965–974.

Seligman, M. E. P. (1998). Afterword—A plea. In P. E. Nathan & J. M. Gorman (Eds.), *A guide to treatments that work* (pp. 568–572). New York: Oxford University Press.

Shapiro, D. A., Firth-Cozens, J., & Stiles, W. (1989). A question of therapist's differential effectiveness: A Sheffield psychotherapy project addendum. *British Journal of Psychiatry, 154*, 383–385.

Smith, M. L., Glass, G. V., & Miller, T. I. (1980). *The benefits of psychotherapy.* Baltimore: Johns Hopkins University Press.

Snyder, C. R., Michael, S. T., & Cheavers, J. S. (1999). Hope as a psychotherapeutic foundation of common factors, placebos and expectancies. In M. A. Hubble, B. L. Duncan, & S. Miller (Eds.), *The heart & soul of change: What works in therapy* (pp. 179–200). Washington, DC: American Psychological Association.

Spence, D. P. (1993). Traditional case studies and prescriptions for improving them. In N. E. Miller, L. Luborsky, J. P. Barber, & J. P. Docherty (Eds.), *Psychodynamic treatment research: A handbook for clinical practice* (pp. 37–52). New York: Basic Books.

Stein, D. M., & Lambert, M. J. (1995). Graduate training in psychotherapy: Are therapy outcomes enhanced? *Journal of Consulting and Clinical Psychology, 63*, 182–196.

Stiles, W. B., & Shapiro, D. A. (1994). Disabuse of the drug metaphor: Psychotherapy process-outcome correlations. *Journal of Consulting and Clinical Psychology, 62*, 942–948.

Stiles, W. B., Shapiro, D. A., & Elliott, R. (1986). "Are all psychotherapies equivalent?" *American Psychologist, 41*, 165–180.

Strupp, H. H. (1976). Themes in psychotherapy research. In J. L. Claghorn (Ed.), *Successful psychotherapy* (pp. 3–23). New York: Brunner/Mazel.

Strupp, H. H. (1993). The Vanderbilt Psychotherapy Studies: Synopsis. *Journal of Consulting and Clinical Psychology, 61*(3), 431–433.

Sullivan, H. S. (1953). *The interpersonal theory of psychiatry.* New York: Norton.

Talley, P. F., Strupp, H. H., & Butler, S. F. (Eds.). (1994). *Psychotherapy research and practice: Bridging the gap.* New York: Basic Books.

Tallman, K., & Bohart, A. C. (1999). The client as a common factor: Clients as self-healers. In M. A. Hubble, B. Duncan, & S. D. Miller (Eds.), *The heart & soul of change: What works in therapy* (pp. 91–131). Washington, DC: American Psychological Association.

Tasman, A. (1993). Setting standards for psychotherapy training: It's time to do our homework. *Journal of Psychotherapy Practice and Research, 2*, 93–95.

Wallerstein, R. S. (1993). Psychoanalysis as science: Challenges to the data of psychoanalytic research. In N. E. Miller, L. Luborsky, J. P. Barber, & J. P. Docherty (Eds.), *Psychodynamic treatment research: A handbook for clinical practice* (pp. 96–108). New York: Basic Books.

Wampold, B. E. (2001). *The great psychotherapy debate: Models, methods, and findings.* Mahwah, NJ: Lawrence Erlbaum Associates.

Warner, L. K., Herron, W. G., Javier, R. A., Patalano, F., Sisenwein, F., & Primavera, L. H. H. (2001). A comparison of dose-response curves in cognitive behavioral and psychodynamic psychotherapies. *Journal of Clinical Psychology, 57*, 63–73.

Zuroff, D. C., Blatt, S. J., Sotsky, S. M., Krupnick, J. L., Martin, D. J., Sanislow, C. A., III, & Simmens, S. (2000). Relation of therapeutic alliance and perfectionism to outcome in brief outpatient treatment of depression. *Journal of Consulting and Clinical Psychology, 68*, 114–124.

CHAPTER

2

Optimizing Outcome Through Prediction and Measurement of Psychological Functioning

Michael J. Lambert
Robert D. Hunt
Brigham Young University

David A. Vermeersch
Loma Linda University

In recent years, government agencies, professional organizations, third-party payers, and consumers have been placing increased pressure on mental health service providers to be more accountable for the services they render. In response to this increased pressure, many clinicians and mental health service agencies have begun to implement quality management systems in their clinical practices (Barkham et al., 2001; Beutler, 2001; Kordy, Hannöver, & Richard, 2001; Lambert, Hansen, & Finch, 2001; Lueger et al., 2001). Quality management systems are designed to ensure that patients are being provided with high-quality treatment at an affordable cost (i.e., cost-effective treatment). There are two fundamental components of quality management systems that provide a basis for optimizing patient treatment outcomes: the prediction of patient treatment response and the measurement of patient change throughout the course of psychotherapy.

The ability to predict which patients will respond to a given type of therapy will help optimize outcome by allowing therapists to modify their intervention strategies or reassign to a different type of treatment those patients who are predicted to respond poorly to a given type of therapy. This in turn will help clinicians allocate time, effort, and resources more efficiently. In fact, several predictors of outcome have been identified and are commonly used as selection criteria in brief therapy (Lambert & Anderson, 1996). Some of these predictor variables have received considerable empirical support, suggesting that they are indeed helpful in distinguishing between patients who will and those who will not respond to a given treatment.

Measurement with psychometrically sound instruments that are appropriate for each patient will also help optimize outcome. The particular outcome measure that is used can influence conclusions about the effectiveness of therapy. In fact, certain measures are more likely to demonstrate patient improvement than other measures. Therefore, it is extremely important that appropriate instruments are used for measuring outcome. By selecting and implementing instruments appropriately, clinicians can effectively adapt the length, type, and focus of therapy in response to measures of patient improvement, thereby producing the best possible outcomes. Furthermore, if core batteries of instruments aimed at assessing outcome for different patient populations are developed and implemented by clinicians and researchers, understanding of the psychological conditions and therapy processes associated with these patient populations will increase. This in turn will facilitate the development of improved treatments, which will ultimately result in better outcomes.

In light of the potential for prediction and measurement of treatment response to enhance patient outcomes, clinicians and researchers may benefit from becoming familiar with research regarding predictors and measures of outcome. Thus, in this chapter we begin with a discussion of the theoretical work and empirical findings related to predictors of outcome. Second, we discuss theoretical, conceptual, and methodological issues related to the measurement of patient outcome. Finally, we discuss efforts to order outcome measurement.

PREDICTORS OF OUTCOME

According to theorists of various orientations (e.g., Sifneos, 1987), successful short-term therapy depends largely on which patients are selected to receive this type of treatment. However, there is sometimes disagreement both within and between the theoretical and empirical literature as to which patients are suitable candidates for short-term therapy. That is, the specific patient characteristics that are used to generate inclusion–exclusion criteria and that predict good–poor outcome have not been well established. Despite this lack of consensus, a few themes have emerged with regard to patient characteristics as predictors of outcome. In a review of the literature, Lambert and Anderson (1996) identified the following patient characteristics as the most commonly cited ways to predict final outcome: severity of disturbance, motivation, capacity to relate, ego strength, psychological mindedness, focality of problem, response to trial therapy, and early response to therapy. All of these patient characteristics are aspects of psychological health or disturbance that can impact treatment planning, psychotherapy processes, and final patient outcome. We consider theoretical perspectives and empirical findings regarding each of these patient characteristics as they relate to final outcome here.

Severity of Disturbance

Severity of disturbance is the most commonly cited predictor of outcome in both the theoretical and research literature (Lambert & Anderson, 1996). The majority of theorists who advocate brief therapy interventions recommend excluding severely disturbed patients from treatment. Actively psychotic individuals, as well as those who have a history of psychotic decompensation, are almost always excluded from brief therapy (Barber & Crits-Christoph, 1991; Bauer & Kobos, 1987; Davanloo, 1980; Malan & Osimo, 1992). Most theorists also recommend that individuals with severe characterological problems be excluded (e.g., borderline or antisocial), including those with intense dependency needs (Garfield, 1989; Mann, 1991), individuals with paranoid personality disorder (Pollack, Flegenagimer, & Winston, 1991), and those who rely on defenses such as denial and withdrawal (Binder & Strupp, 1991; Garfield, 1989; Klein, 1985). Furthermore, psychosomatic complaints (Klein, 1985; Mann, 1991), substance dependence (Bauer & Kobos, 1987), impulse control disorders (Barber & Crits-Christoph, 1991; Sifneos, 1987), and entrenched negativism and hostility (Binder & Strupp, 1991) have been cited as grounds for exclusion. Some theorists recommend excluding patients with severe mood disorders such as those with bipolar disorder (Ursano & Hales, 1986) or those who are at risk for suicide (Klein, 1985). Finally, organic brain damage and cognitive deficits have been suggested by some theorists as grounds for exclusion (Klein, 1985; Ursano & Hales, 1986).

According to Lambert and Anderson (1996), the finding in general outcome research that severity of disturbance is negatively correlated with outcome can be extended to brief therapy as well. Nevertheless, Lambert and Anderson (1996) found several differences between the theoretical and research literature regarding severity of disturbance. According to these researchers, few studies have been aimed at verifying the belief that patients with psychosis should be excluded from brief therapy. Among the studies that exist, most show that psychotic patients do not respond as well as nonpsychotic patients (Malan & Osimo, 1992). However, this finding does not mean that psychotic patients do not benefit from brief therapy or that they should be excluded. In fact, some studies suggest that psychotic patients can be effectively treated with highly structured brief group therapy (Kamas, 1991). Patients who do not have personality disorders have better outcomes and show more improvement than patients with personality disorders (Hoglend, 1993). Nevertheless, structured approaches seem to provide promise for treating patients with borderline personality disorder

(Shearin & Linehan, 1992). Structured approaches may extend the length of therapy; however, such approaches seem able to produce significant improvement more quickly than long-term therapy.

Brief therapy seems effective for a variety of other personality disorders as well, including avoidant, dependent, histrionic, passive aggressive, and obsessive–compulsive personality disorders (Winston et al., 1991). However, patients with narcissistic, antisocial, or paranoid personality disorders have not responded well to brief therapy. Although the findings are mixed, patients who are severely depressed (McLean & Taylor, 1992), as well as those who are diagnosed with substance dependence (Carroll, Rounsaville, & Gawin, 1991), have been successfully treated with brief therapy. Insufficient research exists regarding the effectiveness of brief therapy for bipolar disorder, suicide risk, and organic brain damage. Thus, conclusions cannot yet be drawn regarding these conditions.

Anderson and Lambert (2001) studied the influence of severity of disturbance on how many sessions are required to reach clinically significant (CS) change. These researchers tracked 75 clients in outpatient therapy with the Outcome Questionnaire (Lambert et al., 1996). When data from this study were combined with those from a similar study (Kadera, Lambert, & Andrews, 1996), a significant positive relation between time to reach CS change and initial distress level was found. A survival analysis indicated that clients with higher levels of initial distress took eight more sessions to reach 50% CS change (i.e., the session at which half of the patients with higher levels of initial distress met criteria for CS change) than clients with lower levels of initial distress. The results of this analysis are presented in Fig. 2.1. The patients involved in this study had similar levels of distress to those in other outpatient clinics (Lambert et al., 1996).

Motivation to Change

The second most frequently cited predictor of outcome is motivation (Lambert & Anderson, 1996). According to theorists, the type of motivation that is most predictive of outcome in brief therapy is motivation to change (Marmor, 1979). Benjamin (1991) noted that motivation to change involves willingness to reflect on thoughts, emotions, and behaviors and to incorporate new thoughts, emotions, and behaviors. Motivation to change has been assessed in a variety of ways (Sifneos, 1987). However, theorists do not agree on how much emphasis to place on motivation to change when using it as a selection criterion, largely due to the fact that it is a patient quality that can change once therapy has begun.

Many studies seem to support motivation to change as a predictor of outcome. For example, pretreatment motivation has been linked to 4- and 5-

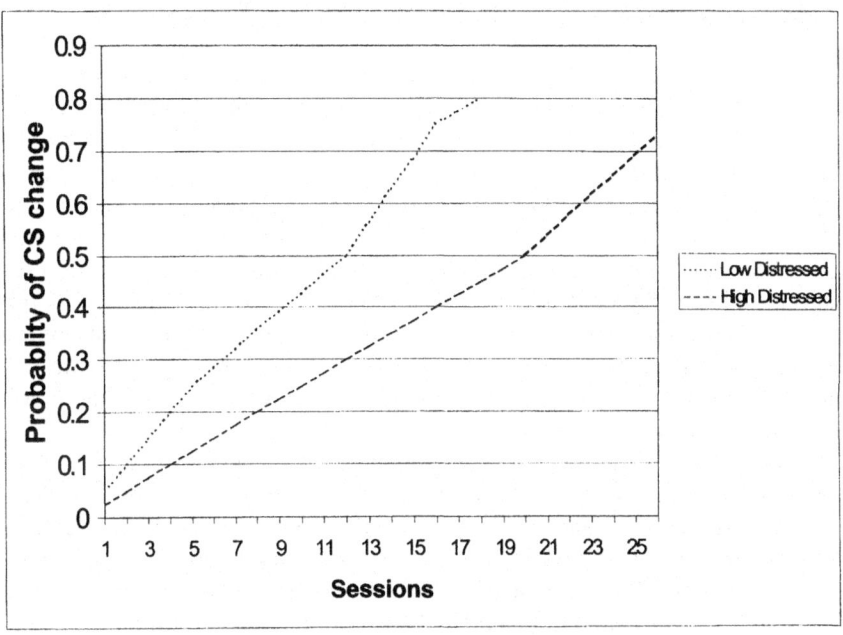

FIG. 2.1. Percentage of initially more and less disturbed patients achieving clinically significant change following specified "doses" of psychotherapy. Adapted from Anderson and Lambert (2001). Reprinted with permission.

year follow-up (Hoglend, 1993). Patient involvement, which reflects motivation, has also been cited as predictive of outcome. In a comprehensive review, Orlinsky, Grawe, and Parks (1994) found a significant positive relation between motivation and outcome in 14 of 28 studies. They also found, in a review of 15 studies, a significant positive relation between patient involvement and good outcome in 92% of patients. Other researchers have not found a significant relation between motivation and outcome (Piper, deCarufel, & Szkrumelak, 1985). Some researchers report that motivation may play a moderating role between certain therapist actions (e.g., exploratory actions and supportive techniques) and outcome (M. J. Horowitz, Marmar, Weiss, DeWitt, & Rosenbaum, 1984). Thus, prejudicial therapist actions (e.g., therapist rejection of patient, lack of empathy, authoritarianism) should be considered when excluding patients on the basis of motivation.

According to some researchers (Bauer & Kobos, 1987; Garfield, 1989; Malan, 1976), the time at which motivation is assessed may also influence the value of motivation as a predictor. Most of these researchers agree that motivation is more predictive when assessed after several sessions (e.g., three sessions) of therapy than when assessed after the first session.

Capacity to Relate

Capacity to relate is the third most cited selection criterion, with more than half of brief therapy theorists reviewed identifying it as an important factor that modifies outcome (Lambert & Anderson, 1996). Capacity to relate has been variously defined as the ability to engage, the ability to form a therapeutic alliance, the maturity of object relations, the capacity for basic trust, and the capacity for intimacy. Some theorists view the capacity to relate as the most important criterion and claim that it is especially important in dynamic therapy (Bauer & Kobos, 1987). Capacity to relate is usually determined by how the patient relates to the therapist and by the quality of the patient's external relationships (Baker, 1991). Good capacity to relate can be indicated by a variety of factors such as being willing to confide in and be influenced by others (Bauer & Kobos, 1987; Klein, 1985).

Several studies support capacity to relate as a selection criterion. Positive correlations have been found between good outcome and the ability to quickly form a good relationship with the therapist (Strupp, 1981), relationship maturity and stability (Piper et al., 1985), the quality of object relations (Piper, Azim, McCullum, & Joyce, 1990), the quality of interpersonal relations at pretreatment (Hoeglend, 1993), and having a confidant (Moos, 1990). Negative correlations have been found between good outcome and social dysfunction (Stotsky et al., 1991), negative contributions to the therapeutic relationship (Horowitz et al., 1984), and amount of family conflict (Moos, 1990). Although the relation between capacity to relate and outcome has not been supported in some studies (Malan, 1976), after reviewing 15 studies that provided information on the topic, Lambert and Anderson (1996) reported that the relation between capacity to relate and outcome generally seems to be supported by the literature.

According to Orlinsky et al. (1994), who conducted a comprehensive review of the process and outcome research, self-reports of extratherapy relationship quality do not produce findings as strong as those achieved when in-session patient ratings of the quality of the therapeutic relationship are used. The therapist's actions and theoretical orientation may influence the utility of the patient's capacity to relate to predict outcome, suggesting that some procedures are more effective than others at overcoming this patient deficit.

Ego Strength

Ego strength was mentioned as an essential capacity by half of the theorists reviewed by Lambert and Anderson (1996). Ego strength is usually viewed as the ability to cope with both internal and external stress (Bauer &

Kobos, 1987; Malan & Osimo, 1992). Ego strength can be indicated by several factors, including a patient's education and occupation (Marmor, 1979), response to a challenge from the therapist (Davanloo, 1980), and responsibility, autonomy, and emotional maturity (Strupp, 1981).

Most studies support the relation between ego strength and outcome (Piper et al., 1985). In a study by M. J. Horowitz et al. (1984), ego strength played a moderating role between certain therapist actions (i.e., therapist exploration and support) and outcome. Psychological health sickness, a variable similar to ego strength, was found to be significantly related to outcome in 22 of 34 (66%) studies (Luborsky, Crits-Christoph, Mintz, & Auerbach, 1988). Those with low ego strength do not respond well to unstructured approaches (Lambert, Bergin, & Collins, 1977) but do appear to respond well to supportive approaches (Piper et al., 1990). Furthermore, whether or not individuals with high ego strength respond to unstructured approaches may depend on their tolerance for and the number of interpretations made by the therapist (Piper et al., 1990). Although ego strength seems to predict outcome in brief therapy, little is known about which aspects of ego strength account for this relation or whether patients with low ego strength are better suited for long-term therapy or more structured approaches rather than short-term therapy.

Psychological Mindedness

Psychological mindedness is a commonly cited selection criterion, with almost half of the theorists identifying psychological mindedness as an important predictor of outcome. Psychological mindedness involves several factors, including the capacity for introspection (Davanloo, 1980), curiosity about the self (Baker, 1991), the ability to communicate thoughts and feelings to others (Bauer & Kobos, 1987), and the capacity for abstract thought (Sifneos, 1987). Dynamic theorists emphasize the capacity for insight as the most important indicator of psychological mindedness (Marmor, 1979).

Although some studies have demonstrated a relation between psychological mindedness and outcome (Strupp, 1980), most studies have failed to support psychological mindedness as a predictor of outcome (Piper et al., 1985). For example, Orlinsky et al. (1994) reported that 70% of 79 studies did not show a significant relation between psychological mindedness and outcome. Furthermore, some studies report that high levels of self-focus are associated with psychopathology, especially if the self-focus is negative (Ingram, 1990). It is important to note, however, that psychological mindedness has been shown to be negatively correlated with attrition in brief dynamic therapy (McCallum & Piper, 1990). Overall, psychological mindedness does not seem very useful as a predictor of outcome.

Focality of Problem

Nearly half of the theorists reviewed by Lambert and Anderson (1996) mentioned focality of problem (i.e., the tendency for a patient's problems to be localized) as a predictor of outcome. Their reasoning stems from the belief that identification of a focal problem allows therapists to allocate their efforts more effectively. However, theorists do not agree on how to differentiate one focal problem from another.

Few studies have been reported on the relation between focality and outcome. In one study involving brief psychodynamic therapy, focality was not significantly related to outcome (Piper et al., 1985). Conversely, good outcomes were not achieved in two cases in which the therapist could not identify a focal problem (Malan & Osimo, 1992). Although there is some evidence to suggest that lack of focality may be associated with attrition, it is also likely true that it is important to allow patients time to identify the focal problem on their own or at least collaboratively with the therapist. Due to the lack of research in this area, no definite conclusions can be made about the utility of focality as a selection criterion.

Response to Trial Therapy

Response to trial therapy, another predictor of outcome proposed by theorists (Lambert & Anderson, 1996), involves providing a representative sample of a particular treatment to a patient for the purpose of ascertaining the patient's likely response to that therapy if it was provided in its entirety. Most theorists who support response to trial therapy or trial interpretations as useful outcome predictors are psychodynamically inclined (e.g., Bauer & Kobos, 1987; Binder & Strupp, 1991; Malan & Osimo, 1992). Increased motivation is one indicator of a positive response to trial therapy, whereas a negative response might include anxiety and confusion. Although assessing a patient's response to trial therapy can be time consuming, information gleaned from a trial treatment may not only assist in assessing a patient's appropriateness for a specific type of treatment, but it may also assist in providing the most appropriate referral to a given patient. According to Lambert and Anderson (1996), a few studies support using a patient's response to trial therapy to predict outcome (Davanloo, 1980). However, other researchers have not found such a relation (Piper et al., 1985). Given these mixed findings, more studies are needed to better understand the relation between response to trial therapy and outcome.

Early Response to Therapy

An additional related predictor of outcome that is not specified by theoreticians but is receiving increased empirical support is early response to therapy. Early response to therapy can be assessed by measuring a patient's improvement or deterioration (by comparing a patient's pretreatment score on an outcome measure with his or her expected score on the measure following a session of psychotherapy) regularly during the first few sessions of therapy. Although little consensus has been reached regarding how to define and measure early response, several studies have found that early positive response is positively correlated with better outcomes (e.g., Tang & DeRubeis, 1999).

In one study, Haas, Hill, Lambert, and Morrell (2002) measured early response by comparing each patient's session-by-session Outcome Questionnaire (Lambert et al., 1996) total scores (which are derived by totaling scores on the Subjective Distress, Interpersonal Relations, and Social Role subscales) to a normative set of expected response curves. With the use of this method, they found that patients who were early positive responders had better outcomes at termination and up to a 2-year follow-up than those who were not early positive responders. Furthermore, and perhaps in contrast to clinical beliefs, it appears that patient deterioration early in the course of treatment is predictive of poor final outcome. For example, multiple studies (Haas et al., 2002; Lambert et al., 2002) have shown that clients who worsen early in the course of treatment have approximately a one in four chance of obtaining a reliable (i.e., improving by more points on an outcome measure than can be attributed to measurement error) or clinically significant change (i.e., reliably changing and moving into a functional range on an outcome measure) if no corrective actions are taken. It is not known whether early positive response is due to specific or to nonspecific factors. However, because most specific factors (i.e., specific treatment interventions) are introduced or thought to take effect later in therapy, nonspecific treatment factors, in interaction with patient characteristics, seem to be largely responsible for the early response phenomenon. Studies in this area are promising and suggest that early response to treatment is a predictor of outcome across therapies, including brief dynamic therapy.

Summary

Although brief therapy has been shown to be effective (Anderson & Lambert, 1995), the patient characteristics most predictive of outcome are not yet well established (Lambert & Anderson, 1996). Nevertheless, it is reasonable to conclude that several of the aforementioned patient characteristics (i.e., severity of disturbance, motivation to change, ego strength, capacity to relate, and early response to therapy) have repeatedly been shown to be correlated with brief therapy outcome. Severe disturbance is associated with less improvement and poorer outcomes in both brief and longer term therapy. Nevertheless, many patients who are severely disturbed can benefit from brief therapy. Severely disturbed patients improve most when treatments are problem focused, structured, both individual and group, and capable of being extended. Motivation to change seems quite useful as a selection criterion, especially when motivation is assessed after several sessions of therapy. Ego strength also seems predictive of outcome. Nevertheless, improvement can be achieved even with patients who have low ego strength, especially when the therapy is structured or supportive (or both) rather than expressive. Both motivation and ego strength can be moderating factors between a therapist's exploratory and supportive actions and outcome (Horowitz et al., 1984). Capacity to relate also seems to be useful in selecting patients for brief therapy, especially when patient ratings of the therapy process are used. Early response to therapy is also predictive of outcome at termination and up to 2 years follow-up. On the other hand, psychological mindedness, focality, and response to trial therapy have yet to be supported by the evidence as outcome predictors. However, low levels of psychological mindedness may be associated with attrition, and the lack of support for focality and response to trial therapy may just be due to the lack of research in these areas. Thus, research aimed at better understanding these and other variables associated with outcome is needed.

Studies on patient characteristics common in those who show little improvement or poor outcomes would also be informative. Moreover, because several of the predictors reviewed previously are abstract and lack precise definitions, further effort should be aimed at clarifying these constructs. Because long-term treatment outcomes are best predicted by severity of disturbance, motivation to change, ego strength, capacity to relate, and early response to treatment, patients who are highly distressed, unmotivated to change, lack ego strength, have difficulty in relating to others (particularly the therapist), and deteriorate early in the treatment process are not likely to benefit from long-term treatment that is unstructured. Although it is arguable that such patients would not, by extension, respond to brief therapy as well, it is also possible that brief therapy that is structured, goal oriented, and employs multiple interventions and modalities may be the treatment of choice for such difficult cases.

Clinicians glean information about a patient's standing on each of the aforementioned predictor variables from many sources (e.g., behavioral observation, patient verbal report, reports of significant others, testing). Understanding information gathered from these sources requires varying degrees of clinical judgment. Although clinical judgment obviously has a place in predicting which patients will or will not likely respond to a particular therapy, studies have repeatedly indicated that predictions are most accurate when empirical data are emphasized in the process of formulating predictions. Therefore, we strongly recommend that clinicians utilize sound measures that are aimed at assessing a patient's standing on the aforementioned predictor variables in their attempts to determine which patients will or will not respond to a particular therapy. In addition to the role of measurement in the prediction of psychotherapy outcome, the second component of quality management systems that provides a basis for optimizing psychotherapy outcome is the measurement of patient change throughout the course of psychotherapy. Thus, in the next section we discuss some of the theoretical, conceptual, and methodological issues related to the measurement of patient outcome, as well as attempts to bring order to outcome measurement.

OUTCOME MEASUREMENT

The history of outcome measurement dates back to the 1920s (Lambert, Christensen, & DeJulio, 1983). Since that time, the importance, development, and use of outcome measures have continued to increase. However, although the use of outcome measures has increased, the focus of outcome research has evolved and generally broadened over time. Modern efforts at assessing outcome largely began in reaction to a study conducted by Eysenck (1952), which concluded that 74% of patients, drawn from 24 studies and diagnosed with neurosis, were found to make progress considered equivalent to a similarly diagnosed group of individuals who received no treatment over a 2-year time period. Following this study, a large body of research was directed toward determining whether psychotherapy assists patients beyond the improvements that can be expected from existing social supports and inner homeostatic mechanisms. Once psychotherapy, at a global level, was established as an effective treatment, outcome research began to focus more on differences in effectiveness between therapies. Although this area of inquiry continues to be a focus of outcome research, the literature to date suggests that different therapies, including dynamically oriented therapies, are equally effective in treating most problems.

A new focus of research is the use of outcome data throughout the course of treatment for the purpose of improving patient outcomes. To this end, many researchers have developed and implemented feedback systems that provide clinicians with ongoing data regarding a particular patient's response to treatment (Barkham et al., 2001; Beutler, 2001; Kordy, Hannöver, & Richard, 2001; Lambert et al., 2001; Lueger et al., 2001). One quality of these feedback systems is that they are able to be utilized by clinicians who practice from any theoretical orientation, including dynamically oriented therapists. The rationale behind these systems is that clinicians can, if needed, adapt their treatment approach in response to feedback regarding patient progress. Many feedback systems have recently been developed, and some have been shown to significantly improve patient outcomes, particularly those of patients who are predicted (based on their early poor response to therapy) to drop out of therapy prematurely or have a poor final outcome (Lambert et al., 2002). Furthermore, in addition to providing regular feedback to clinicians, some researchers are beginning to explore the effects of providing regular feedback based on outcome data to patients and clinical supervisors. As can be seen, the focus of outcome research has broadened from postmortem analyses (i.e., analyses of pre–post change following patient termination from treatment) of outcome data for the purpose of demonstrating treatment effectiveness to a real-time application of outcome data for the purpose of enhancing patient outcomes.

THE UNIQUE TASK OF OUTCOME MEASUREMENT

The ability to accurately assess patient response to treatment throughout the course of therapy is directly related to the quality and appropriateness of the measures being used for this purpose. Kirshner and Guyatt (1985) noted that of the thousands of psychological tests that have been published to date, most have been specifically designed to serve one or more of the following purposes: discrimination, prediction, and evaluation. A *discriminative measure* is one that is used for the purpose of distinguishing between individuals or groups on the basis of an underlying dimension when no external criterion or gold standard is available. Intelligence tests such as the Wechsler Adult Intelligence Scale (Wechsler, 1997) and personality tests such as the Minnesota Multiphasic Personality Inventory (MMPI; Hathaway, McKinley, & Butcher, 1990) are examples of discriminative measures. Discriminative measures are often used as diagnostic instruments because they are specifically designed to discriminate between different individuals (based on their scores on a measure) at a single point in time.

A *predictive measure* is one that is used for the purpose of classifying individuals into categories when a gold standard is available, either concurrently or prospectively, to determine whether individuals have been classified correctly. This type of measure is generally used as a screening instrument to identify which specific individuals have or will develop a target condition. When a measure is used to assist in assessing whether or not a patient is appropriate for a specific type of treatment (e.g., using a measure to assess a patient's ego strength for the purpose of predicting whether he or she will be able to meaningfully participate in brief dynamic therapy), it is being used for predictive purposes. The Child Abuse Potential Inventory (Milner, 1989) is another example of a predictive measure in that it is designed to detect individuals who are at an increased risk of committing abusive acts in the future.

An *evaluative measure* is one that is used for the purpose of measuring change over time (e.g., pretreatment and posttreatment, weekly change over the course of treatment) in an individual or group on the dimension(s) of interest. Tests designed to assess treatment benefits or outcomes are examples of evaluative measures. Outcome measures, then, are quite different from discriminative and predictive measures because they are designed to measure intraindividual change over time via repeated administrations rather than to discriminate between different individuals at a single point in time (Kirshner & Guyatt, 1985).

It is important to note that measures are often used, either appropriately or inappropriately, for some combination of the aforementioned purposes. For example, a measure may be used to assist in determining a patient's appropriateness for a specific type of treatment (i.e., predictive purpose) and then subsequently used to track that patient's progress throughout the course of treatment and status at termination (i.e., evaluative purpose). Although this is justified in cases in which a measure has demonstrated utility in serving multiple purposes, such a practice often represents an application of a measure for a purpose for which that measure was not designed and may lead to the inaccurate assessment of a patient. For example, Froyd, Lambert, and Froyd (1996) reported the MMPI to be among the 10 most frequently used self-report measures of outcome (i.e., evaluative purpose) despite the fact that the MMPI was specifically designed for diagnostic purposes (i.e., discriminative purpose). The MMPI is not an appropriate instrument for measuring outcome because it contains many items that are not sensitive to changes in patients receiving treatment, is excessively long, and is relatively expensive (Froyd et al., 1996). As this example suggests, it is extremely important that care is taken when selecting instruments to measure patient response to treatment.

Qualities of Good Outcome Measures

Given the importance of outcome measurement, clinicians would benefit from being aware of the qualities associated with sound outcome measures. The development of selection criteria (i.e., characteristics of instruments that will lead to the most accurate measurement of patient change) for outcome measures has received increased attention in recent years, largely due to the greater emphasis that managed care has placed on accountability for services rendered (Trabin, 1995). Because professional practices may come to rely heavily on the demonstration of measured effects of treatments, it is imperative that outcome measures possess characteristics that will lead to the most accurate reflection of patient improvement. Some authors (e.g., Pilkonis, 1997) have proposed selection criteria for instruments aimed at measuring changes in symptomatology associated with a specific disorder (e.g., major depressive disorder) or a major diagnostic category (e.g., personality disorders). Others have focused on the development of universally accepted selection criteria that can be applied to the evaluation of any outcome measure (Lambert, Horowitz, & Strupp, 1997; Newman & Ciarlo, 1994). Although there are some differences between the selection criteria proposed by various authors, there appears to be considerable overlap as well.

Synthesizing and building on the available literature, Lambert et al. (1997) suggested that the following 13 criteria consistently emerge as an appropriate means of selecting methods and measures of outcome: relevance to target group; simple, teachable methods; use of measures with objective referents; use of multiple respondents; psychometric strengths and the availability of norms; low measure costs relative to its use; understanding by nonprofessional audiences, easy feedback, and uncomplicated interpretation; useful in clinical services; compatibility with a variety of clinical theories and practices; the possibility of multiple administrations; comprehensiveness; ties to a diagnostic classification system (e.g., *Diagnostic and Statistical Manual of Mental Disorders–IV*, American Psychiatric Association, 2000); and sensitivity to change. Attention to the aforementioned criteria will increase the likelihood of selecting an outcome measure that provides the most accurate reflection of patient improvement. Accurate assessment of patient improvement will, in turn, allow clinicians to demonstrate treatment effectiveness more convincingly and alter treatment strategies in response to patient change if needed. Moreover, the use of good outcome measures will lead to more reliable and valid research findings, which may further our understanding of the therapy process. Conversely, the use of inappropriate, unreliable, or invalid measures will contribute to the failure to find patient benefit.

BRINGING ORDER TO OUTCOME MEASUREMENT

Despite the fact that the history of outcome measurement dates back to the 1920s, outcome research is characterized by an extreme lack of consensus, consistency, and organization regarding appropriate methods and measures for assessing outcome. Much of this confusion stems from the fact that literally thousands of different outcome measures are being used. For example, in a review of outcome studies published in 20 major journals between 1983 and 1988, Froyd et al. (1996) identified 1,430 distinct measures that had been applied in 348 studies. Many of the instruments used in these studies (e.g., MMPI) were applied inappropriately in that they were not designed to be used as outcome measures. In addition to this problem, many of the outcome instruments that are being used are researcher developed or one-item instruments. For example, Meier and Davis (1990) reviewed outcome studies published in 1967, 1977, and 1987 in the *Journal of Counseling*

Psychology and reported that about one third of the scales were developed or modified by the investigator, and the most frequent number of items per scale was one. The chaos in outcome measurement also stems from the fact that treatment is often multifaceted and that change is a multidimensional phenomenon (Ogles, Lambert, & Masters, 1996). Furthermore, some confusion may be due to the tendency for values and theoretical orientations to influence decisions about what is a desirable outcome (Bergin, 1980). Moreover, in a meta-analysis, Miller and Berman (1983) found that the source of measurement (e.g., client, therapist, other) often influences conclusions about the effectiveness of treatment and contributes to the lack of correlation between different measures of the same construct.

The chaos in outcome research makes it difficult for researchers to compare and integrate the results from different studies and draw sound conclusions. Consequently, it is disheartening to clinicians who are attempting to apply research findings or to select appropriate measures for assessing treatment effectiveness. This frustration causes clinicians to lose confidence in research and thus to be less likely to apply research findings in practice. In response to these concerns, several attempts have been made to bring order to the diversity and chaos found in outcome measurement (e.g., Elliot, 1992; Lambert, 1983; Lambert, Ogles, & Masters, 1992; McGlynn, 1996; Newman, Ciarlo, & Carpenter, 1999; Waskow & Parloff, 1975). In the following, we review two recent efforts to organize outcome measurement.

Core Battery Conference at Vanderbilt University

The 1994 American Psychological Association–sponsored Core Battery Conference held at Vanderbilt University was in large part a descendant of the 1970 Outcome Measures Project (OMP). The OMP, which was sponsored by the National Institute of Mental Health, was a conference involving expert therapy researchers in an attempt to identify a standard set of instruments (core battery) that could be used in all psychotherapy outcome studies, regardless of the setting or type of therapy (Waskow & Parloff, 1975). The success of the OMP in reaching this goal was limited by (a) a failure to address specific patient populations and (b) a lack of conceptualization regarding relevant domains of functioning (L. M. Horowitz, Strupp, Lambert, & Elkin, 1997).

Lessons learned from the OMP and from the subsequent attempts to establish a core battery stimulated discussion at the 1992 meeting of the Society for Psychotherapy Research. Forty psychologists and psychiatrists volunteered to pursue the idea of a core battery. All of the major theories of therapy and all of the major treatment modalities were represented in this group. These researchers, who specialized in anxiety, mood, or personality disorders, attempted to address the first limitation of the OMP by focusing separately on these three types of disorders. Moreover, they limited their discussions to nonpsychotic adults. They addressed the second limitation of the OMP by identifying essential domains of functioning that should be tapped by a core battery. Then, at the 1993 Society for Psychotherapy Research meeting, the group discussed four broad questions: (a) "What should a core battery look like?"; (b) "What needs to be measured?"; (c) "What criteria should be adopted in selecting measures?"; and (d) "What specific instruments should be included in the core battery?" (L. M. Horowitz et al., 1997, p. 20).

The preceding events led to the 1994 American Psychological Association–sponsored Core Battery Conference at Vanderbilt University. Prior to the conference, each of 15 experts in the area of measurement was asked to "... draft a manuscript on some issue that he or she considered important in developing consensus in the evaluation of outcome" (Horowitz et al., 1997, p. 21). Then, at the conference, each of these 15 experts was assigned to either a group focusing on anxiety disorders, a group focusing on mood disorders, or a group focusing on personality disorders. This division allowed each group to discuss each of the four questions in terms of its diagnostic category. After discussing each question separately, the three groups came together to discuss each question collectively to compare their responses (L. M. Horowitz et al., 1997).

Answers to the four questions can be seen in the general conclusions that were drawn from the manuscripts written by the participants and the conference itself. First, core batteries are needed to maximize progress toward effective treatments. Second, a core battery manual could include a universal battery appropriate for all disorders, general batteries appropriate for each diagnostic grouping (e.g., anxiety disorders), and specific batteries appropriate for disorders within those groupings (e.g., panic disorder). Third, the general content domains essential for a universal battery are "symptomatic states, social role functioning, and interpersonal functioning" (Lambert et al., 1997, p. 492). Fourth, the qualities essential for each core battery include "outstanding psychometric properties, multiple data sources [patient, therapist, family members, and independent raters], objective referents, pantheoretical [and pantreatment] assumptions, and sensitivity to change" (Lambert et al., 1997, p. 492). Fifth, necessary but perhaps not sufficient batteries could be developed to which researchers in various settings would add additional measures. Sixth, consensus on specific instruments to be included was not reached because of issues such as allegiance, familiarity, autonomy, and theoretical orientation (Lambert et al., 1997).

Although much was accomplished at the 1994 conference, further work is needed. Namely, a consensus must be reached regarding the specific instruments to be included in universal, general, and specific core batteries. If the development of core batteries is further pursued, the first step would likely be for a panel of experts to scale the criteria for selecting instruments in terms of importance. Second, the panel of experts should examine all available instruments that could be used to assess each of the essential domains. Third, these experts should rate each instrument on how well it meets each of the criteria for selection. Then the experts' ratings could be averaged across raters for each criterion, and a weighted sum across criteria then should be computed for each instrument. Finally, the weighted sums could be used to rank the instruments in each domain according to quality. A core battery could then be created by using the highest scoring instrument in each of the domains. This strategy can be used to select universal, general, and specific core batteries by using domains and criteria for selecting instruments that are appropriate for each of these three core battery types (L. M. Horowitz et al., 1997).

A Scheme for Organizing and Conceptualizing Outcome Measurement

In addition to the efforts aimed at developing core batteries, attempts have been made to bring order to outcome measurement by developing schemes for organizing or conceptualizing outcome measurement (e.g., Newman et al., 1999). Such schemes are less rigid than core batteries in that they are based on instrument qualities that can be considered when deciding which instruments to use rather than being based on a collection of specific instruments. These instrument qualities are important ways in which instruments differ. Consideration of such differences will aid clinicians and researchers in selecting appropriate instruments for their specific needs. An example of an organizational and conceptual scheme can be seen in the work of Ogles et al. (1996). Their scheme is based on several reviews of the psychotherapy outcome literature (Bergin & Lambert, 1978; Lambert et al., 1983; Lambert, Shapiro, & Bergin, 1986) and has undergone several revisions (Lambert, 1983; Lambert, Masters, & Ogles, 1992; Lambert, Ogles, et al., 1992). This scheme was designed to guide clinicians and researchers in the process of instrument selection and evaluation, remind them of the possibilities within the field of measurement, and help them select instruments that adequately assess each facet of the domain of interest. In short, such schemes help clinicians and researchers conceptualize outcome measurement more clearly and organize it more efficiently and effectively and thus help further the field of outcome measurement.

The scheme developed by Ogles et al. (1996) involves five dimensions: content, social level, source, technology, and time orientation. The *content dimension* reflects whether the instrument measures behavioral, cognitive, or affective faculties. The *social level dimension* reflects the degree to which the instrument assesses a client's internal attributes as opposed to interpersonal adjustment and social role adjustment. The *source dimension* reflects the source of the outcome information (i.e., client self-report, therapist rating, relevant others, trained observers, and institutional reference). The *technology dimension* reflects the format of the data (i.e., how specific the questions are, how many questions there are, and how and why the data is collected). The technology dimension is based on four general categories (global questions, specific questions, observation of behavior, and status). The status category is based on demographic information (e.g., whether the patient is employed or has been hospitalized). The *time orientation dimension* reflects the degree to which the instrument attempts to measure a stable trait-like characteristic versus an unstable state-like characteristic.

According to Ogles et al. (1996), each outcome instrument can be rated and classified on all five dimensions. For example, the Beck Depression Inventory (Beck, Ward, Mendelson, Mock, & Erbaugh, 1961) is mainly affective in terms of content, intrapersonal in terms of social level, a self-report measure in terms of source, specific in terms of technology, and state-like in terms of time orientation. Clinicians and researchers can select instruments by considering the five dimensions in terms of their unique needs. When they do so, they will be more likely to select appropriate measures and thus will be able to collect more accurate data (Ogles et al., 1996).

CONCLUSIONS

In this chapter, we discussed two important components of quality management systems that provide a basis for optimizing patient treatment outcomes: the prediction of patient treatment response and the measurement of patient change throughout the course of psychotherapy. We discussed several predictors of outcome that have been used as selection criteria in brief therapy. Several of the theoretical beliefs regarding such predictors have been confirmed by empirical findings. Based on the literature, severity of disturbance, motivation to change, ego strength, capacity to relate, and early positive response to therapy seem at least moderately correlated with therapy outcome (Lambert & Anderson, 1996; Haas et al., 2002). On the other hand, psychological mindedness, focality, and response to trial therapy have yet to be demonstrated as useful predictors of outcome. Regardless of which predictors are used, when a patient is predicted to respond poorly to brief therapy it does not necessarily mean that the patient will not benefit from brief therapy or that the patient would respond better to long-term treatment. In fact, brief therapy that is structured and goal oriented and that employs multiple interventions and modalities may be the treatment of choice for such difficult cases (Lambert & Anderson, 1996). If clinicians and researchers become familiar with the research to date and with future research involving predictors of outcome, they will be able to make more accurate decisions about matching therapy interventions with patient variables and thereby improve outcomes.

We also discussed the importance of measuring outcome and the qualities associated with outcome measures. Outcome measures differ in several ways from diagnostic and other instruments. In addition, outcome measures differ in terms of quality. Several qualities seem to be associated with good outcome measures. Clinicians and researchers who select high quality instruments that are appropriate for their needs will be able to monitor patient change more accurately as well as better understand treatment processes. Furthermore, information regarding patient response to treatment can be regularly provided to clinicians and used to improve outcomes of patients.

Finally, we discussed the chaos found in outcome measurement and two of the attempts that have been made to bring order to outcome measurement. The chaos in outcome measurement stems from several sources and makes it difficult for researchers to compare and integrate the results from different studies and draw sound conclusions. Consequently, it is disheartening to clinicians who are attempting to apply research findings or to select appropriate measures for assessing treatment effectiveness. Despite attempts to establish a core battery (e.g., the Core Battery Conference at Vanderbilt University), these efforts have not identified which instruments should be used. Although much has been accomplished through these efforts, much remains to be done. There have also been efforts to help clinicians and researchers organize and conceptualize outcome measurement. For example, Ogles et al. (1996) developed a scheme that can be used to select and evaluate outcome measures. Both of these methods of bringing order to outcome measurement seem fruitful. However, the number of benefits achieved through either method will be closely tied to the number of clinicians and researchers that utilize them. The increased order in outcome measurement that can be achieved with either method would accelerate our understanding of therapy processes and treatment techniques.

As seen in this chapter, significant advances have been made in the prediction of patient treatment response and in the measurement of patient change throughout the course of therapy. These advances have contributed to the development of quality management systems, which have integrated information from these two areas in an effort to ensure that patients receive high quality treatment. Nevertheless, there continues to be a great need for researchers and clinicians to identify, refine, and apply methods of enhancing outcome through assessment performed both prior to and throughout the course of treatment. These methods need to be continually evaluated and refined so that the benefits patients receive from psychotherapy can be maximized.

REFERENCES

American Psychiatric Association. (2000). *DSM-IV-TR: Diagnostic and statistical manual of mental disorders* (4th ed., Text Revision). Washington, DC: Author.

Anderson, E. M., & Lambert, M. J. (1995). Short-term dynamically oriented psychotherapy: A review and meta-analysis. *Clinical Psychology Review, 9*, 1–13.

Anderson, E. M., & Lambert, M. J. (2001). A survival analysis of clinically significant change in outpatient psychotherapy. *Journal of Clinical Psychology, 57*, 875–888.

Baker, H. S. (1991). Shorter-term psychotherapy: A self-psychological approach. In P. Crits-Christoph & J. P. Barber (Eds.), *Handbook of short-term dynamic therapy* (pp. 287–322). New York: Basic Books.

Barber, J. P., & Crits-Christoph, P. (1991). Comparison of the brief dynamic therapies. In P. Crits-Christoph & J. P. Barber (Eds.), *Handbook of short-term dynamic therapy* (pp. 323–356). New York: Basic Books.

Barkham, M., Margison, F., Leach, C., Lucock, M., Mellor-Clark, J., Evans, C., Benson, L., Connell, J., Audin, K., & McGrath, G. (2001). Service profiling and outcomes benchmarking using the CORE-OM: Toward practice-based evidence in the psychological therapies. *Journal of Consulting and Clinical Psychology, 69*, 184–196.

Bauer, P. B., & Kobos, J. C. (1987). *Brief therapy: Short-term psychodynamic intervention*. London: Aronson.

Beck, A. T., Ward, C. H., Mendelson, M., Mock, J., & Erbaugh, J. (1961). An inventory for measuring depression. *Archives of General Psychiatry, 4*, 561–571.

Benjamin, L. S. (1991). Brief adaptive psychotherapy. In P. Crits-Christoph & J. P. Barber (Eds.), *Handbook of short-term dynamic therapy* (pp. 248–286). New York: Basic Books.

Bergin, A. E. (1980). Psychotherapy and religious values. *Journal of Consulting and Clinical Psychology, 48*, 95–105.

Bergin, A. E., & Lambert, M. J. (1978). The evaluation of therapeutic outcomes. In S. L. Garfield & A. E. Bergin (Eds.), *Handbook of psychotherapy and behavior change* (pp. 139–189). New York: Wiley.

Beutler, L. E. (2001). Comparisons among quality assurance systems: From outcome assessment to clinical utility. *Journal of Consulting and Clinical Psychology, 69*, 197–204.

Binder, J. L., & Strupp, H. H. (1991). The Vanderbilt approach to time-limited dynamic psychotherapy. In P. Crits-Christoph & J. P. Barber (Eds.), *Handbook of short-term dynamic therapy* (pp. 137–165). New York: Basic Books.

Carroll, K. M., Rounsaville, B. J., & Gawin, F. H. (1991). A comparative trial of psychotherapies for ambulatory cocaine abusers: Relapse prevention and interpersonal psychotherapy. *American Journal of Drug and Alcohol Abuse, 17*, 229–247.

Davanloo, I. I. (1980). *Short-term dynamic psychotherapy*. Northvale, NJ: Aronson.

Elliot, R. (1992). A conceptual analysis of Lambert et al.'s conceptual scheme for outcome assessment. *Journal of Counseling and Development, 70*, 535–537.

Eysenck, H. J. (1952). The effects of psychotherapy: An evaluation. *Journal of Consulting Psychology, 16*, 319–324.

Froyd, J. E., Lambert, M. J., & Froyd, J. D. (1996). A survey and critique of psychotherapy outcome measurement. *Journal of Mental Health, 5*, 11–15.

Garfield, S. L. (1989). *The practice of brief psychotherapy*. New York: Pergamon.

Haas, E., Hill, R. D., Lambert, M. J., & Morrell, B. (2002). Do early responders to psychotherapy maintain treatment gains? *Journal of Clinical Psychology, 58*, 1157–1172.

Hathaway, S. R., McKinley, J. C., & Butcher, J. N. (1990). *Minnesota Multiphasic Personality Inventory–2* (2nd ed.). Minneapolis: University of Minnesota Press.

Hoglend, P. (1993). Suitability for brief dynamic psychotherapy: Psychodynamic variables as predictors of outcome. *Acta Psychiatrica Scandinavica, 88*, 104–110.

Horowitz, L. M., Strupp, H. H., Lambert, M. J., & Elkin, I. (1997). Overview and summary of the core battery conference. In H. H. Strupp, L. M. Horowitz, & M. J. Lambert (Eds.), *Measuring patient changes in mood, anxiety, and personality disorders: Toward a core battery* (pp. 11–54). Washington, DC: American Psychological Association.

Horowitz, M. J., Marmar, C. R., Weiss, D. S., DeWitt, K. N., & Rosenbaum, R. (1984). Brief Psychotherapy of bereavement reactions. *Archives of General Psychiatry, 41*, 438–448.

Ingram, R. E. (1990). Self-focused attention in clinical disorders: Review and a conceptual model. *Psychological Bulletin, 107*, 156–176.

Kadera, S. W., Lambert, M. J., & Andrews, A. A. (1996). How much therapy is really enough? A session-by-session analysis of the psychotherapy dose-effect relationship. *Journal of Psychotherapy: Practice and Research, 5*, 1–20.

Kamas, N. (1991). Group therapy with schizophrenic patients: A short-term, homogeneous approach. *International Journal of Group Psychotherapy, 41*, 33–48.

Kirshner, B., & Guyatt, G. (1985). A methodological framework for assessing health indices. *Journal of Chronic Diseases, 38*, 27–36.

Klein, R. (1985). Some principles of short-term group therapy. *International Journal of Group Psychotherapy, 35*, 309–329.

Kordy, H., Hannöver, W., & Richard, M. (2001). Computer-assisted feedback-driven quality management for psychotherapy: The Stuttgart-Heidelberg model. *Journal of Consulting and Clinical Psychology, 69*, 173–183.

Lambert, M. J. (1983). Introduction to the assessment of psychotherapy outcome: Historical perspective and current issues. In M. J. Lambert, E. R. Christensen, & S. S. DeJulio (Eds.), *The assessment of psychotherapy outcome* (pp. 3–32). New York: Wiley.

Lambert, M. J., & Anderson, E. M. (1996). Assessment for the time-limited psychotherapies. In L. J. Dickstein, M. B. Riba, & J. M. Olvham (Eds.), *Review of psychiatry* (pp. 23–42). Washington DC: American Psychiatric Press.

Lambert, M. J., Bergin, A. E., & Collins, J. L. (1977). Therapist-induced deterioration in psychotherapy. In A. S. Gurman & A. M. Razin (Eds.), *Effective psychotherapy: A handbook of research* (pp. 452–481). New York: Pergamon.

Lambert, M. J., Christensen, E. R., & DeJulio, S. S. (Eds.). (1983). *The assessment of psychotherapy outcome*. New York: Wiley.

Lambert, M. J., Hansen, N. B., & Finch, A. E. (2001). Client-focused research: Using client outcome data to enhance treatment effects. *Journal of Consulting and Clinical Psychology, 69*, 159–172.

Lambert, M. J., Hansen, N., Umphress, V., Lunnen, K., Okiishi, J., Burlingame, G., Huefner, J., & Reisinger, C. (1996). *Administration and scoring manual for the Outcome Questionnaire (OQ–45.2)*. Wilmington, DE: American Professional Credentialing Services.

Lambert, M. J., Horowitz, L. M., & Strupp, H. H. (1997). Conclusions and recommendations. In H. H. Strupp, L. M. Horowitz, & M. J. Lambert (Eds.), *Measuring patient changes in mood, anxiety, and personality disorders: Toward a core battery* (pp. 491–502). Washington, DC: American Psychological Association.

Lambert, M. J., Masters, K. S., & Ogles, B. M. (1992). Measuring counseling outcome: A rejoinder. *Journal of Counseling and Development, 70*, 538–539.

Lambert, M. J., Ogles, B. M., & Masters, K. S. (1992). Choosing outcome assessment devices: An organizational and conceptual scheme. *Journal of Counseling and Development, 70*, 527–532.

Lambert, M. J., Shapiro, D. A., & Bergin, A. E. (1986). The effectiveness of psychotherapy. In S. L. Garfield & A. E. Bergin (Eds.), *Handbook of psychotherapy and behavior change* (3rd ed., pp. 157–211). New York: Wiley.

Lambert, M. J., Whipple, J. L., Vermeersch, D. A., Smart, D. W., Hawkins, E. J., Nielsen, S. L., & Goates, M. K. (2002). Enhancing psychotherapy outcomes via providing feedback on client progress: A replication. *Clinical Psychology and Psychotherapy, 9*, 91–103.

Luborsky, L., Crits-Christoph, P., Mintz, J., & Auerbach, A. (1988). *Who will benefit from psychotherapy?* New York: Basic Books.

Lueger, R. J., Howard, K. I., Martinovich Z., Lutz, W., Anderson, E. E., & Grissom, G. (2001). Assessing treatment progress of individual clients using expected treatment response models. *Journal of Consulting and Clinical Psychology, 69,* 150–158.

Malan, D. H. (1976). *The frontier of brief psychotherapy.* New York: Plenum.

Malan, D. H., & Osimo, F. (1992). *Psychodynamics, training, and outcome in brief psychotherapy.* Boston, MA: Butterworth-Heinemann.

Mann, J. (1991). Time-limited psychotherapy. In P. Crits-Christoph & J. P. Barber (Eds.), *Handbook of short-term dynamic therapy* (pp. 17–44). New York: Basic Books.

Marmor, J. (1979). Short-term dynamic psychotherapy. *American Journal of Psychiatry, 136,* 149–155.

McCallum, M., & Piper, W. (1990). A controlled study of the effectiveness and patient suitability for short-term group psychotherapy. *International Journal of Group Psychotherapy, 40,* 431–452.

McGlynn, E. A. (1996). Setting the context for measuring patient outcomes. In D. M. Steinwachs, L. M. Flynn, G. S. Norquist, & E. A. Skinner (Eds.), *Using client outcomes information to improve mental health and substance abuse treatment* (pp. 19–32). San Francisco: Jossey-Bass.

McLean, P., & Taylor, S. (1992). Severity of unipolar depression and choice of treatment. *Behavior Research Therapy, 30,* 443–451.

Meier, S. T., & Davis, S. R. (1990). Trends in reporting psychometric properties of scales used in counseling psychology research. *Journal of Counseling Psychology, 37,* 113–115.

Miller, R. C., & Berman, J. S. (1983). The efficacy of cognitive behavior therapies: A quantitative review of the research evidence. *Psychological Bulletin, 94,* 39–53.

Milner, J. (1989). Additional cross-validation of the Child Abuse Potential Inventory. *Journal of Consulting and Clinical Psychology, 57,* 219–223.

Moos, R. H. (1990). Depressed outpatients' life contexts, amount of treatment, and treatment outcome. *Journal of Nervous and Mental Disorders, 178,* 105–112.

Newman, F. L., & Ciarlo, J. A. (1994). Criteria for selecting psychological instruments for treatment outcome assessments. In M. E. Maruish (Ed.), *The use of psychological testing for treatment planning and outcome assessment* (pp. 98–110). Hillsdale, NJ: Lawrence Erlbaum Associates.

Newman, F. L., Ciarlo, J. A., & Carpenter, D. (1999). Guidelines for selecting psychological instruments for treatment planning and outcome assessment. In M. E. Maruish (Ed.), *The use of psychological testing for treatment planning and outcomes assessment* (2nd ed., pp. 153–170). Mahwah, NJ: Lawrence Erlbaum Associates.

Ogles, B. M., Lambert, M. J., & Masters, K. S. (1996). *Assessing outcome in clinical practice.* Needham Heights, MA: Allyn & Bacon.

Orlinsky, D. E., Grawe, K., & Parks, B. K. (1994). Process and outcome in psychotherapy: Noch einmal. In A. E. Bergin & S. L. Garfield (Eds.), *Handbook of psychotherapy and behavior change* (4th ed., pp. 270–376). New York: Wiley.

Pilkonis, P. A. (1997). Measurement issues relevant to personality disorders. In H. H. Strupp, L. M. Horowitz, & M. J. Lambert (Eds.), *Measuring patient changes in mood, anxiety, and personality disorders: Toward a core battery* (pp. 371–388). Washington, DC: American Psychological Association.

Piper, W. E., Azim, H. E., McCallum, M., & Joyce, A. (1990). Patient suitability and outcome in short-term individual therapy. *Journal of Consulting and Clinical Psychology, 58,* 475–481.

Piper, W. E., deCarufel, F. L., & Szkrumelak, N. (1985). Patient predictors of process and outcome in short-term individual psychotherapy. *Journal of Nervous and Mental Disorders, 173,* 726–733.

Pollack, J., Flegenagimer, W., & Winston, A. (1991). Brief adaptive psychotherapy. In P. Crits-Christoph & J. P. Barber (Eds.), *Handbook of short-term dynamic therapy* (pp. 199–219). New York: Basic Books.

Shearin, E. N., & Linehan, M. M. (1992). Patient-therapist ratings and relationship to progress in dialectical behavior therapy for borderline personality disorder. *Behavior Therapy, 23*, 730–741.

Sifneos, P. E. (1987). *Short-term dynamic psychotherapy.* New York: Plenum.

Stotsky, S., Glass, D., Shea, T., Pilkonis, P., Collins, J. F., Elkin, I., Watkins, J. T., Imbers, S. D., Leber, W. R., Mayer, J., & Oliveri, M. E. (1991). Patient predictors of response to psychotherapy and pharmacotherapy: Findings in the NIMH treatment of depression collaborative research program. *American Journal of Psychiatry, 148*, 997–1008.

Strupp, H. H. (1980). Success and failure in time-limited psychotherapy: Comparison 3. *Archives of General Psychiatry, 37*, 831–841.

Strupp, H. H. (1981). Toward the refinement of time-limited dynamic psychotherapy. In S. H. Budman (Ed.), *Forms of brief therapy* (pp. 219–225). New York: Guilford.

Tang, T. Z., & DeRubeis, R. J. (1999). Reconsidering rapid early response in cognitive behavioral therapy for depression. *Clinical Psychology: Science and Practice, 6*, 283–288.

Trabin, T. (1995). Making quality and accountability happen in behavioral healthcare. *Behavioral Healthcare Tomorrow, 4*, 5–6.

Ursano, R. J., & Hales, R. E. (1986). A review of brief individual psychotherapies. *American Journal of Psychiatry, 143*, 1507–1512.

Waskow, I. E., & Parloff, M. B. (1975). *Psychotherapy change measures.* Rockville, MD: National Institute of Mental Health.

Wechsler, D. (1997). *WAIS–III administration and scoring manual.* San Antonio, TX: The Psychological Corporation.

Winston, A., Pollack, J., McCullough, L., Flegenheimer, N., Kestenbaum, R., & Trujillo, M. (1991). Brief psychotherapy of personality disorders. *Journal of Nervous and Mental Disorders, 179*, 188–193.

CHAPTER

3

The First Interview

Bonnie A. Rudolph
Texas A&M International University

The psychodynamic reader will appreciate the combination of dread and delight experienced during the writing of this chapter: delight to focus on such an important, yet relatively neglected phase of therapy, its initiation, and fear because there are so many different factors to consider when studying therapists' tasks within the first interview. Furthermore, I have always identified as an integrationist with no particular allegiance to psychodynamic theory. Motivated by these conflicting feelings, I reviewed theory and research on the conduct of the first interview of brief therapy and brief psychodynamic psychotherapy. As the psychodynamic brief therapy literature is extensive, and brief psychotherapy research is wide ranging and complex, this was an ambitious undertaking. Furthermore, as any psychotherapy process researcher knows all too well, there is scant support for linking a single therapist task or technique with positive therapy outcome (Bergin & Garfield, 1994). Still, expert clinicians and sophisticated therapy researchers continue to believe in the clinical significance of certain therapeutic tasks.

 The task analysis approach used throughout this book has particular merit for trainees developing psychotherapy skills (Rudolph, Craig, Leifer, & Rubin, 1998). Within this particular chapter, the approach is to identify and define specific first-interview tasks. Experience as a teacher of graduate trainees in clinical psychology and as a researcher of trainee skill acquisition confirm that clear definition of first-interview tasks facilitates trainee task enactment and self-evaluation. Ambiguity about expectations for task performance has been reported by trainees (Rosenbaum, 1984), and although a modest amount of anxiety may enhance learning, unnecessary anxiety due to lack of clear definition can and should be avoided (Smelson, Kordon, & Rudolph, 1997). Examples from video and audio recordings of first interviews are particularly useful in displaying the tasks and their typical sequence. Trainees can practice and then master the sequence with greater sensitivity to the nuances of particular therapeutic relationships.

LIMITATIONS

The purpose of this chapter is to describe how the brief psychodynamic psychotherapist may sensitively and productively conduct the first interview with adult or near-adult individuals who seek help of their own accord. This chapter describes typical tasks a brief psychodynamic psychotherapist might enact when conducting a first interview with an individual. Modifications would certainly be needed when interviewing couples, families, or children. Although these therapeutic formats are important and increasingly common in psychotherapy practice, they are not the focus of this chapter. Other limitations in application also apply. The tasks suggested here are appropriate with patients who seek psychotherapy of their own volition. Patients mandated to participate in psychotherapy necessitate variations in therapist tasks as well as a significant alteration in the therapist's role that substantially affect the process of the interview. Naturally, patients who are actively psychotic also require a different interview process and therapist stance.

The context in which the first interview is conducted also influences the appropriateness of the tasks described here. These tasks do not fit every context! They are not designed to be part of a mental status exam or a forensic exam. There are excellent treatments of these types of interviews elsewhere (Meloy, 1989; Schwartz, 1989).

It is important to note here that the first interview with patients with communicative disabilities also requires important modifications in therapist tasks and interview processes. Increasingly psychotherapists are providing services to patients who are hearing impaired, use sign language, or experience speech impediments. How the therapist conducts these first interviews is particularly important and warrants sensitive and thoughtful study. Cultural differences between the patient and the therapist in the first interview should also influence the tasks of the therapist. If there are differences between the patient and therapist in race, culture, social class, language, or sexual orientation they must be responded to sensitively in the first interview. One fundamental purpose of the first interview is to provide the patient with a safe and trustworthy setting for self-exploration. Therefore, it is essential that differences, which could handicap or limit the creation of this safe setting for the patient, are discussed with sensitivity and respect. Thus, it is clear that "one size does not fit all" when discussing first-interview tasks. However, certain categories of tasks or factors are, with some notable exceptions, universally present in "good" first psychotherapy interviews and are probably linked to positive therapy outcomes. I return to this point later.

Another set of limitations deserves comment: the basic resources supporting the interview. One may wish to take these for granted, but as a trainer having supervised over a hundred therapy trainees, I've learned to take little for granted about even the basics of the first interview. To adequately conduct the first interview, one should have a quiet, private, ventilated room with a door that closes. One should have few or no interruptions and the privacy and confidentiality of the exchanges should be communicated and safeguarded. It is essential that there be clarity between therapist and patient as to how any record of the interview is going to be made and with whom, if anyone, this record will be shared. There should be an adequate and comfortable seating arrangement that is consistent with the cultural background of the patient. The space of the room should be welcoming and convey a tone of sanctuary, again within the cultural context of the participants.

Last, there should be adequate time allotted for this first interview. There are a number of different tasks and processes that must occur for the interview to be truly productive. Sufficient time is required to accomplish these various tasks. At least 60 min should be allotted for the first interview; 75 is definitely preferable. Research supports this practice. For example, longer first interviews reduce attrition from psychotherapy (Tryon, 1990), and more adequate and comprehensive interviews are associated with longer versus shorter first interviews (Vayo, Liton, & Jersell, 1995).

The Person of the Psychotherapist

The focus on the tasks of the first interview in this chapter is not meant to diminish the importance of the person of the psychotherapist. How the therapist enacts tasks is critical in communicating to patients what therapy is and is not about. It is fundamental to the development of rapport and a therapeutic alliance. The traits, dispositions, and states of the therapist will certainly influence the manner in which and the times in which interview tasks are performed. These tasks may be thought of as the vehicle used to transverse the time and terrain of the first interview; the therapist must still plot and correct the course of the journey. Therapist energy, attention, skill, experience, and confidence will influence the quality of the journey as well as the destination reached.

Therapist attitudes or qualities conducive to successful therapy processes and outcomes have been discussed in the literature since Freud. The reader is referred to Sullivan (1954); Rogers (1951); and Beutler, Machado, and Neufeldt (1994) in Bergin and Garfield (1994) for thoughtful discussions. The focus here is on the specific brief psychotherapy literature concerning useful and productive attitudes of the brief therapist. Flegenheimer (1982) suggested that the brief therapist be experienced in the provision of long-term therapy to maximize the quick learning of brief therapy models. However, he noted, "Ideally, the trainee coming to learn brief therapy should have the knowledge and skills acquired from many years of experience with long-term therapy while not having become habituated to any of his or her own techniques" (Flegenheimer, 1982, p. 14). He also stated, "In some ways it is easier to teach brief therapy to a novice in psychotherapy, because he or she has much less to unlearn" (Flegenheimer, 1982, p. 15).

Desirable Brief Therapist Attitudes or Qualities

The qualities or attitudes that seem most productive for the brief psychodynamic psychotherapist to possess are summarized as follows. The therapist should be:

1. *Alert:* The therapist is rested, watchful, active, and attentive to the patient and the interview process, both overt and covert.
2. *Reflective:* The therapist ponders and thinks carefully; does not operate on "automatic pilot"; is able to offer a new perspective or view of interview content or process, or both.
3. *Empathic:* The therapist identifies with and understands the feelings and communications of the patient.
4. *Respectful:* The therapist shows consideration or esteem for the patient and offers considerate treatment.
5. *Genuine:* The therapist is sincere, honest, and authentic.
6. *Open:* The therapist has no barriers obstructing reception of the patient's communications, verbal and nonverbal, explicit and implicit.
7. *Engaged:* The therapist actively undertakes the tasks of the interview.
8. *Expectant:* The therapist looks forward to the therapeutic work and its success as something probable or certain.

With practice, the brief therapist comes to possess a certain presence and poise in the first interview. This is often described by observers as calmness, gentle constancy, or "centeredness." Interestingly, the word *poise* is defined as "to bring into or hold one's balance or equilibrium" (*Webster's Dictionary and Thesaurus*, 1999). In a first interview in which so much is unknown and unfamiliar, therapist maintenance of a sense of balance is usually perceived as competence by the patient.

THE FIRST INTERVIEW: AN ABBREVIATED REVIEW

The first interview of psychotherapy has been the topic of books (Benjamin, 1969; Budman, Hoyt, & Friedman, 1992; Craig, 1989; Sullivan, 1954), chapters (Matarazzo, 1965; Rudolph et al., 1991; Sanavio, 1998), journal articles (Adams, Peircy, & Jurich, 1991; Cornell, 1986; Eisenthal & Lazare, 1976; Rudolph et al., 1993; Tryon, 1990), and dissertations and clinical research projects (Jenkins, 1982; Kordon, 1995; Leonardi, 1996). A few authors have provided older reviews on research and the anatomy of the first interview (Matarazzo, 1965, 1978; Wiens & Matarazzo, 1983) and more recent literature reports on specific structured interviews linked to the *Diagnostic and Statistical Manual of Mental Disorders* (Hersen & Turner, 1994).

Within this literature, there has been some discussion of phases of the first interview (Benjamin, 1969; Craig, 1989; Kanfer & Scheft, 1988; Sullivan, 1954). Some literature on therapist tasks has also begun to appear (Hill, 1989; Ivey, 1971, 1988; Rudolph et al., 1993; Sanavio, 1998). However, thorough study of therapist tasks in the initial interview for brief psychotherapy is still lacking, especially within the brief psychodynamic literature. As psychotherapy process research and treatment manuals become increasingly popular, this lack will hopefully be addressed. This chapter also adds to the literature.

Although delineating therapist tasks in the first interview of brief therapy has not been their particular focus, psychodynamic theorists have written extensively about selection criteria (Horowitz, 1986; Klerman, Weissman, Rounseville, & Chevron, 1984; Malan, 1976; Sifneos, 1992), setting and maintaining the focus (Davanloo, 1980; Sifneos, 1992), therapist activity (Bellak, 1984; Bloom, 1997; Davanloo, 1980), attention to therapist–patient interactions and dynamics (Luborsky, 1984; Sifneos, 1992; Strupp & Binder, 1984), and creation, maintenance, and repair of the therapeutic alliance (Crits-Christoph & Barber, 1991; Luborsky & Mark, 1991; Pinsker, Rosenthal, & McCullough, 1991; Sullivan, 1954).

IDENTIFICATION OF FIRST INTERVIEW THERAPIST TASKS

Psychodynamic brief therapy writers, starting with Alexander and French (1946) and leading up to the more recent works of Strupp and Binder (1984); Luborsky (1984); Horowitz (1986); Pinsker, Rosenthal, and McCullough

TABLE 3.1
Psychodynamic Therapist Tasks for the First Interview

Number Brief Dynamic Theorists Endorsing (N)	Task Description
20	Set a goal or focus
15	Reformulate presenting problem into central theme
15	Offer interpretations
12	Investigate patient relationships
	a. With others
	b. With self
12	Take a history: Comprehensiveness, or focus varies
10	Confront negative transference
9	Establish a safe environment for patient self-disclosure
6	Assess level of crisis and/or assess patient suitability
7	Focus on interaction between patient and therapist
7	Confront defenses
6	Communicate expectation of hard work
6	Quantify and define phenomenon
5	Watch for countertransference
2	Understand and communicate how symptoms fit into patterns or themes

Note. Psychodynamic theorists surveyed: Strupp & Binder (1994); Davanloo (1980); Horowitz, Bellak, & Small (1965); Pinsker, Rosenthal, & McCullough (1991); Lewin (1970); Pollack, Flegenheimer, & Winston (1991); Klerman et al. (1984); Baker (1991); Bloom (1997); Smith-Benjamin (1991); Gustafson (1986); Luborsky (1984); Bauer & Kobos (1987); Malan (1976); Crits-Christoph & Barber (1991); Mann (1973); Sifneos (1992); Wolberg (1965); Alexander & French (1942).

(1991); and Pollack, Flegenheimer, and Winston (1991) were reviewed. The review particularly focused on each writer's recommendations concerning tasks in the first interview of brief psychodynamic psychotherapy. Fourteen different tasks were identified that were mentioned by at least 2 of the 20 dynamic psychotherapy writers reviewed. These psychodynamic therapist tasks and the writers reviewed are listed in Table 3.1.

A second literature search was then conducted using PsycINFO and Medline databases to identify scales and measures evaluating therapist tasks in clinical interviewing and tasks of the first interview of nondynamic models of brief psychotherapy. Nondynamic models were included because so few measures were found in the psychodynamic literature. A second list was generated from this database. It is noteworthy that only two published measures that listed specific tasks for the first interview were located: the Assessment Interview Skill Deployment Inventory-Revised (Rudolph et al., 1998) and the Diagnostic Interview Rating Scale developed by Bogels et al. (1995) in the Netherlands.

A third brief review of the counseling psychology literature for therapist tasks produced the work of Ivey (1992), which includes listings of counselor tasks but no particular focus on the first interview; the work of Hill (1989) using response modes; and general books on interviewing (Hersen & Van Hasselt, 1998), which cover basic processes but identified few specific therapist tasks.

A Plethora of Tasks

Combination of the reviews of these three areas resulted in 346 tasks noted by various psychodynamic and nondynamic writers and researchers of therapist actions or tasks in the first interview of brief psychotherapy. This list was then checked over for redundancies, commonalities, and uniqueness and a refined list of 173 tasks recommended by both nondynamic and dynamic brief theorists was generated. The 173 tasks were sorted into six categories, five of which were previously used to assess tasks of therapists in training during initial interviews (Rudolph et al., 1998). The previous categories used were structuring tasks, facilitation of patient participation and disclosure tasks, collect data and pursue inquiry tasks, professional conduct tasks, and alliance-building tasks (Rudolph et al., 1991). A sixth category, focusing tasks, was added to reflect the specific category of clarifying a specific goal or objective for the subsequent therapy. This six-category system had no category that had less than 20 tasks within it and alliance building and focusing categories had the most tasks with 38 and 41 tasks, respectively. Sorting the tasks identified in the first interview brief therapy literature into these categories was difficult and readers may contact me if they would like a copy of the categories. The sorting process primarily helped me in refining the initial listing of first-interview tasks to reduce redundancies and served as a handy organizer for reflection.

Comparison of the brief dynamic tasks listed in the parsimonious Table 3.1 with the plethora of cross-theory categorized tasks was an interesting endeavor. Due to space limitations, I only note a few points here. Structuring tasks appear to be less emphasized within the dynamic task listing than in cross-theory task listing, whereas alliance-building qualities are implied in many of the dynamic tasks. Focusing tasks appear very important in both listings. Furthermore, the six-category system is consistent with dynamic tasks, although the application to dynamic tasks seems less useful due to the shorter list of tasks.

A Revised Approach to Therapeutic Tasks: Therapeutic Clusters

The category system of sorted tasks seemed unsatisfactory for the purposes of this chapter because it was developed to evaluate graduate psychology trainee actions in first interviews conducted at various practicum sites using all types of therapy approaches and with no distinction between long- and short-term formats. After repeated review of these tasks and their categorization, I re-sorted them into new categories referred to as clusters. I propose these clusters represent therapeutic events in the first interview of brief psychotherapy. This new clustering of the first-interview tasks takes into account the developmental processes that occur in the first interview of brief therapy. The first task cluster is called *set the stage and structure the interview*, the second is *initially engage the patient in participation and problem disclosure*, the third is *deepen exploration and emotional expression*, the fourth is *reflection and naming*, and the fifth is called *clarify and test the focus*. A cluster named *forge a therapeutic alliance* appeared to be a "megatask" in that just about every therapist task could fit into this cluster as well as into one of the five others.

It seemed logical to conceptualize forge a therapeutic alliance as a megafactor for several reasons. Since Borden (1979), the alliance has been conceptualized as containing three aspects: the bond, the goals, and the tasks. Also, if there is to be a second therapy interview, then beginning creation of a working alliance as a result of the first interview would seem highly important, if not essential. Furthermore, if one of the goals of the first interview for psychotherapy is to create a safe and trustworthy sanctuary then forging an alliance between patient and therapist cannot be separated from this outcome. Likewise, as patients interact with the brief therapist in the first interview, they begin to use new or underutilized relationship skills that, ipso facto, contribute to the therapeutic alliance. Aside from these practical considerations, the rationale was supported by ubiquity of the therapeutic alliance as a fundamental concept in all forms of psychotherapy (Borden, 1979) and research findings that strength of the therapeutic alliance consistently predicts therapy outcome (Horvath & Greenberg, 1994). The six proposed therapeutic task clusters of the first interview of brief psychotherapy and their approximate sequence are depicted in Fig. 3.1. The sixth megafactor, forge a therapeutic alliance, is set off to the side in the figure.

The first cluster, set the stage and structure the interview, would include such dynamic tasks from Table 3.1 as establish a safe environment for patient self-disclosure and assess level of crisis and/or assess patient suitability. Initially engage the patient in participation and problem disclosure would include such dynamic tasks as investigate patient relationships and take a history. Deepen exploration and emotional expression includes the dynamic tasks of quantify and define phenomenon and focus on interaction between patient and therapist, whereas reflection and naming includes such dynamic tasks as confront defenses, offer interpretations, and understand and communicate how symptoms fit into patterns or themes. Clarify and test the focus involves such dynamic tasks as set a goal, reformulate presenting problems into a central theme, and confront negative transference.

3. FIRST INTERVIEW

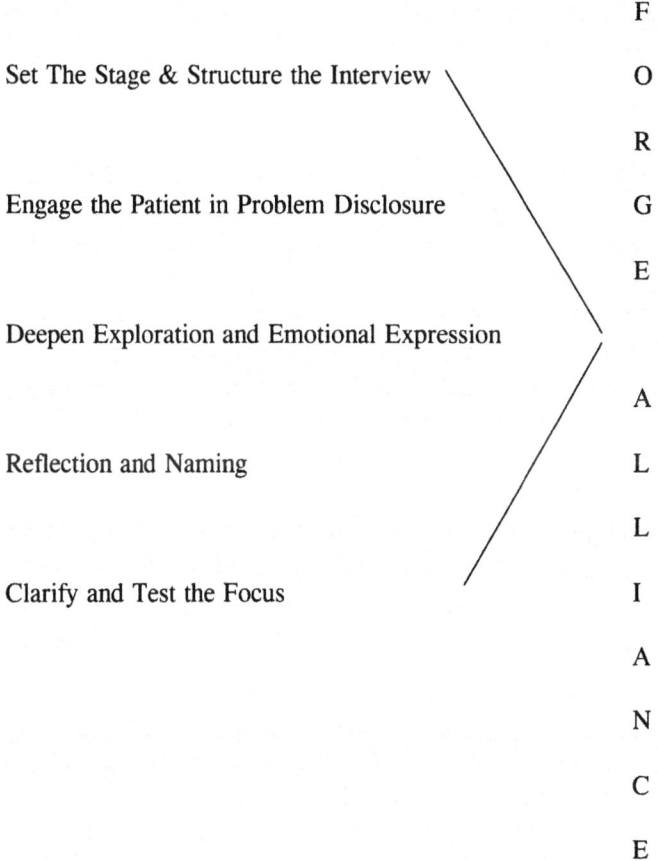

FIG. 3.1. First interview task clusters and Forging a Therapeutic Alliance megafactor.

Elaboration of the Proposed Six Task Clusters

To further describe this model of the first interview for brief therapy, each therapeutic cluster is individually defined and representative tasks for each cluster are listed. I begin with the beginning.

Setting the Stage and Structuring the Interview. The therapeutic cluster *setting the stage and structuring the interview* is defined as those tasks the therapist utilizes to orient the patient to the interview purposes, limitations, and processes. Therapists' tasks to manage transitions, interruptions, disclosures, and passage of interview time are also included within this cluster. Therapists' tasks having to do with discussion of various contextual influences on the interview such as agency policies, referral questions, insurance coverage, and any cultural or lifestyle differences between therapist and patient also fit into this cluster.

A representative sampling of therapist tasks contributing to this cluster includes the following:

- The therapist discusses the purpose(s) of the interview.
- The therapist communicates confidentiality and limits to it.
- The therapist provides a safe and ample environment for patient disclosure.
- The therapist smoothly handles changing from one topic to another.
- The therapist actively encourages patient communication.
- The therapist encourages discussion of any cultural and lifestyle differences between patient and therapist.
- The therapist alerts the patient to time passage and the impending end of the interview.
- The therapist forecasts efforts required for successful therapeutic work.
- The therapist summarizes the content or process of the interview.
- The therapist arranges for further therapeutic contact with the patient.
- The therapist closes the interview and manages leave taking.

The tasks within this factor are therapeutic because they convey to the patient that the therapist is knowledgeable and comfortable in conducting therapeutic work and establishing an initial therapeutic relationship. These tasks also create the framework within which the therapeutic work may be carried out. The structure reduces patient anxiety and communicates to the patient the therapist's competence and confidence. Research on the importance of the patient's perception of the therapist as competent is abundant (Sloan, Staples, Cristol, Yorkston, & Whipple, 1975; Strupp, Fox, & Lessler, 1969).

Initial Engagement of the Patient and Disclosure of Problems. This cluster refers to therapist tasks that help the patient begin to actively participate in the first-interview process and facilitate initial patient disclosures about problems. Tasks incorporated within this factor typically occur at the beginning of the first interview, usually right after the therapist has set the stage and oriented the patient to interview purposes and limitations. Therapist tasks involving both initial open-ended and closed questions also belong here.

A representative sampling of therapist tasks for this cluster include the following:

- Therapist inquires as to the reason the patient sought help at this time.

- Therapist inquires into the patient's presenting problem.
- Therapist responds with empathy to patient disclosures.
- Therapist uses paraphrase to assure accurate understanding and convey careful attending.
- Therapist conveys warmth, acceptance, and support as patient discloses.
- Therapist attempts a variety of approaches to engage the reticent patient.
- Therapist encourages patient to elaborate on important material.
- Therapist invites patient reactions to initiating and orienting phase of interview.
- Therapist encourages patient to take initiative in the first phase of the interview.

It is hypothesized that this category of therapist tasks is therapeutic because it directly involves initial facilitation of patient participation in the interview process. High patient engagement or involvement in psychotherapy has been linked to positive treatment outcomes (Strupp, 1973; Orlinsky & Howard, 1986). In addition, these therapist tasks make a metacommunication to the patient. They implicitly convey the message, "You have valuable information to offer in our work and you must actively participate in the interview for our work to be successful." These therapist tasks help the patient understand his or her essential role in the therapy and facilitate and reward the patient's initial enactment of it. The reduction of ambiguity for the patient that these therapy tasks engender is probably also therapeutic and "remoralizing." Tryon (1986) developed a system to measure patient engagement and has linked it to patients staying in therapy for more than 10 sessions. This task cluster directly relates to facilitating patient engagement, which reduces attrition and enhances therapy success.

Deepen Exploration and Emotional Expression. Brief psychodynamic theorists all emphasize the importance of therapist facilitation of patient exploration of material and helpful expression of emotions. This therapeutic cluster is defined here as the category of therapist actions or tasks that prompts and subsequently promotes the patient to discuss material to a degree and in a manner that allows examination of it more extensively and with more attention to patient emotional experience than is typical in "normal" social interactions. These therapist tasks are more advanced than those used in the previous cluster because they involve discerning which patient material to further pursue, when, and in what manner.

Representative therapist tasks included within this cluster are the following:

- The therapist asks about the patient's feelings and states of mind.
- The therapist asks the patient to discuss important relationships in his or her life.
- The therapist communicates observation of patient behavior and inquires into its meaning.
- The therapist inquires into the patient's feelings and thoughts about the therapist in the interview.
- The therapist asks the patient to discuss his or her thoughts and feelings about the interview process.
- The therapist inquires into patient dreams, wishes, and fears.
- The therapist asks the patient to report his or her earliest memory.
- The therapist pursues important material and encourages the patient to elaborate.
- The therapist asks the patient to think about how she or he evaluates or regards himself or herself.
- The therapist promotes discussion of the patient's needs from the patient's perspective.
- The therapist inquires into the way the patient relates to himself or herself and to patient self-appraisal and self-talk.
- The therapist inquires into change points in the patient's life.

These tasks are therapeutic precisely because they engage the patient in disclosure and discussion at a level and in a manner that is not usual in social exchanges. Thus, patients have an opportunity to experience the material in a new way, which may facilitate alterations in perceptions and meanings and leads to the fourth cluster of tasks described next.

Reflection and Naming. The therapeutic cluster of reflection and naming is consistently emphasized by brief psychodynamic writers (Davanloo, 1978; Luborsky, 1984). Most dynamic writers address the specific therapist task of therapist-offered interpretations. However, there are a wide range of therapist tasks within this category that contribute to the strength and influence of this therapeutic factor. This task cluster refers to therapist actions or tasks that cast a new or different perspective on patient presented material. Some representative therapist tasks within this cluster are listed following:

- The therapist offers an interpretation of patient material.
- The therapist offers a process observation of patient interview behavior and links it to patient difficulties.

3. FIRST INTERVIEW

- The therapist links past events or relationships to current ones in patient's life.
- The therapist names a feeling implicit in a patient communication but not made explicit by the patient.
- The therapist observes a pattern in the patient's interpersonal relationships and communicates this observation to the patient.
- The therapist repeats an expression of the patient's, giving different emphasis to the phrasing.
- The therapist links a patient reaction to the therapist with patient reactions to other significant people in the patient's present or past.
- The therapist examines the interaction between the patient and the therapist in the here and now of the session and does this out loud.
- The therapist "confronts" a patient's defense (names the patient behavior as defensive and communicates the negative consequences of the defense for patient progress).
- The therapist educates or advises a patient about a condition, treatment, process, or risk.

This cluster of tasks has long been considered therapeutic because it involves the patient in perceiving his or her experience in a different way. This experience sometimes facilitates patient motivation for behavior change as well as shifts in feeling states. Many brief therapists use tasks within this cluster as trial therapy to determine patient suitability.

Clarify and Test the Focus. This therapeutic process or category of therapist tasks has always been associated with brief psychotherapy, psychodynamic and otherwise (Bloom, 1997; Flegenheimer, 1982). It is defined here as the category of tasks in which the therapist clearly communicates a goal, objective, focal theme, conflict, or behavior change in an interpersonal pattern as the aim of the therapeutic work and therapist tasks to seek patient agreement on and commitment to the focus or goal in the subsequent therapy. Some representative therapist tasks within this therapeutic factor are the following:

- The therapist explicitly suggests a focal conflict as the object of therapeutic work.
- The therapist suggests amelioration of a difficulty or problem in the patient's life as the focus or objective of the subsequent therapy.
- The therapist suggests a patient's maladaptive pattern as the focus for therapy.

- The therapist suggests a core conflictual relationship theme as the focus for therapy.
- The therapist suggests an oedipal conflict or derivative as the focus of therapy.
- The therapist paraphrases the patient's goal for therapy such that it is more clear, measurable, and motivating.
- The therapist suggests a symptom to lessen or eliminate as the focus of therapy work.
- The therapist specifically asks the patient if he or she is committed to working on the focal area. Or conversely, the therapist inquires into doubts the patient may have about the focus of the subsequent therapy.
- The therapist inquires into what will be different as a result of therapy.
- The therapist inquires into how the patient's life would be if the problem miraculously disappeared.

Forge a Therapeutic Alliance: The Megafactor Cluster. Many reviews of measures of the therapeutic alliance report a positive correlation between high alliance scores and positive therapy outcomes (Crits-Christoph, 1991; Luborsky, 1984; Marmar, 1990). Forging a therapeutic alliance is important for all forms of therapy (Borden, 1979). For my purposes, this category of therapist tasks refers to all deliberate therapist tasks that create or foster a collaborative partnership between patient and therapist, one in which the efforts of both partners are acknowledged and balanced. Therefore, therapist tasks within this category also include therapist actions to encourage and acknowledge patient initiative and contributions to the work.

Every therapist task in the first interview has the potential of facilitating to the development of an alliance. Indeed, even actions not intended to be therapeutic may effect alliance development in the first interview. This is so because in the first interview both participants are creating first impressions that can be particularly potent for patients who are unfamiliar with professional helpers, therapeutic relationships, and therapeutic collaboration. The therapist knows, in general terms, what to expect in a first interview; the patient typically does not. The patient can also often approach the interview with heightened anxiety. In effect, the patient is being socialized into the role of therapy patient or participant in what is often a highly charged and novel situation. For some patients these circumstances may make the lessons learned more potent. Even when the patient is not especially sensitive to such learning, he or she is learning nonetheless how his or her participation interacts with the actions of this particular therapist. This initial learning sometimes becomes the template for subsequent joint

3. FIRST INTERVIEW 61

therapeutic effort. Some representative therapist tasks in this far-ranging and critical cluster include the following:

- The therapist addresses the patient by his or her name.
- The therapist uses the word *we* and refers to the joint, mutual effort of both patient and therapist.
- The therapist responds empathically to the patient's fears, anxieties, and hesitancies.
- The therapist attends to the patient.
- The therapist acknowledges the patient's feelings.
- The therapist accurately paraphrases the patient's material.
- The therapist asks the patient for feedback on the interview process.
- The therapist gives information the patient needs to proceed therapeutically.
- The therapist forecasts the work the two will do together in subsequent therapy.
- The therapist communicates how she or he can be contacted and the procedures for setting and canceling appointments.
- The therapist invites questions of the patient.

If adequate time is allotted for the first interview of brief therapy, the proposed six therapeutic events should occur. Adequate performance of tasks in each of the six clusters should be correlated with successful first interviews and development of an initial working alliance for the subsequent therapy. Obviously there are some limits to this proposed correlation. These include, for example, that the interview is conducted by a moderately well trained brief psychotherapist who is working with an adult patient who is not psychotic, able to communicate in the same language as the therapist, and seeking help volitionally.

INTERACTION OF THERAPEUTIC CLUSTERS AND PATIENT CONTRIBUTIONS

The sequencing of the task clusters is much less fixed than the ordering in Fig. 3.1 implies. Everything affects everything else in a first interview. Patients greatly influence the processes and outcomes of first interviews as they do psychotherapy as a whole. How much initiative the patients exert and the quality and type of their contributions naturally influence the therapist's tasks and the sequence of their occurrence. Likewise, therapists may elect to perform certain tasks in a different sequence. Although no single therapist task is consistently linked with positive interview outcomes, clusters of tasks, as suggested previously, may comprise therapeutic factors or therapeutic events in the first interview. These first interview therapeutic events may set the tone for the subsequent treatment and may sometimes forecast treatment outcome (Rudolph et al., 1993). The occurrence of these clusters in a first therapeutic interview would certainly be consistent with the finding that typically successful patients experience beginning therapy as remoralizing (Frank, 1973).

Phases of the First Interview

As for the idea of phases existing in first interviews, there is more theory than research supporting this idea (Benjamin, 1969; Craig, 1989; Kanfer & Scheft, 1988; Rogers, 1951; Sullivan, 1954). However, Schneider (1991) did find evidence of phasing of therapist response modes in first interviews of brief collaborative therapy (Rudolph, 1996). Schneider's findings, using a variation of Hill's (1989) therapist response modes system, identified that certain response modes predominated in three phases of the first interview, which Schneider (1991) simply called beginning, middle, and end.

When the proposed six therapeutic clusters described in this chapter are related to the beginning, middle, and end phases of the first interview, the phases can be labeled Phase I, orienting and initiating; Phase II, jointly working to understand; and Phase III, clarifying, contracting, and closing. Indeed, when two audiotapes and transcripts of brief therapy first interviews I conducted over 15 years ago were reviewed, the clusters seemed to account for all therapist tasks in these first interviews and there was a predominance of certain tasks and clusters over the three phases of the first interviews.

In the orienting and initiating phase (the first phase), two categories of tasks predominated: setting the stage and structuring the interview and initially engaging the patient in participation and problem disclosure. In the second phase, working to understand, exploring and emotional expression, reflection and naming, and forging an alliance categories predominated. In the final phase, clarifying, contracting, and closing, clarifying and testing the focus and structuring and setting the stage categories were most prevalent. A graphic presentation of the therapeutic clusters and interview phases is offered in Fig. 3.2. The limited research suggests the first phase is usually longer than the final phase but not nearly as long as the second phase (Schneider, 1991). Typically the longest portion of the interview is the second phase, jointly working to understand.

In this chapter, definitions of the five therapeutic clusters and the megacluster of forging an alliance have been offered and some sample therapist

3. FIRST INTERVIEW   63

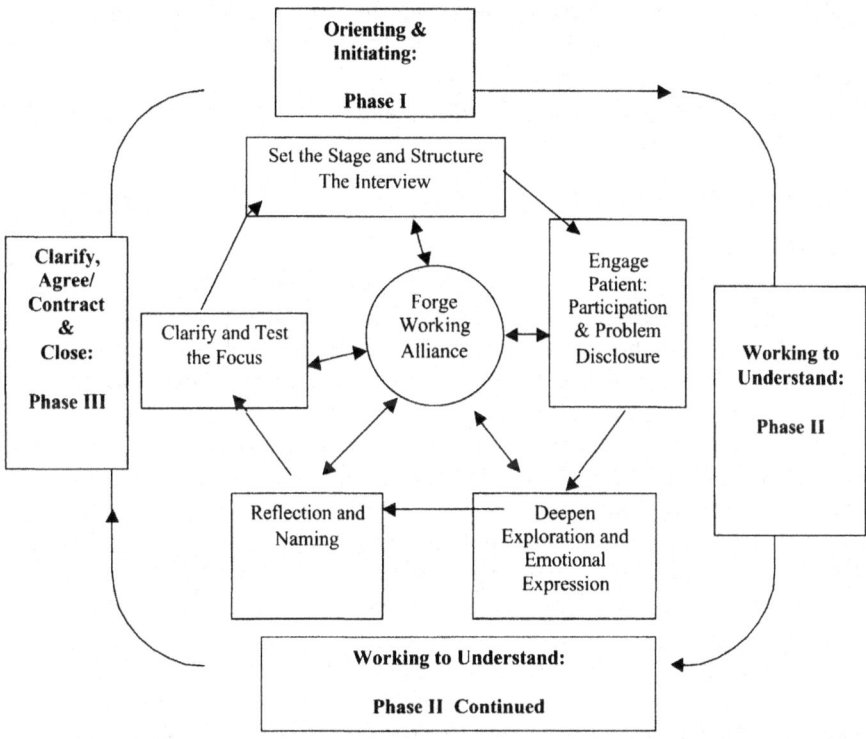

FIG. 3.2. Three phases of first interview encompassing the six task clusters.

tasks for each have been listed. As points of comparison, readers may wish to review the items listed in various measures of therapeutic alliance (Greenberg & Pinsof, 1986) or refer to measures of first interview therapist skills (Bogels et al., 1995; Rudolph et al., 1998).

This organization of therapist tasks into therapeutic clusters is one system and other terms or perhaps even categories are available to capture the initial interview process. For example, Bauer and Kobos (1987) noted four main therapist conceptual tasks in their summary of dynamic theorists: understand the patient's presenting problem, assess the level of crisis, understand the genetic development of the patient's difficulties, and gain a sense of the patient's current life situation and past history. Sifneos (1992) listed five main tasks: assess the presenting problem, obtain a systematic developmental history, use the appropriate selection criteria, formulate a specific dynamic focus for the psychotherapy, and obtain an agreement from the patient to work cooperatively with the therapist to resolve the underlying emotional conflicts. Craig (1989) listed 11 therapist techniques used in diagnostic and clinical interviewing but did not categorize them. However, these authors did not specifically utilize a task-analysis approach when creating their task categories. The clusters proposed here are based on such an approach and appear to have heuristic and research value. Three phases of the first interview for brief therapy have also been labeled and the meager research supporting phases and how they relate to clusters has been discussed.

CONCLUSION

This chapter has attempted to identify first-interview tasks that psychodynamic and brief therapy writers of various theoretical orientations have noted in their published work. However, it must be recognized that what therapists say they do in interviews and what they actually do is not necessarily the same. The increase in therapy manuals and frequent supervision for adherence to the manuals in psychotherapy research studies attest to this fact. To verify that the tasks described in the brief therapy literature are actually the tasks that occur in first interviews, one must record first interviews, transcribe them, and carefully and systematically rate the tasks that are actually carried out. This is very labor intensive, unglamorous research. I wish we did more of it.

Having said that, I assert that the tasks identified in this chapter are important for the first interview of brief psychodynamic psychotherapy. The mere fact that so many brief therapy writers, psychodynamic and otherwise, have written about them lends some credence to their first-interview strength and value. Furthermore, I believe that clusters of tasks, if sufficiently present in the first interview, lead to positive interview outcomes. Obviously, detailed study of first interviews is needed to investigate this claim.

A promising strategy might be to compare first-interview tasks of experienced or expert therapists with novice or less experienced brief therapists. One might expect that expert brief therapists would be more proficient at moving through the sequence of therapist tasks and in deviating from it to best engage a particular patient than less experienced therapists. It may also be that expert therapists are particularly adept at capitalizing on tasks that contribute to multiple therapeutic clusters at once. By comparing expert and novice therapists in the first interview, one could not only study the tasks performed but also the processes of therapist task performance as well. Such task-analysis research may generate other tasks and clusters that are more valid or useful. Certainly, as new therapies develop and as new patient populations are served, other tasks may be identified.

What is clear from the review conducted here is that there are a very large number of first-interview tasks that the brief therapist needs to accomplish. The novice brief therapist need not be set adrift on an uncharted course of abbreviated therapeutic work. The challenge, rather, is selecting which tasks best fit the patient's needs, the training site's mission, and development of trainee skills. By considering the framework of six therapeutic clusters suggested here, as well as the three first interview phases, trainers and trainees may be able to focus their efforts so that all parties enhance their outcomes.

Although this chapter has focused on the what of the first interview, the how or the way in which therapist tasks are enacted cannot be ignored. Likewise, the critical role of the patient and patient task performance in the first interview must be acknowledged. Each patient brings unique strengths and weaknesses to the first visit. These patient qualities act as parameters within which the therapist must operate. However, if we conduct ourselves in this first interview with respect and compassion for the patient, an open mind, and responsive, culturally sensitive behavior, then we have a human encounter that will likely lead to reflection and growth for both participants.

REFERENCES

Adams, J., Peircy, F., & Jurich, J. (1991). Effects of solution focused therapies "formula first session task" on compliance and outcome in family therapy. *Journal of Marital and Family Therapy, 17,* 277–290.
Alexander, F., & French, T. (1946*). Psychoanalytic therapy.* New York: Ronald Press.
American Psychiatric Association. (1994). *Diagnostic and statistical manual of mental disorders DSM–IV* (4th ed.). Washington, DC: American Psychiatric Press.
Bauer, G., & Kobos, J. (1987*). Brief therapy: Short term psychodynamic intervention.* Northvale, NJ: Aronson.
Bellak, L. (1984). Intensive brief and emergency psychotherapy. In L. Grinspoon (Ed.), *Psychiatry update: The American Psychiatric Association annual review* (Vol. 3, pp. 11–24). Washington, DC: American Psychiatric Press.
Bellak, L., & Small, L. (1965). *Emergency psychotherapy and brief psychotherapy.* New York: Grune & Stratton.
Benjamin, A. (1969). *The helping interview* (2nd ed.). Boston: Houghton Mifflin.
Bergin, A. E., & Garfield, S. (Eds.). (1994). *Handbook of psychotherapy and behavior change* (4th ed.). New York: Wiley.
Beutler, L., Machado, P., & Neufeldt, S. (1994). Therapist variables. In A. Bergin & S. Garfield (Eds.), *Handbook of psychotherapy and behavior change* (4th ed., pp. 229–269). New York: Wiley.
Bloom, B. (1997). Bloom's single-session psychotherapy. In B. Bloom, *Planned short-term psychotherapy: A clinical handbook* (2nd ed., pp. 62–83). Boston: Allyn & Bacon.
Bogels, S. M., van der Viuten, P., Blok, G., Kreutzkamp, R., Melles, R., & Shmidt, H. (1995). Assessment and validation of diagnostic interviewing skills for the mental health professions. *Journal of Psychopathology and Behavioral Assessment, 17,* 217–230.
Borden, E. (1979). The generalizability of the psychoanalytic concept of the working alliance. *Psychotherapy: Theory, Research, and Practice, 16,* 252–260.
Budman, S., Hoyt, M., & Friedman, S. (Eds.). (1992). *The first session in brief therapy.* New York: Guilford.

Cornell, W. F. (1986). Setting the therapeutic stage: The initial sessions. *Transactional Analysis Journal, 16*, 4–10.
Craig, R. (Ed.). (1989). *Clinical and diagnostic interviewing*. New York: Aronson.
Crits-Christoph, P., & Barber, J. (1991). Comparison of the brief dynamic therapies. In P. Crits-Christoph & J. Barber (Eds.), *Handbook of short-term dynamic psychotherapy* (pp. 323–352). New York: Basic Books.
Davanloo, H. (Ed.). (1978). *Basic principles and techniques in short-term dynamic psychotherapy*. New York: SP Medical and Scientific Books.
Davanloo, H. (1980). *Short-term dynamic psychotherapy*. Northvale, NJ: Aronson.
Eisenthal, S., & Lazare, A. (1976). Specificity of patients' requests in the initial review. *Psychological Reports, 38*, 739–748.
Flegenheimer, W. V. (1982). *Techniques of brief psychotherapy*. New York: Aronson.
Frank, J. (1973). *Persuasion and healing*. Baltimore: Johns Hopkins University Press.
Greenberg, L. S., & Pinsof, W. M. (1986). *The psychotherapeutic process: A research handbook*. New York: Guilford Press.
Gustafson, J. P. (1986). *The complex secret of brief psychotherapy*. New York: Norton.
Hersen, M., & Turner, S. M. (Eds.). (1994). *Diagnostic interviewing* (2nd ed.). New York: Plenum.
Hersen, M., & Van Hasselt, V. (Eds.). (1998). *Basic interviewing: A practical guide for counselors and clinicians*. Mahwah, NJ: Lawrence Erlbaum Associates.
Hill, C. (1989). *Therapist techniques and client outcomes*. New York: Sage.
Horowitz, M. (1986). *Stress response syndromes* (2nd ed.). New York: Aronson.
Horvath, A., & Greenberg, L. (Eds.). (1994). *The working alliance: Theory, research, and practice*. New York. Wiley.
Ivey, A. (1971). *Microcounseling: Innovations in interviewing training*. Springfield, IL: Thomas.
Ivey, A. (1992). *Managing face to face communication*. Framingham, MA: Munstraing Associates.
Jenkins, W. W. (1982). *The development and evaluation of a scale to rate interview competence*. Unpublished doctoral dissertation. Ann Arbor, MI. U.M.I. 8218911.
Kanfer, F. H., & Scheft, B. K. (1988). *Guiding the process of therapeutic change*. Champaign, IL: Research Press.
Klerman, G. W., Weissman, M. M., Rounseville, B., & Chevron, E. (1984). *Interpersonal psychotherapy of depression (IPT)*. New York: Basic Books.
Kordon, M. (1995). *Towards the reliability of the Global Impressions of the Diagnostic Interview–Revised (GIDI–R): Assessing the global quality of diagnostic interviewing in clinical psychology training programs*. Unpublished clinical research project, #632. Illinois School of Professional Psychology, Chicago.
Leonardi, F. (1996). *Investigation of the reliability of the Assessment Interview Skill Development Inventory*. Unpublished clinical research project, #768. Illinois School of Professional Psychology, Chicago.
Lewin, K. K. (1970). *Brief encounters: Brief psychotherapy*. St. Louis, MO: Green.
Luborsky, L. (1984). *Principles of psychoanalytic psychotherapy: A manual for supportive–expressive treatment*. New York: Basic Books.
Luborsky, L., & Mark, D. (1991). Short-term supportive–expressive psychoanalytic psychotherapy. In P. Crits-Christoph & J. Barber (Eds.), *Handbook of short-term dynamic psychotherapy* (pp. 110–136). New York: Basic Books.
Malan, D. (1976). *A study of brief psychotherapy*. New York: Plenum.
Mann, J. (1973). *Time limited psychotherapy*. Cambridge, MA: Harvard University Press.
Marmar, C. R. (1990). Psychotherapy process research: Progress, dilemmas and future directions. *Journal of Consulting & Clinical Psychology, 58*, 265–272.
Matarazzo, J. D. (1965). The interview. In B. Wolman (Ed.), *Handbook of clinical psychology* (pp. 403–450). New York: McGraw-Hill.
Matarazzo, J. D. (1978). The interview: Its reliability and validity in psychiatric diagnosis. In B. Wolman (Ed.), *Clinical diagnosis of mental disorders* (pp. 47–96). New York: Plenum.

Meloy, J. R. (1989). The forensic interview. In R. Craig (Ed.), *Clinical and diagnostic interviewing* (pp. 269–288). Northvale, NJ: Aronson.

Orlinsky, D., & Howard, K. (1986). Process and outcomes in psychotherapy. In S. Garfield & A. Bergin (Eds.), *Handbook of psychotherapy and behavior change* (2nd ed., pp. 311–381). New York: Wiley.

Pinsker, H., Rosenthal, R., & McCullough, L. (1991). Dynamic supportive psychotherapy. In P. Crits-Christoph & J. Barber (Eds.), *Handbook of short-term dynamic psychotherapy* (pp. 220–247). New York: Basic Books.

Pollack, J., Flegenheimer, W., & Winston, A. (1991). Brief adaptive psychotherapy. In P. Crits-Christoph & J. Barber (Eds.), *Handbook of short-term dynamic psychotherapy* (pp. 199–219). New York: Basic Books.

Rogers, C. (1951). *Client-centered therapy*. Boston: Houghton-Mifflin.

Rosenbaum, D. N. (1984). Evaluation of student performance in psychotherapy. *Journal of Clinical Psychology, 4*, 1106–1110.

Rudolph, B. (1996). *Brief collaborative therapy: A practical guide for practitioners*. Westport, CT: Praeger.

Rudolph, B., Cardella, H., Datz, J., Jochem, J., Kadlec, M., G., Mann, E., Somberg, E., & Stone, M. (1991). Illinois School of Professional Psychology: Brief psychotherapy research project. In L. Beutler & M. Craig (Eds.), *Psychotherapy research: An international review of programmatic studies* (pp. 279–284). Washington, DC: American Psychological Association.

Rudolph, B., Craig, R., Leifer, M., & Rubin, N. (1998). Evaluating competency in the diagnostic interview among graduate psychology students: Development of generic scales. *Professional Psychology: Research & Practice, 29*, 488–491.

Rudolph, B., Datz-Weems, H., Marrie, S., Cusack, A., Beerup, C., & Kiel, S. (1993). Assessment interview processes: A successful and a failed brief therapy. *Psychotherapy in Private Practice, 12*(2), 17–35.

Sanavio, E. (1998). Topography of the first interview. *Behavior and cognitive therapy today. Essay in honor of Hans J. Eysenck* (pp. 229–240). Oxford, England: Elsevier Science, Ltd.

Sifneos, P. (1992). *Short-term anxiety-provoking psychotherapy: A treatment manual*. New York: Basic Books.

Schneider, M. (1991). *Therapist verbal response modes at initiation of brief therapy: A taxonomy*. Unpublished Clinical Research Project #330. Chicago: Illinois School of Professional Psychology.

Schwartz, E. (1989). The Mental Status Exam. In R. Craig (Ed.), *Clinical and diagnostic interviewing* (pp. 269–288). Northvale, NJ: Aronson.

Sloane, R. B., Staples, F. R., Cristol, A. H., Yorkston, N. J., & Whipple, K. (1975). *Psychotherapy versus behavior therapy*. Cambridge, MA: Harvard University Press.

Smelson, D., Kordon, M., & Rudolph, B. (1997). Evaluating the diagnostic interview: Obstacles and future directions. *Journal of Clinical Psychology, 53*, 497–505.

Sullivan, H. S. (1954). *The psychiatric interview*. New York: Norton.

Strupp, H., Fox, R., & Lessler, K. (1969). *Patients view their psychotherapy*. Baltimore: Johns Hopkins University Press.

Strupp, H., & Binder, J. (1984). *Psychotherapy in a new key: A guide to time-limited dynamic psychotherapy*. New York: Basic Books.

Strupp, H. (1973). On the basic ingredients in psychotherapy. *Journal of Consulting & Clinical Psychology, 41*, 1–8.

Tryon, G. (1986). Client and counselor characteristics & engagement in counseling. *Journal of Counseling Psychology, 33*, 471–474.

Tryon, G. (1990). Session depth and smoothness: Relation to the concept of engagement in counseling. *Journal of Counseling Psychology, 37*, 248–253.

Vayo, M., Liton, C., & Jersell, J. (1995). Quality and counselor's intake evaluations as a function of client presenting concern. *Journal of Counseling Psychology, 42*, 100–104.

Webster's dictionary and thesaurus with United States & world atlas. (1999). New York: Nichols Publishing Group.

Wiens, A. N. (1976). The assessment interview. In B. Wiener (Ed.), *Clinical methods in psychology* (pp. 3–60). New York: Wiley.

Wiens, A. N., & Matarazzo, J. D. (1983). Diagnostic interviewing. In M. Herson, A. Kazdin, & A. Bellak (Eds.), *The clinical psychology handbook* (pp. 309–328). Elmsford, NY: Pergamon.

Wolberg, L. (1965). *Short-term psychotherapy.* New York: Grune & Stratton.

CHAPTER

4

Assessing Patient Capacities for Therapy: Psychological-Mindedness and Quality of Object Relations

Anthony S. Joyce
University of Alberta

Mary McCallum
Private Practice, Edmonton, Alberta, Canada

In this chapter, we provide an overview of two patient characteristics and their assessment. The characteristics are representative of important capacities for engaging successfully in short-term dynamic psychotherapy (STDP). *Psychological mindedness* (PM) is a personality trait associated with the patient's capacity to make productive use of the "language" of therapy, that is, to understand and apply the therapist's interventions to the process of resolving personal problems. *Quality of object relations* (QOR) represents a more global personality style associated with the capacity to establish and maintain relationships based on mutuality and autonomy, that is, to establish and maintain a collaborative relationship with the therapist that can allow for the therapy process to occur. The variables derived from PM and QOR assessments have demonstrated empirical relations with measures of the process and outcome of STDP. The assessment procedures also have utility regarding the selection of patients and the prediction of therapy process developments over the course of STDP treatment. The two measures, PM and QOR, are presented in turn. In each section, a representative case is used to demonstrate the features of each assessment and their implications for the treatment process.

PSYCHOLOGICAL MINDEDNESS

Geneviève presented at our Psychiatric Treatment Clinic requesting therapy to address her loneliness and depression. She believed that the root of her unhappiness lay in her failure to form an enduring intimate relationship with a man. She stated that she wanted such a relationship "more than anything else in the world." Approaching age 35, she was fearful that she would also never have a child. Geneviève appeared attractive, bright, and engaging. Attempting to understand the root of her unhappiness, the intake clinician explored Geneviève's history of relationships, including the family history. The history revealed a consistent, lifelong pattern. Each time Geneviève had become close to anyone, she eventually wound up feeling hurt, unappreciated, and betrayed. Those who betrayed her included her parents, school friends, boyfriends, and work colleagues. Her sense of betrayal was heightened by her own tendency to be protective of everyone, beginning with her parents and including her most recent boyfriend.

The intake clinician hypothesized that although Geneviève's stated and conscious desire was to establish an enduring relationship with a man, on an unconscious level she was probably fearful that a relationship would only bring more hurt and disappointment. Her recent relationships with men suggested that an unconscious compromise to the conflict between her wish for and her fear of a relationship had been established. In other words, Geneviève unconsciously behaved in such a way that her wish was partially met and her fear was not stimulated sufficiently to reach conscious awareness. Specifically, Geneviève's recent boyfriends included men who were married, living in another city, or otherwise unavailable. The clinician interpreted to Geneviève that she had chosen men who could be kept at arm's length, that is, with whom she would never become completely vulnerable. In this way, she enjoyed certain aspects of the relationship while simultaneously avoiding the potential for pain if she were to surrender to a truly intimate relationship with an emotionally and physically available partner. The clinician also interpreted that although Geneviève was lonely and depressed, she was also "safe."

The intake clinician debated whether to offer Geneviève a contract of STDP and whether the approach should be primarily supportive or interpretive. To benefit from therapy, Geneviève needed to be receptive to the links between her loneliness and depression and the unconscious process hypothesized in the clinician's formulation. Such receptivity has been called psychological mindedness (Bloch, 1979; Tyson & Sandler, 1971). According to Silver (1983), the capacity for psychological mindedness includes

> The patient's desire to learn the possible meanings and causes of his internal and external experiences as well as the patient's ability to look inwards to psychical factors rather than only outwards to environmental factors ... [and] to potentially conceptualize the relationship between thoughts, feelings, and actions. (p. 516)

Psychological mindedness (PM) is commonly regarded as a desirable attribute of patients being considered for any psychodynamically oriented psychotherapy (e.g., Malan, 1976). The psychologically minded patient shares a commonality with the therapist, that is, they "speak the same language." The psychoanalytic assumptions regarding human behavior and psychopathology form the conceptual template for the therapist's interventions. The psychologically minded patient is held to tacitly employ these same assumptions and is therefore believed to benefit from dynamic therapy by being better able to assimilate and work with the therapist's interpretations. It is also believed that these patients are able to formulate understandings of their own dynamics between and beyond therapy sessions. The therapist could predict Geneviève's likely response in STDP if her level of PM could be determined.

THE PSYCHOLOGICAL MINDEDNESS ASSESSMENT PROCEDURE (PMAP): CONCEPTUAL BACKGROUND

The initial development of the PMAP occurred at McGill University in the early 1980s (McCallum & Piper, 1987). At that time there were few studies that attempted to operationalize PM and investigate its relation with therapy process and outcome (e.g., Kernberg et al., 1972). The results of the studies that did exist were inconsistent and inconclusive. The paucity of the research seemed to reflect ambiguities associated with the definition and measurement of PM.

The term, psychological mindedness, is used interchangeably with a multitude of concepts, for example, insight (Tolor & Reznikoff, 1960), introspection, and self-awareness (Marini & Case, 1994). It has also been associated with other constructs such as alexithymia (Taylor, 1984), personal intelligence (Park, Imboden, Park, Hulse, & Unger, 1992), and private self-consciousness (Fenigstein, Scheier, & Buss, 1975). The nature of the construct of psychological mindedness has been represented as an ability, an interest, and a motive. Finally, approaches to its measurement have involved questionnaires, clinical appraisals (e.g., response to trial interpretations), and the combination of scores from measures of associated variables (see McCallum & Piper, 1997b). Each approach is associated with problems, that is, conceptual overlap with other constructs, rater inference, and indirect measurement.

Informed by previous attempts, we committed ourselves to constructing a reliable and valid measure of PM. Toward that end, we first identified the basic assumptions associated with psychoanalytic theory that would serve as guiding principles for development of the measure. That approach was consistent with our operational definition of PM: *the ability to identify dynamic (intrapsychic) components and to relate them to a person's difficulties.*

Psychoanalytic theory is represented by various schools of thought. Despite the differences and debates among these schools, all psychodynamically oriented psychotherapists share basic assumptions about human behavior and psychopathology (Eagle, 1984). As stated previously, these assumptions guide the language of therapy in that they form the conceptual template for the therapist's interpretations. With the incorporation of these assumptions into our measurement of PM, we believed that the patient's capacity to speak the same language in therapy could be accurately predicted.

The first assumption of psychoanalytic theory is *psychic determinism*, that is, all problems are believed to be determined—at least to some extent—by unconscious processes. The second assumption is that *unconscious motives or their derivatives press for fulfillment*. These motives include wishes, needs, wants, or impulses. Freud's drive theory referred collectively to these unconscious motives as the *id*. In contrast to drive theory, object relations theorists argue that attachment or relationship is the quintessential need of humans. Stated another way, whereas Freud might have argued that infants form an attachment to their mother to procure food, object relations theorists argue that even when amply nourished infants deprived of a caretaker's affection and physical contact fail to thrive and often die (Freud, 1923/1961, 1926/1959).

Regardless of how one conceptualizes motives, dynamic therapists agree that inevitably some needs come into conflict with the frustrating or nongratifying aspects of external reality or their internalized representation. Freud referred to these internalized societal rules and prohibitions as the *superego*. The proscriptions of the superego are made manifest as the experience of anxiety or fear. Object relations theorists describe this counterforce in terms of the internalization or introjection of previous relationship patterns, which may manifest as fears of abandonment or engulfment. When these two conflictual forces (i.e., need and fear) collide, it is theorized that the resulting intrapsychic conflict creates a tension that pushes for resolution. The third assumption of psychoanalytic theory is the ubiquitous presence of *intrapsychic conflict*.

To resolve this conflict, the (ego) defense mechanisms are mobilized. A defensive compromise allows partial expression of the impermissible wish at the same time that anxiety is alleviated. The fourth assumption of psychoanalytic theory states that *conflictual impulses are permitted expression only in a distorted or diminished form after being filtered through self-protective or defensive mechanisms*. Since Freud's earliest writings, several individual defense mechanisms have been conceptualized. Vaillant (1977) developed a hierarchy to categorize the various defense mechanisms. The hierarchy ranges from mature defenses (e.g., humor, altruism, sublimation) through intermediate defenses (e.g., displacement, reaction formation, intellectualization) to immature defenses (e.g., projection, denial, acting out). Contemporary theorists have made an invaluable contribution to clinical work by identifying defense mechanisms exhibited by patients with more primitive personality structures such as borderline or narcissistic disorders (Kohut, 1971). The more primitive defense mechanisms include splitting and projective identification. Notwithstanding the relative maturity of some defense mechanisms, all defenses are conceptualized as being only partially successful in providing a solution to an intrapsychic conflict. Hence, the person remains disturbed in some way by the conflict; this residual disturbance is manifested in either psychiatric symptomatology such as depression or in interpersonal psychopathology such as loneliness.

PMAP: SCALE DESCRIPTION

These four assumptions became the anchors for our psychological mindedness scale. The more a person's understanding of human psychopathology reflects these four assumptions, the more psychologically minded he or she is deemed to be. Following this conceptual development, we constructed a standardized stimulus to test a person's understanding of human psychopathology. The test stimulus consisted of two simulated patient–therapist interactions, which were scripted and videotaped. The use of videotape reflected our goal of assessing PM in a manner that reflected the preferences of contemporary society. We also wanted to insure that the assessment of PM was not confounded with the subjects' educational level and intelligence. Specifically, we did not want to bias the performance of those individuals, especially those with limited formal education, who were often astute about the dynamics of other people but apprehensive about forms or testing.

Each scenario involves an actress patient describing a recent event to her therapist. The event in the first scenario is seeing her ex-husband in a store buying a piece of jewelry. The event in the second scenario is an argument with her new boyfriend about his alleged flirtatiousness with a waitress. The scenarios include verbalizations reflecting dynamic components (e.g., conflictual wishes and fears, defensive maneuvers) and links between internal and external events (e.g., links between cognitions, affects, and behavior). After viewing each interaction, the tape is stopped and the person being assessed is asked, "What seems to be troubling this woman?" The scenario is then replayed (to eliminate possible confounding due to memory differences across respondents) and the person is allowed to elaborate on his or her initial answer.

The PMAP differentiates nine levels of psychological mindedness. Table 4.1 presents the nine levels of the PM dimension and the associated criteria for evaluating the responses of the subject. The person's responses are scored according to how well they reflect the four basic assumptions of psychodynamic theory.

TABLE 4.1
The Nine Levels of Psychological Mindedness

Level	Description
IX	The subject recognizes that despite the use of defenses, the patient remains disturbed by a conflict.
VIII	The subject recognizes that the patient uses defenses to deal with a conflict.
VII	The subject identifies a causal link in which tension (fear, anxiety) motivates an expression.
VI	The subject identifies a causal link in which a conflict generates an expression (an affect, behavior, or cognition).
V	The subject identifies conflictual components of the patient's experience.
IV	The subject recognizes that the motivating force is largely or totally out of the patient's awareness or is unconscious.
III	The subject identifies a causal link between an internal experience of the patient and its resultant expression.
II	The subject recognizes the driving force of an internal experience of the patient.
I	The subject identifies a specific internal experience of the patient.

The criteria for Levels I through III are based on the assumption of psychic determinism. For example, the statement, "Her loneliness is making her feel depressed" meets Level III criteria by clearly attributing the depression to the internal state of loneliness. Level IV criteria require an understanding of unconscious influences. The criteria for Level V, the midpoint of the scale, correspond to the recognition of ambivalence or conflict. An example of a response meriting a Level V rating is, "Well, she wants to be with her husband again, but at the same time she's very angry with him." The criteria for Levels VI and VII reflect the assumption that a conflict generates tension and motivates attempts at resolution. These attempts are, however, seen to be only partially successful. The assumption regarding the use of defense mechanisms to deal with conflict are reflected in the criteria for Levels VIII and IX. An example of a Level IX rating is, "That's sour grapes to say she's 'really better off without him'; I think she really feels that she'd be a lot happier with him." The scoring process results in a single index of psychological mindedness ranging from 1 (*low*) to 9 (*high*). The videotape and manual for application of the scoring criteria became the PMAP (McCallum & Piper, 1987, 1990b, 1996, 1997a).

GENEVIÈVE'S PM SCORE AND RESPONSE TO THERAPY

As a precursor to Geneviève beginning therapy, the intake clinician referred her to the assessment team. She was administered the PMAP. The following was her response to the first scenario, the one in which the actress-patient recounts seeing her ex-husband in a store buying a piece of jewelry.

> She hasn't resolved how the relationship ended; she has some very positive and some very negative thoughts. She seems to get some of her identity from the relationship, the daydream she recounts is of a wonderful occasion. That shows that that's where she gets her happiness. That's why she wants him back, so she'll get her identity back, know who she is. She then snaps out of it, back to reality. She realizes that he was more abusive, not as kind as she'd like to pretend. But she's also not willing to allow herself to feel those feelings. She's trying to distance herself from him emotionally, just as she tried to do so physically in the store. I don't know that she's sure of how she's supposed to feel about how the situation ended. So, deliberately, she's kept it all inside, and has been running from it. She doesn't trust her feelings; her instinct was to run from what appears to be a normal encounter but she didn't follow the instinct, afraid that it wasn't the right instinct, afraid of her own instincts—both to want him and to run from him.

Geneviève obtained the highest possible PM score (9) for this response. Of note was Geneviève's ability to identify a number of the defensive maneuvers employed by the actress-patient on the videotape. Specifically, Geneviève noted that although the daydream brought the patient happiness, it was unrealistic and defensive: "She then snaps out of it, back to reality. She realizes that he was more abusive, not as kind as she'd like to pretend." Geneviève also noted how the patient defended against her own emotions: "She's also not willing to allow herself to feel those feelings. She's trying to distance herself from him emotionally, just as she tried to do so physically in the store." Geneviève also identified what the patient was ultimately defending against: "... afraid that it wasn't the right instinct, afraid of her own instincts—both to want him and to run from him." Clearly, Geneviève's response reflected an appreciation of the concept of intrapsychic conflict. Indeed, she immediately identified the woman's ambivalence: "She has some very positive and some very negative thoughts." Finally, given Geneviève's focus on the link between the patient's troubles and her internal experience, her response also clearly reflected an acceptance of the assumption of psychic determinism. Based on Geneviève's response to the PMAP, she was predicted to be a good candidate for brief dynamic therapy.

The estimate of Geneviève's PM proved to be a good indicator of her response to the process of STDP. She was able to articulate her problems in psychological terms, that is, as deriving from aspects of her own internal functioning rather than attributing their development solely to external factors. The therapist found that his interpretations often served to extend her own rather elegant psychodynamic formulations and could thus be provided only as needed and at appropriate times. In her response to interpretation, Geneviève showed a capacity to contribute additional material, that is, to engage in free association to the meaning of the interpretation in the manner prized by practitioners of psychodynamic therapy. In effect, Geneviève's PMAP response represented her capacity to engage in a process of "work" in STDP.

RESEARCH EVIDENCE SUPPORTING THE IMPORTANCE OF PM IN STDP

Research Populations

The psychometric properties of the PMAP have been investigated with six separate populations. The first involved a nonclinical group of adult volunteers. The other five involved psychiatric outpatients participating in clinical trials of different forms of psychodynamic psychotherapy. The first trial (McCallum & Piper, 1990a) involved a short-term group therapy approach designed for the treatment of patients dealing with chronic issues associated with a significant loss. The next two trials (McCallum, Piper, & O'Kelly, 1997; Piper, Rosie, Joyce, & Azim, 1996) involved intensive group-oriented partial hospitalization programs for patients with comorbid mood and personality disorders. The fourth and fifth clinical trials were similar in that each involved a comparison of interpretive versus supportive forms of short-term, time-limited dynamic therapy. One comparative study (Piper, McCallum, Joyce, Rosie, & Ogrodniczuk, 2001) involved short-term group therapy for complicated grief, whereas the other (Piper, Joyce, McCallum, & Azim, 1998) involved STDP for outpatients with mixed diagnoses.

Psychometric Properties: Construct Validity

Consistently strong interrater reliability has been demonstrated for the PMAP in applications across the various clinical trial studies. This is a notable feature for an assessment that is both easy and quick (10–15 min) to administer. In terms of construct validity, the PMAP has been found to be significantly related to but not redundant with other measures of psychological mindedness (Gough, 1957; Tolor & Reznikoff, 1960). In contrast, the PMAP has proven to be unrelated to possible confounding variables. No significant associations have been obtained with demographic variables such as gender, level of education, age, marital status, or employment status. Similarly, scores on the PMAP have consistently been found to be not significantly related to measures of personality, intelligence, psychiatric symptomatology or distress, diagnosis, use of psychotropic medications, or the incidence of previous psychiatric treatment or hospitalization.

Psychometric Properties: Predictive Validity

We have investigated PM's association with attrition, process (e.g., in-session work), and outcome in each of the five clinical trials. In short-term group therapy for complicated bereavement, PM was predictive of remaining versus dropping out (McCallum & Piper, 1990a). PM was not associated with attrition in the other clinical trials. With regard to the therapy process, PM has consistently been related to working in group forms of dynamically oriented therapy (McCallum & Piper, 1990a; McCallum et al., 1997; Piper, Joyce, Azim, & Rosie, 1994). Finally, PM was found to be predictive of benefit in day treatment (Piper et al., 1994; Piper et al., 1996) and in both interpretive and supportive forms of short-term, time-limited group and individual psychotherapy (Piper et al., 1998, 2001).

The implications of these findings are relatively clear. PM appears to be a trait associated with the patient's ability to engage productively in psychodynamic forms of psychotherapy. Patients of low PM may not speak the same language as an interpretive therapist, thereby impeding their ability to benefit from this approach to therapy. Positive relations between PM and observed work behavior have emerged from studies of various group treatment modalities in which many perspectives on the patient's in-session behavior (the therapist, other members, outside observers) are available. Direct relations between PM and measures of treatment benefit suggest that the trait is associated with positive outcome across a variety of approaches to psychotherapy. Taking these findings as a whole, we believe that PM reflects a general capacity of the patient to make effective use of therapeutic interventions and the therapy process to achieve problem resolution. More recent explorations of our data have aimed at identifying moderating factors that facilitate (e.g., support of a spouse) or impede (e.g., presence of personality disorder) the association between PM and productive therapy process and outcome (e.g., Ogrodniczuk, Piper, Joyce, & McCallum, 2001).

QUALITY OF OBJECT RELATIONS

At the time of the initial assessment for psychotherapy, a formulation of the patient's internal object relations can help establish his or her ability to form a collaborative working relationship with the therapist. A predisposition to establish a relatively trusting give-and-take relationship with an authority figure is an important indicator for a positive therapy process. The object relations formulation can also provide an estimate of the patient's capacity to tolerate frustrations in the therapy relationship, including the termination, and a prediction of other transference reactions that are likely to emerge. During therapy, the formulation can assist with the therapist's comprehension of relational issues emerging in the treatment and the most appropriate intervention strategies to employ with a given patient. These all represent critical considerations when implementing a STDP. The Quality of Object Relations (QOR) assessment was originally developed to quantify a patient characteristic that we believed had an important influence on the treatment approach offered in clinical trial studies of STDP (see Azim, Piper, Segal, Nixon, & Duncan, 1991; Piper, Azim, McCallum, & Joyce, 1990). The QOR assessment also has clinical utility as a tool for patient selection and treatment planning.

QOR ASSESSMENT: CONCEPTUAL BACKGROUND AND SCALE DEVELOPMENT

The development of the QOR assessment was not associated with any of the specific variations of object relations theory (Greenberg & Mitchell, 1983). The conceptual foundation for the measure does, however, include elements that are central to these theories: that is, the motivational importance of the object, the processes of internalization, the development of psychological structure (the "inner world"), and the influence of internal self–other representations on interpersonal behavior. Elements of classical drive theory are also incorporated in the QOR criteria, but the constructs of wish, anxiety, and defense are all expressed in relational terms.

An early version of the QOR assessment was used at the Individual and Group Psychotherapy Unit of the Allan Memorial Institute in Montreal, Canada, as part of the assessment of patients participating in a comparative outcome study of four forms of time-limited individual and group psychotherapy (Piper, Debbane, Bienvenu, & Garant, 1984). Following a clinical interview, the assessor rated the patient on three aspects of interpersonal functioning: the quality of the individual's object choices, the type of relationship (e.g., parasitic, symbiotic, equitable), and the degree of sexual role adjustment. In turn, these ratings were modified versions of selected criteria from the Object Relations scale of the Camarillo Dynamic Assessment Scales (May & Dixon, 1969), an instrument developed in the context of the Menninger Foundation's Psychotherapy Research Project (Robbins, Wallerstein, Sargent, & Luborsky, 1956; Wallerstein, 1986). The QOR ratings were found to be directly associated with desirable process and outcome for time-limited forms of analytically-oriented individual and group psychotherapy (de Carufel & Piper, 1988; Piper, de Carufel, & Szkrumelak, 1985).

Since these early applications, the QOR assessment has undergone substantial development in our psychotherapy research program at the Department of Psychiatry, University of Alberta in Edmonton, Canada. A semistructured interview format was adopted, assessment criteria were defined and detailed, and patient prototypes for different levels of QOR were formulated (Azim et al., 1991). Further modifications occurred through a series of clinical trial studies of the psychodynamically oriented treatments offered to outpatients presenting to the Department. The QOR criteria and scoring procedures were refined to improve conceptual clarity and interviewer reliability. The first major revisions were made prior to a controlled clinical trial (Piper et al., 1990) of interpretive STDP. Further modifications occurred prior to two clinical trials (McCallum et al., 1997; Piper et al., 1996) of time-limited, analytically-oriented partial hospitalization treatment programs for patients with affective and personality disorders. The most recent modification of the QOR assessment was made prior to a recently completed comparative trial (Piper et al., 1998) of interpretive and supportive forms of STDP. The latest application of the measure was in a comparative trial (Piper et al., 2001) of interpretive and supportive forms of short-term, time-limited group therapy for patients presenting with complicated grief.

QOR SCALE DESCRIPTION AND ASSESSMENT PROCEDURES

We define QOR as a person's *internal enduring tendency to establish certain types of relationships* that range along an overall dimension from primitive to mature (Azim et al., 1991). The QOR construct refers to the *recurring pattern* of relationships over the individual's life span rather than to relationships during any one period (e.g., recent interpersonal functioning). The five anchored levels of the QOR dimension (primitive, searching, controlling, triangular, and mature) and their predominant characteristics are presented in Table 4.2.

The patient's QOR is assessed by an experienced clinician during a 1-hour semistructured interview. During the assessment, the interviewer solicits information regarding four areas of functioning. Criteria within each of the five QOR levels are organized in terms of behavioral manifestations, affect regulation, self-esteem regulation, and antecedent (etiological) factors. Criteria regarding *behavioral manifestations* consider the individual's typical patterns of behavior in interpersonal relationships. Criteria regarding *affect regulation* address the kinds of interpersonal relationships the individual unconsciously and consciously wishes for and engages in, both in fantasy and in real action, to reduce anxiety, obtain gratification, or both. In similar fashion, criteria regarding *self-esteem regulation* refer to the wished for, fan-

TABLE 4.2
Predominant Characteristics of the Five Levels
of the Quality of Object Relations Scale

Level	Anchor Point	Predominant Characteristics
Mature	9	The person enjoys equitable relationships characterized by love, tenderness, and concern for objects of both sexes. There is a capacity to mourn and tolerate unobtainable relationships.
Triangular	7	The person is involved in real or fantasized triangular relationships. Competition for one object is inspired by victory over the other object. There is concern for the objects.
Controlling	5	The person engages in well-meaning attempts to control and possess objects. Relationships are characterized by ambivalence. Attempts to control the person are met with defiance or pseudocompliance.
Searching	3	The person is driven to find substitutes for a longed-for lost object. Substitutes provide a short-lived sense of optimism and self-worth, which is followed by disillusionment and the reexperience of loss.
Primitive	1	The person reacts to perceived separation or loss of the object, or disapproval or rejection by the object, with intense anxiety and affect. There is inordinate dependence on the object, who provides a sense of identity for the person.

tasized, and behaviorally expressed interpersonal relationships that enhance self-regard or reduce mortification. Criteria addressing *historical antecedents* address those past events or relationship outcomes thought to be clinically or theoretically predisposing to a given QOR level. The interviewer assigns greater weight to behavioral manifestations because they are observable, experience near, and often manifest during the interview itself. Because they are relatively experience distant and require greater inference to evaluate, affect regulation, self-esteem regulation, and historical antecedents, in that order, are given less weight. Table 4.3 presents the most important criteria from each of the four areas for the five QOR levels.

The interview is roughly divided into three segments in which relationships in the patient's childhood, adolescence, and adulthood are successively the focus of attention. Although encouraging spontaneity of discussion by the patient of relationships during these periods, the interviewer also tries to address certain specific questions. For example, questions are routinely asked about abuse in childhood, falling in love during adolescence, and the experience of stormy relationships in adulthood. Knowledge of the rating criteria informs the interviewer about which areas to pursue in more detail. Table 4.4 presents the critical questions associated with each QOR level for the periods of childhood, adolescence, and adulthood.

TABLE 4.3
Key Criteria for Each Area by QOR Level

Level	No. of Criteria	Key Criterion
Behavioral Manifestations		
Mature	6	Capacity to express love, tenderness and concern for objects of both sexes. This involves an intimate dyadic relationship with at least one object.
Triangular	5	Repetitive involvement in rivalrous triangular relationships, typically with one same sex and one opposite sex, but can also be two same or two opposite sex. (By *rivalrous* we mean that the subject is competing with an object for another object.) The subject is not necessarily aware of this triangulation.
Controlling	5	The participant manifests a repetitive pattern of well-meaning attempts to control an object in a relationship.
Searching	4	The individual appears to "fall in love" with others repeatedly. This may be acted out in actual relationships or remain a part of expressed fantasy. Objects of choice are substitutive and bear psychological and at times a physical resemblance to an original lost object.
Primitive	7	A persistent or repeated pattern of intense, unstable, and destructive relationships with objects characterized by hurting and being hurt.
Affect Regulation		
Mature	3	Capacity to mourn objects and relationships that are not attainable or lost.
Triangular	3	There are feelings of triumph over the third party.
Controlling	4	Affect is characterized by anger, even rage, in reaction to inability to control or possess the object.
Searching	4	Persistent craving and longing for the lost object or the object substitute.
Primitive	5	Preoccupation with destroying or being destroyed by the object manifested by murderous rage and fear of annihilation.
Self-Esteem Regulation		
Mature	1	Based on equitable receiving from and giving to objects.
Triangular	1	Self-esteem is dependent on repeated episodes, in reality or in fantasy, of conquering a third party and acquiring the object, usually in fantasy.
Controlling	1	Self-esteem is maintained by successfully controlling and possessing the object.
Searching	1	Positive self-esteem is dependent on the availability in reality or fantasy of a relationship with a substitute for the lost object.
Primitive	4	Tendency toward idealization or devaluation of objects.

(Continued)

TABLE 4.3
(Continued)

Level	No. of Criteria	Key Criterion
Antecedents		
Mature	1	"Good enough" pre-Oedipal relationships and healthy resolution of the Oedipal complex leading to identification with both parents and choosing a good enough love object.
Triangular	4	The parent of the same sex competes with the individual for the affection of the parent of the opposite sex.
Controlling	3	Inordinate attempts by the caregivers to control the person's actions, thoughts, or feelings.
Searching	2	Experiencing an intensive attachment to a parent or caregiver who became the lost object.
Primitive	3 (multipart)	Traumatization: sexual abuse; physical abuse; parental rejection; premature, sudden, repetitive separations.

Note. QOR = quality of object relations.

Following the interview, the assessor distributes 100 points among the five QOR levels. The weighting is determined by the strength and number of criteria at each level that are met by the patient's contribution to the interview. A simple arithmetic formula is then used to generate an overall score that ranges from 1 to 9; the higher the score the higher the QOR. Scoring procedures and prototypes for each QOR level are described in a manual (Piper, McCallum, & Joyce, 1993) that can be obtained from us.

A VIGNETTE FROM GENEVIÈVE'S THERAPY

Approaching the midpoint of the 20-session therapy, both patient and therapist were feeling positive about the process and eventual outcome of treatment. Geneviève, a single woman in her mid 30s, had presented to the clinic concerned about a series of relationships that had ended badly. She expressed an interest in understanding why she would enter these relationships with high hopes only to encounter strain and eventual hurt and disappointment. The therapist, a male of roughly the same age, found Geneviève to be pleasant, intelligent, and articulate about her concerns and reactions regarding relationships. The transference had been positive from the outset, Geneviève regarding the therapist as an ally and the therapy relationship as collaborative. At the beginning of the 7th session, the therapist announced that he would be away for 2 weeks following the next contact. He

TABLE 4.4
The QOR Assessment: Critical Questions for the Periods of Childhood, Adolescence, and Adulthood

Period to Be Covered	Major Level Criteria to Be Covered				
	Primitive	*Searching*	*Controlling*	*Triangular*	*Mature*
Childhood (family of origin)	Do you remember much abuse or disorder in your childhood?	Was there a major event that changed the course of your childhood?	How would you describe your parents in terms of their being controlling of your thoughts, feelings, or behavior?	Was there anything special or unique about your relationship with your (opposite sex parent) that you did not share with your (same sex parent)?	In what ways did members of your family express love and concern for each other?
Adolescence: Period of transition (peers, parents)	Tell me about any incident you can recall where you felt hurt or betrayed by peers at school or socially.	Were there any times as a teen or young adult where you found yourself falling in love? How did those experiences turn out?	How did you engage in rebellion as a teen or young adult?	Can you tell me about any incident where you and another were both vying for the attention of a third person? How did that work out?	Were there things about your high school friends that irritated you? How did it affect your relationships?
Adulthood (partners, children)	In what way would you say your intimate relationships have been stormy or hurtful?	Looking back over your relationships, have they been a bit like a roller coaster, lots of ups and downs?	Do you find yourself taking care of your partner, sort of looking out for him or her, trying to help him or her with his or her problems?	How would you say you've been competitive with people that you are close to?	Do you have good male and female friends?

intended this communication to be of the "housekeeping" variety and believed the patient received it in this spirit. During the session, however, the therapist observed a change in the patient's demeanor—Geneviève began to avoid eye contact, her voice became softer, and her contributions became marked by frequent pauses and tangential content. Putting his observation into words, the therapist inquired if the patient was aware of any change in her behavior or feelings. She denied she was behaving or feeling in a way that "was different from any other time I've been with you." The therapist persisted, asking if Geneviève had any feelings about his announcement; again, she denied this was so, claiming, "we all need a holiday." Some tension was evident as the session ended.

Geneviève was 20 min late for the next session. She described a situation at work that had resulted in a significant increase in her duties and a need for her to be at the office on the upcoming weekend. That her colleagues were not being saddled with extra labor was clearly a source of upset and irritation. The patient uncharacteristically restricted herself to a rehashing of the situation; the therapist felt he had little opportunity to ask questions or make comments linking the material to previous discussions. At the close of the hour, he noted that they would meet for their next session 3 weeks hence. Geneviève responded with a curt "Fine" and left with some haste.

At this juncture, the challenge for the STDP therapist is twofold: first to understand what is happening in the therapy relationship and second to intervene in such a way that the process is clarified and Geneviève's awareness of how she functions in close relationships is increased. The first task requires that the therapist have a clear conception of the patient's internal object relations, that is, the representations of self and other in relationships that Geneviève has internalized through past experiences with important others in her life. These representations are assumed to function as a "script" the individual attempts to follow in current relationships. Although the script allows for some predictability in relational functioning, the person may rigidly adhere to forms of interpersonal behavior that are maladaptive. The therapist believes that this interpersonal script is being enacted in the therapy relationship. The second task, intervening to clarify and facilitate insight into the meaning of the therapy transaction, requires that the therapist attends to Geneviève's interpersonal patterns and facilitates a "corrective relational experience." The QOR assessment procedure provides the clinician with a useful resource for effectively engaging in both tasks.

GENEVIÈVE'S ORIGINAL QOR FORMULATION

Geneviève was assigned an overall QOR score of 5.8. This was well above the midpoint of the scale (4.5) that has routinely been employed to subdivide treatment samples into low QOR (more primitive) and high QOR (more mature) patients. In terms of the five QOR levels, the assessor saw Geneviève as having the following profile: primitive, 10 points; searching, 10 points; controlling, 25 points; triangular, 40 points; and mature, 15 points. The patient was seen to most resemble the prototypic triangular case, reflecting issues associated with Oedipal conflicts and competition. In addition, Geneviève shared a number of features with the prototypic controlling case. The assessor provided a narrative formulation highlighting the historical influences associated with Geneviève's QOR profile.

The Narrative Formulation

As a child and into her teens, Geneviève enjoyed a unique alliance with her father against her mother. He would invariably take her side against her mother whenever questions about her misbehavior arose. She also enjoyed the "special trips" with him on his sales route, even if they entailed time off from school or clashed with her mother's plans. In Geneviève's later childhood and adolescence her mother apparently became threatened by this alliance; Geneviève and her mother began to compete for the father's attentions. The mother's resentment at her husband's indulgence of the daughter increased, and Geneviève was made the target of this anger. The escalation of friction further elicited the father's intervention and protection of Geneviève. In her teens, her mother threatened to send Geneviève away to boarding school, an intention her father opposed. The mother eventually gave up and had been rejecting of her daughter since that time.

Geneviève described initially feeling good that she had "won my way" over her mother. She had enjoyed playing her parents against one another to obtain privileges. However, Geneviève felt increasingly anxious when she and her mother were together, in anticipation of her mother's next retaliation. The distance between them grew as she became aware of how she was much more comfortable in the company of her father. Nevertheless, she periodically felt sadness over the lack of a relationship with her mother. She also began to feel guilty for enjoying her close relationship with her father and thereby contributing to the problems in her parents' marriage. She spoke of feeling pity for her mother and described attempts at reconciliation that only highlighted how distant they had become. Geneviève was unaware of her anger at her father for never completely protecting her from her mother or for never truly choosing her and abandoning the mother.

As an adult, Geneviève describes feeling more comfortable with men than with women. When with couples, she focuses her attention on the man and interacts in a coy, flirtatious fashion; that is, she attempts to recreate her role as "daddy's little girl." Men tend to intervene to be chivalrous, for example, offering her advice regarding work concerns. Their attention to her irritates their partners. Other women find her to be competitive and tend to snub her.

Geneviève describes feeling guilty for winning the favor of these male friends. She expresses sadness over the lack of female friendships and anger at the women who were rejecting of her "for no good reason."

The controlling aspects of Geneviève's object relations emerged in the context of her special relationship to her father. Although unequivocally indulgent, her father was also a stern advocate of order and consistency. He emphasized rules and tended to enforce these with rather harsh disciplinary actions, for example, sending Geneviève to her room without dinner when she objected to his scheduling of her homework activity. In her teens, her special relationship with her father was punctuated by clashes over her autonomy. She described these as her "rebellious" years; rather than yield to delinquent behavior, however, Geneviève was a "quiet revolutionary" who engaged in school truancy, violation of curfews, and dressing in a manner designed to provoke her father. On these occasions, the father relied on psychological intimidation to "keep her in line"; that is, he would express disapproval and disappointment, thus threatening her with a withdrawal of his affection. Geneviève developed a rigid self-control to avoid the dangerous consequences of spontaneous action when in her father's presence. As an adult, Geneviève periodically struggles with feelings of inadequacy and worries about "screwing up." At these times, she assumes the role of an experienced and helpful advisor for her friends; that is, her own attempts at control are well intentioned. However, the recipients of her advice tend to feel patronized, much as she would when given directives by her father. When others complain, Geneviève feels unappreciated, criticized, and angry about her failure to control the other person.

Relational Meaning of the Therapy Event

With his knowledge of the QOR formulation, the therapist considered the meaning of the therapy event in the context of Geneviève's controlling and triangular object relations. He suspected that Geneviève's reaction had likely reflected two co-occurring possibilities. First, he suspected that his being away demonstrated that as an object important to supporting her self-regard, he was outside of her control. Consequently, she would have been angry and experienced his absence as a rejection of her as flawed. Second, he suspected that she perceived his absence from her as a moving towards another; that is, she would imagine a rival was involved in the pursuit of his attentions. The QOR formulation thus provided a number of working hypotheses to consider when he and Geneviève reconvened the therapy after his absence.

The therapist had noted aspects of her controlling style earlier in the therapeutic relationship. For example, she had frequently recommended books on popular psychology for him to read to "continue your development." At the beginning of the session following the therapist's absence, the patient referred to scheduling problems with work colleagues that she had found irritating. The therapist asked if his perception that she had been irritated with his announcement 3 weeks previously was correct; Geneviève responded, "indeed it was—I was quite put out." She went on to say that she had already blocked off time for her sessions, and that his "vacation" had upset these plans; she also reported she was angry that he "hadn't discussed with me beforehand that you'd be away." At the same time, she noted that it was "ridiculous" that she had been so upset and that she "simply couldn't bring myself" to comment on the situation in the session preceding the therapist's absence. The therapist confronted the patient at this point, noting that the reference to her feelings as "ridiculous" was her attribution, whereas the therapy contract encouraged her to talk about whatever mattered to her regardless of the value she placed on it. Geneviève protested that the disappointment and anger implied she was "weak" and she'd be "embarrassed" to show herself this way to him. The therapist replied that these feelings were her "natural response" to a change in "a relationship you clearly find important" and thus legitimate to examine in a therapeutic manner. The therapist also observed that the discussion had moved from the patient's efforts to place the therapist under her control to the detrimental effects of her own rigid self-control. Geneviève agreed this represented an important focus for further examination.

At this point, the triangular elements of her relational functioning emerged more clearly. Geneviève abruptly shifted topics and manner, coyly asking about how the therapist had enjoyed his "escape from work." The therapist noted that she seemed at once curious and anxious and encouraged her to articulate the thoughts and feelings that lay behind her inquiry. Her casual reply was, "Oh, I was just wondering where you went, who you were with, that sort of thing." The therapist directed her to describe what she imagined about his absence. The patient paused, and then, in a rush, described a fantasy that the therapist had "run off" to offer a "special" course of intensive therapy to another woman patient. Geneviève's manner during this description was flirtatious. The therapist, knowing that her imaginings had no correspondence with the reality of his trip to a professional conference, asked how this fantasy was related to her behavior prior to the break. The patient stated, "I couldn't stand it" that the therapist might be more interested in spending time with "another woman." She had portrayed her workload as she did for two reasons: first by way of competing with the therapist to show that "I honor my commitments," and second by way of competing with the fantasized rival patient to show that she had a greater need for his "special attention."

After conveying her fantasy about the therapist's absence, Geneviève alluded to being troubled by "mixed-up feelings." She reported feeling guilty that she had expected the therapist to be exclusively available to her, and anxiety should the therapist ever develop a picture of her as demanding and difficult. The therapist interpreted the contrast between the reality and the patient's fantasy view of the therapeutic relationship. On the reality side, the relationship represented a collaboration oriented to understanding Geneviève's interpersonal dynamics; on the fantasy side, the patient had represented the two of them as lovers involved in an exclusive relationship. The patient was surprised by this analogy but agreed that it seemed to fit her experience. The therapist then mused aloud about similar dynamics operating in her early relationships with her parents; the patient ruefully agreed that she had brought a number of these into the therapeutic relationship. She went on to make links to similar experiences in her intimate relationships as an adolescent and adult. At the end of a session that was notable for the degree of patient insight, she proclaimed, "It was a good thing you went away when you did!"

In this example, the QOR formulation helped the therapist to develop working hypotheses regarding the strain that developed in the therapeutic alliance. During the subsequent session, the therapist was alert to cues from the patient that had a bearing on these hypotheses and was able to interpret the related dynamics in the relationship accordingly. The patient's level of QOR allowed for the development and maintenance of a reasonably good collaborative relationship and therefore some capacity to tolerate the interpretive focus. The understanding Geneviève acquired regarding what was transpiring for her in the transference paved the way for some useful insights into her usual patterns of relational functioning. How would Geneviève appear if she presented as a patient of more primitive object relations? How would the therapy event be interpreted? How would the therapist's strategy in the subsequent session be different?

GENEVIÈVE'S ALTERNATE QOR FORMULATION

For our hypothetical presentation of Geneviève as a low-QOR patient (Geneviève B), the QOR assessment resulted in an overall score of 3.2. This score is well below the midpoint of the scale (4.5) demarcating low (more primitive) and high QOR (more mature) patients. In terms of the five levels, the following profile was provided for Geneviève B: primitive, 40 points; searching, 30 points; controlling, 15 points; triangular, 10 points; and mature, 5 points. The patient was thus seen to most resemble the prototypic primitive case, reflecting issues associated with identity concerns and object constancy. In addition, Geneviève B shared a number of features with the prototypic searching case. Once again, the assessor's narrative formulation is reviewed followed by a presentation of the therapist's use of the formulation to understand the patient's response to his absence and to determine his intervention strategy.

The Narrative Formulation

Dynamics associated with the primitive level of QOR were established during Geneviève B's early childhood. From a very young age, Geneviève B had experienced sexual and physical abuse from her father. Her mother was somewhat inadequate and felt helpless to prevent the abuse or protect her daughter; she consequently withdrew from Geneviève B, an action that was experienced by the young girl as a maternal rejection. The early relationships Geneviève B developed with peers ended prematurely because of the frequent moves associated with father's employment problems. Consequently, the only sense of self Geneviève B developed as a child was as an object to be used; her sense of relationships was that they were transitory and impermanent. She had never experienced positive self-esteem in her early relational transactions. The patient's only defense against despair and helplessness was to egocentrically assume responsibility for the chaos in her life and blame for her parents' abuse. This afforded her some semblance of control. She nonetheless remained dependent on her parents to define her identity, although the messages were invariably negative. Her rage over the abuse and deprivation was contained and dissipated through the use of splitting and projective identification. Geneviève B's basic needs for nurturance, security, and stability remained unmet during her childhood, but she survived.

As an adult, Geneviève B remains preoccupied with destroying or being destroyed in relationships. She oscillates between fears of her own rage and of being annihilated if the other abandons her. Her yearnings to be dependent continue to motivate her interactions. As a result, she alternates between being clingy or defensively distant from others. She has a history of choosing partners who are excessively indulgent at the beginning of the relationship, thus meeting Geneviève B's more narcissistic needs. As the relationships progress and Geneviève B falls more under their control, her partners' abusive qualities begin to emerge. Again seeking to have some sense of control, Geneviève behaves in a manner that is provocative of this abusiveness, exacerbating the instability in the relationship. In addition to the rage these partners bring to the relationship, Geneviève B's reliance on projective identification means they will also act out her rage. The partners only partially serve the function of meeting her needs for nurturance, security, and stability. Because she fears her own striving for dependency, Geneviève B often sabotages the relationships to maintain a sense of her own separateness.

Dynamics associated with the searching level of QOR operate in similar fashion to the primitive pattern described previously but in somewhat muted form. The searching dynamics were largely precipitated by father's abrupt abandonment of the family when Geneviève B was age 9. Even though the relationship had been marked by abuse, the preteen Geneviève B defensively viewed her father's inappropriate involvement with her as something "special." To combat the feelings of powerlessness she had experienced with father's abuse, Geneviève B had unconsciously harbored the hope that she could transform her father, moving him to recognize the damage his behavior had caused her and becoming a devoted, caring object. His sudden departure dashed these unlikely dreams from ever being realized. Her mother eventually established a common-law relationship with another man, someone who worked hard to establish a good relationship with Geneviève B. Although she appreciated his efforts, she kept herself aloof from him, believing it unlikely any kind of special intimacy could be established with him. In her current adult life, Geneviève B unconsciously awaits the return of the lost father but in the form she never had, that is, the caring man devoted to healing her injuries. When entering a new relationship, Geneviève B's perceptions are intensely romantic; a unique, special bond is believed to exist with the new partner. She experiences a sense of excitement, optimism, feelings of completeness, and passion during this initial stage of infatuation and idealization. She remains buoyant as long as the other is indulgent of her; at the same time, she feels vulnerable to loss, rejection, or abandonment. To contend with these anxieties, Geneviève B attempts to distance herself from contact either psychologically (e.g., by being silent) or physically. She also projects her fear of rejection onto the other person and then complains that the person should be more attentive and caring. Eventually, the relationship moves toward a sour ending, leaving Geneviève B feeling pessimistic, dejected, and filled with longing for the devoted, caring other she perceived at the outset. Geneviève B escapes this dysphoria by quickly becoming enamored with another new object.

Relational Meaning of the Therapy Event

The therapist understood that Geneviève B had idealized him somewhat during the early sessions of therapy. She had commented frequently on his capacity to understand her "like no one else" and on how much she had gained from his observations. He was alert to any indication that the patient might experience disillusionment, suspecting that a different side of her character would be revealed as a result. The therapy had been characterized by more therapist emphasis on supportive interventions in response to the patient's perceived fragility.

Based on his understanding of Geneviève B's QOR, the therapist recognized that his announcement of a 2-week absence had represented a traumatic abandonment for the patient. In therapy, Geneviève B had felt listened to and nonjudgmentally validated by another, perhaps for the first time in her life. The therapist's attention to the boundaries of the relationship meant she had felt safe from intrusion; his supportive encouragement had allowed her to feel permitted to express her own views. The therapist's announcement had destroyed her perception that therapy represented her salvation and that she was the therapist's "special patient," and she found herself struggling with intense rage toward the therapist for his "betrayal." As in the past, however, she assumed responsibility for the collapse of the relationship, choosing to believe that the therapist "needed the break" because she had proven too needy and demanding. Fearing a confirmation of these beliefs, she had defensively distanced herself following the announcement and subsequently by coming late to the next session and precluding any contribution on his part.

Following the break, Geneviève B began the session by announcing that she had scheduled an appointment with a new therapist. As she described looking forward to this meeting, the therapist was aware of the comparisons she was drawing that were unfavorable to him. He raised the issue of his "abandonment" by wondering aloud if his announcement had felt "sudden" to the patient and whether she had felt "profoundly hurt" by the interruption to the therapy his absence had caused. When she affirmed that this was so, the therapist noted that she perhaps felt safe enough to explore the issue because he had, after all, "returned to her." He encouraged Geneviève B to speak about other relationship experiences that had represented a betrayal or empathic failure. He reflected the affect that was associated with these experiences, that is, her agonizing loneliness and self-negation. He also emphasized that in contrast to her experience of her parents, he continued to maintain his interest in her well-being and commitment, as her clinician, to the success of the therapy relationship.

The patient suddenly began to cry; through her tears, she described the deep disappointment she had felt when their work had to be "put on hold" for the therapist's absence. The announcement and subsequent absence had apparently underscored the patient's inability to "hold" the therapist and therapy in her internal world until the sessions resumed in reality. Her response highlighted how important the therapist was to her as a nurturant object and the therapy was to her as a source of self-esteem. The therapist acknowledged this and emphasized that their work together had indeed been productive. He stated that this work could reasonably be expected to continue to be productive. He suggested that working toward the patient's goals and concluding the therapy as contracted would be of substantially greater benefit than searching for another candidate for the "ideal therapist" role. The discussion turned to an examination of Geneviève B's expectations of the other person in her relationships and how much these were tied to an archaic and irrational view of her relationship with her biological father. The patient became tearful again after the therapist gently pointed out that the loss of what she had never had with her father had at some point to be grieved. "Letting go" of this dream and her search for a substitute was framed as a process that would lead Geneviève B to true independence. This discussion highlighted the reality of the eventual termination of the therapy when a similar "letting go" would be required. The therapist stated, "Together, we can insure that the experience will be a positive one." He stressed that the termination represented an opportunity to experience an ending that could be beneficial rather than devastating to Geneviève B's self-regard. The patient ended the session by indicating that she would not keep her appointment with the alternate clinician and that she felt recommitted to her therapy.

In this alternative scenario, the patient had an intensely affective response to the therapist's absence. Her profound difficulty managing this response reflected the characteristics of the primitive QOR level, and her efforts to find a substitute object reflected aspects of the searching QOR level. The major task for the therapist was to attend to this emotional upheaval and provide a corrective relational experience. Less important was providing an interpretive understanding of what had transpired or facilitating the patient's insight into her relational style. Consequently, this alternative scenario required that the therapist assume a more supportive stance with the patient than in the previous example.

Summary. The patient's QOR can have a major influence on the nature of the therapeutic interaction—even ostensibly similar occurrences during treatment can have radically different meanings as a function of the patient's QOR level. The QOR assessment can improve the clarity of the therapist's formulation of the patient's object relations and assist in determining the meaning of relational phenomena arising in the treatment process. In turn the therapist has a basis for developing technical strategies that make sense in terms of the patient's capacities for healthy relationships and the goals for treatment.

RESEARCH EVIDENCE SUPPORTING THE IMPORTANCE OF QOR IN STDP

Reliability and Construct Validity

Considerable information regarding the interjudge reliability, concurrent validity, and predictive validity of the QOR assessment has emerged from the five clinical trial studies of psychotherapy conducted in Edmonton. This information is detailed in Piper and Duncan (1999). Interjudge reliability has improved steadily with successive modifications of the measure. In the most recent investigation, the comparative study of short-term group therapy for complicated grief, the average intraclass correlation coefficient was .83, indicating high reliability (Piper et al., 2001). In general, QOR has been found to be independent of demographic and historic characteristics of the patient. The construct has also not been found to be related to Axis I conditions. As one would expect, patients with lower QOR scores (i.e., less than 4.5) tend to be more likely to have an Axis II diagnosis than patients with higher QOR scores (equal to or greater than 4.5), although the two dimensions have been shown to be far from synonymous. For example, in the controlled trial of STDP (Piper et al., 1990), 45% of the low-QOR patients received a personality disorder diagnosis compared with 17% of the high-QOR patients. In similar fashion, low QOR has a greater likelihood of being associated with greater symptomatic disturbance on outcome variables assessed at pretherapy, but these relationships have not been found to be strong, that is, correlation coefficients of .3 or less. In sum, QOR represents a relatively pure measure of an important construct that is independent of demographic and clinical variables commonly assessed as patient characteristics.

Predictive Validity

The QOR variable has been found to be a strong predictor of therapy process and outcome in STDP. In the controlled trial of STDP (Piper et al., 1990), QOR was directly associated with ratings of the therapeutic alliance provided by both the patient and therapist. QOR was also directly related to favorable therapy outcome on measures of general psychiatric symptoms at posttherapy, and on measures of individual goals for treatment at posttherapy and 6-month follow-up (Piper, Azim, Joyce, McCallum, Nixon, & Segal, 1991). In the comparative trial of individual and supportive forms of STDP (Piper et al., 1998; Piper, Joyce, McCallum, Azim, & Ogrodniczuk, 2002), QOR was directly related to the patient rated therapeutic alliance during the critical early third of treatment. QOR was also directly related to favorable outcome in interpretive therapy but virtually unrelated to outcome in supportive therapy. In the comparative trial of the short-term group therapies (Piper et al., 2001), we did find evidence for a true interaction with form of therapy: high-QOR patients improved more in interpretive than supportive therapy, whereas the reverse held for low-QOR patients. This finding was specific to the measures of complicated grief that were targeted by the interventions. Across these studies, then, the implication is that high QOR represents an important selection criterion for interpretive forms of STDP. The high-QOR patient's history of meaningful give-and-take relationships appears to allow for the establishment of a strong collaboration with the therapist and greater readiness to make use of the interpretive approach.

There is also evidence that QOR serves as a moderator of important relations between technique and process in STDP. The relation between the extent to which the therapist uses transference interpretations and the average level of the therapeutic alliance or treatment outcome has differed depending on the level of QOR (Ogrodniczuk, Piper, Joyce, & McCallum, 1999; Piper, Azim, Joyce, & McCallum, 1991). Significant negative relations between the frequency of transference interpretations and alliance or outcome were found for the high-QOR patients in the controlled trial (Piper et al., 1990). Based on these findings, the therapists providing interpretive therapy in a subsequent trial were instructed to be more judicious in their use of transference-focused technique. The average frequencies of these interventions in the interpretive therapies of the comparative trial (Piper et al., 1998) were substantially lower than in the controlled trial. Negative relations between the frequency of transference interpretations and alliance or outcome were again identified in the comparative trial data, in this instance for the low-QOR patients. Taken together, these findings suggest that high- and low-QOR patients differ in their degree of tolerance for a transference-focused approach. Because of their capacity for mutuality in relationships, high-QOR patients may be able to make use of the therapist's transference observations. These patients can thus tolerate a greater frequency of transference interpretations during sessions. Low-QOR patients, in contrast, appear to be more reactive to the perceived criticism or deprivation represented by interpretations of transference. Tolerance of this technical approach is correspondingly much lower among these patients. For each type of patient, the findings suggest a certain optimal use of these interventions beyond which the technique can prove detrimental.

Similarly, the relation between the extent to which the therapist provides "accurate" transference interpretations and the average level of the therapeutic alliance or treatment outcome has differed depending on the level of QOR (Piper, Joyce, McCallum, & Azim, 1993). "Accurate" in this sense is defined as the "correspondence" between the interpretation's content and the content of the initial formulation of the patient's problem; that is, it represents a measure of therapist consistency (Joyce & Piper, 1996). For this variable, a direct relation with treatment outcome was found for high-QOR patients, whereas inverse relations were found with the alliance and outcome for low-QOR patients. In essence, transference interpretations are beneficial to the high-QOR patient when used sparingly and with accuracy to the central problem. For the low-QOR patient, an accurate transference interpretation appears to represent a form of injury. In effect, the use of transference-oriented interventions with the low-QOR patient is problematic, whether the index is frequency or accuracy of the transference focus.

These findings concerning the extent of use and accuracy of transference interpretations have received support in independent studies from Norway (Høglend, 1993a, 1993b; Høglend & Piper, 1995).

The findings previously summarized indicate that an interpretive therapy approach is an appropriate match for the high-QOR patient. These patients appear to be responsive to the demands of the therapy, that is, pressure on the patient to talk, encouraging the exploration of uncomfortable emotions, and making use of the therapy relationship to demonstrate relational patterns. The findings also suggest that a more supportive approach might be of benefit for the low-QOR patient. An explicit indication of this emerged from an analysis of the pattern of change in the alliance over the course of STDP treatment. An increasing pattern of the therapist-rated alliance over the course of therapy was found to be directly related to favorable outcome for low-QOR patients (Piper, Boroto, Joyce, McCallum, & Azim, 1995). This suggests that low-QOR patients may be more in need of forming a gratifying relationship with the therapist than exploring their pattern of nongratifying relationships in therapy. Findings from other investigators also suggest the validity of this perspective (e.g., Høglend, 1993a, 1993b; Horowitz, Marmar, Weiss, DeWitt, & Rosenbaum, 1984).

CONCLUDING COMMENTS

Our objective in this chapter was to demonstrate that the PMAP and QOR assessments are useful tools not only for research on psychotherapy but also for the clinical activities of assessing, preparing, and working with patients in STDP. The measures provide valid indications of the patient's appropriateness for the therapy approach or when certain technical modifications (e.g., a more supportive emphasis) may be required. The measures can also provide information that is useful to the formulation of therapeutic strategy at times when the alliance may be under strain and a premature termination is threatening. Moreover, we believe that both systems can readily be incorporated into the clinician's routine. The PMAP is a very brief assessment that has great appeal to subjects and can be used with high reliability. The QOR assessment can be easily combined with the initial relational history interview conducted with patients being considered for psychotherapy.

Our investment in the development of the PMAP and QOR assessments has been a learning experience of high quality. We have also been pleased that the measures have demonstrated a strong ability to predict the process and outcome of therapy. Our work with these measures has underscored the profound value of using psychoanalytic constructs in the effort to understand and treat patients. The two procedures are systematic representations of central analytic principles that have a direct theoretical relevance to psychotherapy as practiced, that is, psychic determinism and defensive functioning in the case of the PMAP, internalization and the influence of object relations on behavior in the case of the QOR assessment. Even if these assessment procedures are not employed in a complete fashion by the clinician, we are certain that the principles they embody represent a gold standard for comprehending and helping others struggling with the human condition.

ADDENDUM: THE CASE OF JUNE

In this addendum, we consider the levels of PM and QOR exhibited by the patient June, as presented in the transcript of her second therapy session. Although June was not assessed with either of the measures, indications of her PM and QOR are reflected throughout the transcript. Obviously, a complete appraisal of her PM or QOR is not possible. By applying the criteria of the two measures to the content of the transcribed psychotherapy session, however, we can speculate on June's PM and QOR. Content in support of our observations is noted by reference to the line in the transcript from each session, for example (2–6) refers to line 6 from the transcript for session 2.

To begin with PM, one of the major themes of the session is June's irritability: "I get irritated, but I don't know why" (2–6). An estimate of June's PM can be formulated by how she addresses this problem of irritability during the session. The reader can familiarize him or herself with the criteria for the nine levels of the PMAP (Table 4.1). For the criteria at each level, the reader can substitute "June" for "the subject" and "the patient." For example, "June identifies a specific internal experience of herself" (Level I), or "June recognizes that she is engaging in a defensive maneuver" (Level VIII). A review of the PMAP indicates that June easily and immediately meets the criterion for the first level. She focuses on her own internal experiences: "I just seemed to go on, you know, not happy, not sad, just went on" (2–2). In terms of knowing what she wants (Level II), June is initially rather vague: "I let people walk all over me, I don't like it, and yet I won't do anything about it" (end of 2–16). She is hinting at the fact that she wants to be more assertive, to stop letting people walk all over her. It is only later at Section 2–24 when she clearly states her wish and thereby meets the criterion of Level II: "That's what annoys me, I know she knows I'm going to say yes. And I haven't got the guts to turn around and say, No. And I wish I had" (2–24). In addition to identifying her wish, June also exhibits in this statement an appreciation of the causal associations between her internal and external experiences (Level III) as well as the conflicted nature of her internal experiences (Level V). There are frequent instances throughout the transcript where June demonstrates an appreciation of some inner conflict, for example, "Yeah, I get annoyed but don't say anything about it" (2–18). It is evident that June also meets the criterion for Level IV: "... but the feelings are always there, so it may be it did trigger something off I don't know" (end of 2–10). This statement suggests that June is aware that her feelings are being triggered by something outside of her awareness.

With regard to the scale's higher levels, June acknowledges very early in the session that she is engaging in defensive maneuvers. Referring to the previous session, she states, "I seemed to sort of block it out a bit at first" (2–2). In terms of the problem of her irritability, she is also aware of her use of the defense of displacement: "... and I just took it out on everybody" (2–3). June's appreciation of her own defenses suggests a high level of PM, garnering a rating of 8 on the 9-point PMAP scale. June does not identify the fear that is associated with her conflicted internal experience (Level VII). The therapist explores June's fear of what might happen if she were to say no to her sister regarding babysitting her children (2–25). June hints at the fear of her sister's anger (2–34) and her fear of being replaceable (2–26). However, the true basis of her fear does not become clear in this session. Nevertheless, June displays high PM during this dialogue with her therapist.

Regarding the dimension of QOR, the transcript does offer insights into June's current relationships with family members. By reviewing Tables 4.2 through 4.4, the reader can appreciate that the QOR assessment relies on information from the subject's entire relationship history. Unfortunately, there is no material describing June's romantic relationships or her earlier relationships with her family, that is, before she was diagnosed with diabetes. Nevertheless, the material that is provided is certainly informative about her QOR. The parents are presented as concerned and involved on one hand yet overprotective and somewhat intrusive on the other. June's conflicted response to her parents, especially her father, is identified in section 2–86: "We're all big enough now to be able to look after our health. But we still feel in front of them ... like little kids. He doesn't ... consciously he's never made us feel like that, but there's something about what he says, there is something there that makes you think, well hold on, we can't do that in front of him."

June's description of her relationship with her parents is consistent with the antecedents for the Controlling level of the QOR dimension (see Tables 4.2–4.4). Although she feels loved and cared for by them, June also feels infantalized and controlled by them. She becomes secretive to avoid their disapproval (2–85) and also to protect them (2–84): "I don't like smoking with family, because I know it hurts them." She rebels against their control by displaying a lack of healthy self-care, for example, "oh I didn't eat for one day, and then I had some whiskies and a few fags, another Chinese take-away" (2-59). The manner in which June's rebellion manifests itself actually serves to underscore her irresponsibility. In turn, this irresponsible self-care behavior would unwittingly serve as an invitation to her parents to continue their intrusive, overprotective stance with her.

The health-threatening, if not life-threatening, consequences of her rebellion might also suggest the presence of more primitive aspects in June's object relations. However, we do not have precise information about criteria consistent with the Primitive level. What we do know further supports the criteria for the Controlling level. Specifically, despite her resentment, June continues to feel very responsible for her sister and her sister's children. Indeed, as the therapist says, "You're much more responsible with other people than you are to yourself, aren't you" (2-56)? Furthermore, although June does not have a current boyfriend, she assumes that a romantic relationship would be characterized by him being "under [her] feet" (2-65). That assumption prompts the therapist to clarify that, "A boyfriend isn't like a dog, where you just looked after him.... He'd actually have to have responsibility for you too" (2-66). The transcript thus suggests that June tends to engage in caretaking of others, a stance that is consistent with the behavioral criteria for the Controlling level.

REFERENCES

Azim, H. F. A., Piper, W. E., Segal, P. M., Nixon, G. W. H., & Duncan, S. (1991). The Quality of Object Relations scale. *Bulletin of the Menninger Clinic, 55,* 323–343.

Bloch, S. (1979). Assessment of patients for psychotherapy. *British Journal of Psychiatry, 135,* 193–208.

de Carufel, F. L., & Piper, W. E. (1988). Group psychotherapy or individual psychotherapy: Patient characteristics as predictive factors. *International Journal of Group Psychotherapy, 38,* 169–188.

Eagle, M. (1984). *Recent developments in psychoanalysis.* New York: McGraw-Hill.

Fenigstein, A., Scheier, M. F., & Buss, A. H. (1975). Public and private self-consciousness: Assessment and theory. *Journal of Consulting and Clinical Psychology, 43,* 522–527.

Freud, S. (1923/1961). The ego and the id. *Standard Edition, 19,* 1–66.

Freud, S. (1926/1959). Inhibitions, symptoms, and anxiety. *Standard Edition, 20,* 75–174.

Gough, H. G. (1957). *California psychological inventory.* Palo Alto, CA: Consulting Psychologists Press.

Greenberg, J. R., & Mitchell, S. A. (1983). *Object relations in psychoanalytic theory.* Cambridge, MA: Harvard University Press.

Høglend, P. (1993a). Suitability for brief dynamic psychotherapy: Psychodynamic variables as predictors of outcome. *Acta Psychiatrica Scandinavica, 88,* 104–110.

Høglend, P. (1993b). Transference interpretations and long-term change after dynamic psychotherapy of brief to moderate length. *American Journal of Psychotherapy, 47,* 494–507.

Høglend, P., & Piper, W. E. (1995). Focal adherence in brief dynamic psychotherapy: A comparison of findings from two independent studies. *Psychotherapy, 32,* 618–628.

Horowitz, M. J., Marmar, C. R., Weiss, D., DeWitt, K. N., & Rosenbaum, R. (1984). Brief psychotherapy of bereavement reactions: The relationship of process to outcome. *Archives of General Psychiatry, 41,* 438-448.

Joyce, A. S., & Piper, W. E. (1996). Dimensions and predictors of patient response to interpretation. *Psychiatry, 59,* 65-81.

Kernberg, O., Burstein, E., Coyne, L., Applebaum, H., Horowitz, L., & Voth, H. (1972). Psychotherapy and psychoanalysis: Final report of the Menninger Foundation's Psychotherapy Research Project. *Bulletin of the Menninger Clinic, 36,* 1-275.

Kohut, H. (1971). *The analysis of the self: A systematic approach to the psychoanalytic treatment of narcissistic personality disorders.* New York: International Universities Press.

Malan, D. H. (1976). *The frontier of brief psychotherapy.* New York: Plenum.

Marini, Z., & Case, R. (1994). The development of abstract reasoning about the physical and social world. *Child Development, 65,* 147-159.

May, P. R. A., & Dixon, W. J. (1969). The Camarillo Dynamic Assessment Scale. I: Measurement of psychodynamic factors. *Bulletin of the Menninger Clinic, 33,* 1-35.

McCallum, M., & Piper, W. E. (1987). *Manual for the Psychological Mindedness Assessment Procedure.* Unpublished manuscript. Department of Psychiatry, University of Alberta, Edmonton, Alberta, Canada.

McCallum, M., & Piper, W. E. (1990a). A controlled study of effectiveness and patient suitability for short-term group psychotherapy. *International Journal of Group Psychotherapy, 40,* 431-452.

McCallum, M., & Piper, W. E. (1990b). The psychological mindedness assessment procedure. *Psychological Assessment: A Journal of Consulting and Clinical Psychology, 2,* 412-418.

McCallum, M., & Piper, W. E. (1996). Psychological mindedness. *Psychiatry: Interpersonal and Biological Processes, 59,* 48-64.

McCallum, M., & Piper, W. E. (1997a). The psychological mindedness assessment procedure. In M. McCallum & W. E. Piper (Eds.), *Psychological mindedness: A contemporary understanding* (pp. 27-58). Mahwah, NJ: Lawrence Erlbaum Associates.

McCallum, M., & Piper, W. E. (Eds.). (1997b). *Psychological mindedness: A contemporary understanding.* Mahwah, NJ: Lawrence Erlbaum Associates.

McCallum, M., Piper, W. E., & O'Kelly, J. G. (1997). Predicting patient benefit from a group oriented evening treatment program. *International Journal of Group Psychotherapy, 47,* 291-314.

Ogrodniczuk, J. S., Piper, W. E., Joyce, A. S., & McCallum, M. (1999). Transference interpretations in short-term dynamic psychotherapy. *Journal of Nervous and Mental Disease, 187,* 572-579.

Ogrodniczuk, J. S., Piper, W. E., Joyce, A. S., & McCallum, M. (2001). Using DSM Axis II information to predict outcome in short-term individual psychotherapy. *Journal of Personality Disorders, 15,* 126-138.

Park, L. C., Imboden, J. B., Park, T. J., Hulse, S. H., & Unger, H. T. (1992). Giftedness and psychological abuse in borderline personality disorder: Their relevance to genesis and treatment. *Journal of Personality Disorders, 6,* 226-240.

Piper, W. E., Azim, H. F. A., Joyce, A. S., & McCallum, M. (1991). Transference interpretations, therapeutic alliance and outcome in short-term individual psychotherapy. *Archives of General Psychiatry, 48,* 946-953.

Piper, W. E., Azim, H. F. A., Joyce, A. S., McCallum, M., Nixon, G. W. H., & Segal, P. S. (1991). Quality of object relations vs. interpersonal functioning as predictors of therapeutic alliance and psychotherapy outcome. *Journal of Nervous and Mental Disease, 179,* 432-438.

Piper, W. E., Azim, H. F. A., McCallum, M., & Joyce, A. S. (1990). Patient suitability and outcome in short-term individual psychotherapy. *Journal of Consulting and Clinical Psychology, 58,* 475-481.

Piper, W. E., Boroto, D. R., Joyce, A. S., McCallum, M., & Azim, H. F. A. (1995). Pattern of alliance and outcome in short-term individual psychotherapy. *Psychotherapy, 32,* 639-647.

Piper, W. E., Debbane, E. G., Bienvenu, J. P., & Garant, J. (1984). A comparative study of four forms of psychotherapy. *Journal of Consulting and Clinical Psychology, 52,* 268–279.

Piper, W. E., de Carufel, F. L., & Szkrumelak, N. (1985). Patient predictors of process and outcome in short-term individual psychotherapy. *Journal of Nervous and Mental Disease, 173,* 726–733.

Piper, W. E., & Duncan, S. C. (1999). Object relations theory and short-term dynamic psychotherapy: Findings from the Quality of Object Relations scale. *Clinical Psychology Review, 19,* 669–685.

Piper, W. E., Joyce, A. S., Azim, H. F. A., & Rosie, J. S. (1994). Patient characteristics and success in day treatment. *Journal of Nervous and Mental Disease, 182,* 381–386.

Piper, W. E., Joyce, A. S., McCallum, M., & Azim, H. F. A. (1993). Concentration and correspondence of transference interpretations in short-term psychotherapy. *Journal of Consulting and Clinical Psychology, 61,* 586–595.

Piper, W. E., Joyce, A. S., McCallum, M., & Azim, H. F. A. (1998). Interpretive and supportive forms of psychotherapy and patient personality variables. *Journal of Consulting and Clinical Psychology, 66,* 558–567.

Piper, W. E., Joyce, A. S., McCallum, M., Azim, H. F. A., & Ogrodniczuk, J. S. (2001). *Interpretive and supportive psychotherapies: Matching therapy and patient personality.* Washington, DC: American Psychological Association Press.

Piper, W. E., McCallum, M., & Joyce, A. S. (1993). *Manual for assessment of quality of object relations.* Unpublished manuscript. Department of Psychiatry, University of Alberta, Edmonton, Alberta, Canada.

Piper, W. E., McCallum, M., Joyce, A. S., Rosie, J. S., & Ogrodniczuk, J. S. (2001). Patient personality and time-limited group psychotherapy for complicated grief. *International Journal of Group Psychotherapy, 51,* 525–552.

Piper, W. E., Rosie, J. S., Joyce, A. S., & Azim, H. F. A. (1996). *Time-limited day treatment for personality disorders.* Washington, DC: American Psychological Association.

Robbins, L. L., Wallerstein, R. S., Sargent, H. D., & Luborsky, L. (1956). The psychotherapy research project of The Menninger Foundation: Orientation, rationale, design, concepts, sample use of method. *Bulletin of the Menninger Clinic, 20,* 221–278.

Silver, D. (1983). Psychotherapy of the characterologically difficult patient. *Canadian Journal of Psychiatry, 28,* 513–521.

Taylor, G. J. (1984). Alexithymia: Concept, measurement, and implications for treatment. *American Journal of Psychiatry, 141,* 725–732.

Tolor, A., & Reznikoff, M. (1960). A new approach to insight: A preliminary report. *Journal of Nervous and Mental Disease, 130,* 286–296.

Tyson, R. L., & Sandler, J. (1971). Problems in the selection of patients for psychoanalysis: Comments on the application of the concepts of "indications," "suitability," and "analysability." *British Journal of Medical Psychology, 44,* 211–228.

Vaillant, G. E. (1977). *Adaptation to life.* Boston: Little, Brown.

Wallerstein, R. S. (1986). *Forty-two lives in treatment: A study of psychoanalysis and psychotherapy.* New York: Guilford.

PART

II

DETERMINING AND MAINTAINING A FOCUS

CHAPTER

5

Outcomes and Factors Related to Efficacy of Brief Psychodynamic Therapy

Stanley B. Messer
Amelia H. Kaplan
Rutgers University

This chapter reviews the evidence on outcome and the major factors contributing to progress and outcome in brief psychodynamic therapy (BPT). Our aim in the first of the two main sections of this chapter is to address the question of whether BPT is an effective form of therapy. In doing so, we present two types of outcome studies: meta-analysis, which aggregates the results of many studies that compare BPT to treated or untreated groups, and more recent individual studies that compare BPT to other brief therapies or to long-term psychoanalytic therapy.

In the second section, we present the empirical literature on three salient factors related to therapeutic progress and outcome in BPT. The first factor, which we explore in some depth, is the role of therapists' adherence to a psychodynamically formulated focus and its effect on progress and outcome. The second factor is patient suitability: Among diagnostic groups that have been studied empirically, who is best served by these methods? Diagnoses reviewed include depression, opiate dependency, bulimia, panic disorder, psychosomatic disorder, and personality disorder. The third area examined is "the dose-effect relationship," that is, the relationship of number of therapy sessions to percentage of patients improved. Finally, we suggest areas for future investigation and pose questions for the reader's reflection.

EVIDENCE ON OUTCOMES OF BRIEF PSYCHODYNAMIC THERAPY

Meta-Analysis

In this procedure individual findings from a large number of studies are aggregated by employing a common metric known as an effect size. Effect size expresses the difference between the means of treated versus untreated groups compared in standard deviation units. Much of this research is on mixed diagnostic groups. There have been three meta-analyses of brief psychodynamic therapy: Svartberg and Stiles (1991), Crits-Christoph (1992), and Anderson and Lambert (1995), each employing somewhat different criteria for selecting studies.

The Svartberg and Stiles (1991) meta-analysis included 19 studies appearing between 1978 and 1988, many of which were seriously flawed from both methodological and clinical standpoints (see Messer & Warren, 1995). Svartberg and Stiles defined their inclusion criteria as group designs that included BPT along with either a no-treatment control or an alternative group, or both, and two of the following: the underlying theory of the approach was psychodynamic, the stated goal was the acquisition of insight or the achievement of personality change, and the techniques emphasized interpretation and transference. In addition, there had to be a conceptually planned brief duration of treatment of fewer than 40 sessions.

BPT showed a small but significant superiority to the no-treatment condition at termination of therapy, but this advantage had disappeared by 1-year follow-up. However, those studies that included such a follow-up averaged only 6.8 sessions in duration, which the authors pointed out (and the dose-effect relationship studies described later confirms) were not enough time for BPT to show its benefits. Compared with alternative approaches such as behavioral or cognitive therapy, BPT was inferior at posttreatment, equivalent at 6-month follow-up, and inferior at 1-year follow-up.

The Crits-Christoph (1992) meta-analysis was more exacting in the selection of studies than that of Svartberg and Stiles (1991): Only two studies overlapped and almost all of the studies in Crits-Christoph (1992) appeared after 1988. The selection criteria were use of a specific form of BPT as represented in a manual-like guide (a criterion that has become de rigueur in comparative studies); the comparison of BPT and either a waiting list control condition, an alternative therapy, medication, or a nonpsychiatric treatment (such as a self-help group, drug counseling, or low contact treatment); and the study's provision of the information necessary to calculate effect sizes. Two other important criteria were a minimum of 12 sessions and therapists who were experienced in conducting BPT. The outcome measures compared included target symptoms, general level of psychiatric symptoms, and social functioning. The results of the meta-analysis of the 11 studies reviewed indicated that BPT demonstrated large effects compared to the waiting list control, slight superiority to the nonpsychiatric treatments, and equal effects to other psychotherapies and medication.

A third meta-analysis by Anderson and Lambert (1995) included 26 studies, 10 of which overlapped with those in the Crits-Christoph (1992) review. BPT was found to be superior to no treatment and equivalent to alternative therapies. BPT showed a small but significant superiority to the alternative treatments when follow-up was conducted after more than 6 months. In brief, according to the two more representative meta-analyses, being in BPT is much better than not being in therapy, but is no better and no worse than being in other bona fide therapies such as cognitive behavior therapy or receiving medication. It is possible that longer-term follow-up would reveal differences among these therapies.

Luborsky et al. (2002) performed a meta-analysis of 17 meta-analyses (known as a *mega-analysis*) comparing active treatments including BPT with each other. There was only a small and nonsignificant effect size ($d = .20$) due to treatment effect, which shrank even further ($d = .12$) when corrected for researcher theoretical allegiance. Messer and Wampold (2002) argued that even these small effects are an overestimate of the true difference, which is close to zero. Luborsky et al.'s results were very similar to those of Grissom (1996) who meta-analyzed 32 meta-analyses of comparative treatments. These meta-analyses reinforce the Crits-Christoph (1992) and Andersen and Lambert (1995) findings of no differences among bona fide therapies (i.e., those that have a considerable theoretical, empirical and clinical literature to back them up).

Individual Studies Comparing BPT to Other Brief Therapies and to Long-Term Therapy

Several randomized controlled trials comparing BPT to other therapies have appeared since the last meta-analysis in 1995. In general, these have supported the results of the meta-analyses. In one, BPT was compared to supportive therapy for patients with mixtures of depression, anxiety, low self-esteem, and interpersonal conflict (Piper, Joyce, Azim, & McCallum, 1998). Both treatment groups showed significant improvement according to statistical and clinical criteria but did not differ from each other. At 6-month and 12-month follow-up, improvement was maintained, again with no difference between treatments (Piper, McCallum, Joyce, Azim, & Ogrodniczuk, 1999).

In two other studies, depressed patients were treated with either 8 or 16 sessions of either cognitive-behavioral or psychodynamic-interpersonal therapy. In the first (Shapiro, Barkham, Rees, Hardy, Reynolds, & Startup, 1994), there were substantial gains that were maintained at 3-month and 1-

year follow-up with few differences between the therapies (Shapiro et al., 1995). The more severely depressed patients improved more with 16 versus 8 sessions. In a replication of this study (Barkham et al., 1996), gains in both treatments were large and approximately equivalent. However, gains were not maintained as well by patients in this study as in the earlier one, probably due to the greater severity of their depression. Overall, clients again did better in 16- versus 8-session therapy.

To summarize, these individual studies show equivalence of different kinds (but not different lengths) of brief therapy, reflecting the modal finding of other controlled comparisons, meta-analyses, and the Luborsky et al. (2002) mega-analysis.

In a comparison of short-term ($M = 22$ sessions) to long-term ($M = 76$ sessions) psychoanalytic therapy, outcomes were equivalent. However, according to the cost–benefit analysis of time expenditure by both therapists and patients, short-term therapy was superior (Piper, Debbane, Bienvenu, & Garant, 1984).

In brief, the studies of outcome largely converge on the conclusion that BPT is an effective form of therapy compared to waitlist controls, that it is as effective but no more so than other bona fide therapies, and that it is more cost effective than long-term psychoanalytic therapy. We turn now to a consideration of the factors of focality, diagnosis, and number of sessions as predictors of progress and outcome in BPT.

FACTORS RELATED TO OUTCOME IN BRIEF PSYCHODYNAMIC THERAPY

The Importance of Focus in Progress and Outcome

The question of whether therapist adherence to a psychodynamic focus correlates with treatment progress and outcome is significant particularly for short-term psychodynamic therapy in which the brevity of treatment requires an early and well-articulated focus (Messer, 2001b). In general, brief therapists have adhered rigorously to a focal theme that is formulated at the outset of therapy (e.g., Binder, 1977; Malan, 1976a). The question then turns to whether the empirical literature supports the value of such adherence.

What Is a Focus?

Malan (1976b), a pioneer in the development of the BPT drive or structural model, described "focality" (p. 11) as the therapist's attempt to address the patient's "basic neurotic conflict" (p. 13). The therapist must first derive a psychodynamic formulation of the patient's problems and then use this guiding conception strategically to devise and offer interventions to the patient (e.g., interpretations, clarifications, reflections, etc.). The therapist's adherence to the focus has also been referred to as accuracy, congruence, suitability, compatibility, correspondence, and correctness (Piper, Joyce, McCallum, & Azim, 1993). Drawing on the writings of Menninger (1958), Malan (1976a, 1976b) used a schematic of two triangles as a conceptual framework for formulating a person's dynamics and as a way to guide treatment focus. The *triangle of conflict* describes the relationship among impulses or feelings, defenses against them, and the anxiety or other inhibitory affects such as shame or guilt that occur when the defense fails. The *triangle of person* refers to interpersonal relationships from the patient's past, in the present, and with the therapist (i.e., the transference). Interventions regarding impulses, defenses, and consequent anxiety are made in connection with the figures on the triangle of person.

Malan (1976b) correlated therapist interpretations along the lines of the focus with treatment outcome. *Interpretation* was defined as "any intervention in which the therapist suggests or implies an emotional content in the patient over and above what the patient has already said" (Malan, 1976b, p. 213). He found a moderate relationship between focality of interventions and therapeutic outcome. Although he was one of the first to study empirically therapist focal adherence, his study had several methodological problems such as using therapist notes dictated from memory rather than session transcripts as his main data source and no control groups.

Several other methods have been developed subsequently to formulate a patient's core problems as elaborated on by Eells and Lombart (chap. 6, this volume). The psychometric properties and construct validity of these methods have been described in a review by Barber and Crits-Christoph (1993) and in a book edited by Eells (1997). One of the most thoroughly studied ways of formulating a focus is the core conflictual relationship theme method (CCRT; Luborsky & Crits-Christoph, 1990). In this approach, independent judges derive a formulation from transcripts of patient narratives based on three components: the person's wishes, needs, feelings, or all of these toward others; the other's responses; and the subsequent reactions of the person.

Another approach to formulation of a focus is the Plan Diagnosis Method, later renamed the Plan Formulation Method (PFM; Curtis, Silberschatz, Weiss, Sampson, & Rosenberg, 1988). Based on a cognitive psychoanalytic theory developed by Weiss, Sampson, and the Mt. Zion Psychotherapy Research Group (1986), patients are said to have developed unconscious pathogenic beliefs in childhood and enter therapy with the intent of disconfirming and changing such beliefs. The PFM requires raters to define the patient's plan, which is the set of conscious or unconscious beliefs patients have for disconfirming their pathogenic beliefs and behavior patterns. Using material from the first few sessions, raters define the patient's plan by identifying patient goals, perceived obstacles to achieving the goals (or pathogenic beliefs), tests of the therapist to confirm or disconfirm the beliefs, and insights about the pathogenic beliefs (see Eells & Lombart, chap. 6, this volume, for further elaboration of the CCRT and PFM). Adherence, or plan compatibility, is measured by the Plan Compatibility of Intervention Scale (Weiss, Sampson, & the Mt. Zion Psychotherapy Research Group, 1986).

One example of defining a focus is found in the case of June, who reported many instances where things felt "incomplete." She also felt "not cared about," worthless, and rejected and came to believe that she didn't deserve proper care. This theme affected both her own ability to care for herself as well as to elicit and receive care from others: Instead of accepting care, she rejected it. Therefore, just as she had ceased to attend to herself, so had others stopped caring for her. Focal interpretations might center on her core conflicts about self-care, including identifying her self-fulfilling prophecy and interpreting why she resists self-care.

Relation of Focal Adherence to Outcome

Crits-Christoph, Cooper, & Luborsky (1988) used the CCRT method to examine the relationship of accuracy of therapist interpretations, as measured by their agreement with the CCRT, to outcome. For the 43 patients studied, they found a moderately strong, statistically significant relationship between accuracy of interpretation and treatment outcome. In particular, focal accuracy of the patient's main wishes and responses from others reliably predicted the best treatment results. The authors concluded that a helpful therapeutic strategy is to focus on the patient's stereotypical patterns of needs and wishes as well as responses of others rather than limit the focus to the patient's typical responses to others.

In one of the earlier studies to suggest that focal adherence may be related to outcome, Horowitz, Marmar, Weiss, DeWitt, and Rosenbaum (1984) studied 52 bereaved patients to look for relations between therapist actions and outcome. They found that greater efforts on the part of the therapist to clarify the focus of treatment were related to improved patient relationships. However, the authors cautioned that, given the number of correlations they performed, the result might have been due to chance.

Some studies have examined patient characteristics, including the focal suitability of patients' problems, as essential variables in the relation between focus and outcome. In a group of 22 patients treated with BPT, clinical judges rated the degree to which the patients' problems could be encompassed within an oedipally-toned circumscribed focus (Høglend & Heyerdahl, 1994). The oedipal features included problems in competition and achievement, rivalry, problems with authority figures, fear of responsibility, inhibited anger, and guilt over sexual intimacy. Patients for whom such a circumscribed conflict could be clearly identified had the most favorable dynamic change in a 4-year follow-up.

Piper et al. (1993) examined the effect of patient characteristics on the relation between focal transference interpretations and outcome. They were particularly interested in patients' level of *quality of object relations* (QOR), which is defined as a person's internal enduring tendency to establish certain types of relationships ranging from primitive to mature. Earlier work (Piper, Azim, Joyce, & McCallum, 1991) demonstrated that the concentration of transference interpretations, regardless of focality, was inversely proportional to measures of alliance and outcome in high-QOR patients such that a high dose of transference interpretations was associated with worse outcome for such patients.

In the Piper et al. (1993) study, they again examined the relationship between concentration or number (quantity) of focal transference interpretations and outcome. In addition, they studied correspondence or accuracy (quality) of adherence to dynamic focus of transference interpretations with outcome. Focal correspondence was based on formulations devised by the therapist after the patient's first two sessions, and independent raters judged the extent of the correspondence. The researchers found that a patient's characteristic QOR plays a significant role in mediating the effect of therapist transference interpretations. For high-QOR patients, greater focal correspondence of transference interpretations was associated with better outcome but only when delivered at low concentration or dosage. For low-QOR patients, the greater the concentrations of focal transference interpretations the lower were both alliance and outcome measures.

Using data from separate studies in Edmonton, Canada and Oslo, Norway, Høglend and Piper (1995) also examined the relationship between focal adherence and QOR. The process for finding a focus differed between teams. In Edmonton, dynamic formulations were derived solely by the therapist, whereas in Oslo it was by consensus of the therapist with several clinicians who observed an interview with the patient. In both studies focal adherence was associated with positive outcome in high-QOR patients and negatively associated with outcome in low-QOR patients. Such findings reinforce the evidence that maintaining a focus consistent with the dynamic formulation is associated with good outcome for patients with a high quality of object relations as long as the dose of transference interpretations is not too high.

These results suggest the important clinical implication that knowing a patient's level of QOR can help clinicians determine what level of focal adherence to employ. Although it is often posited that lower functioning clients need more structured treatment, a less focused therapy in which patients are enabled to speak with less emphasis on specific focal content may actually be indicated for low-QOR patients. Being thus less restricted may allow them to build trust in the relationship.

Relation of Focal Adherence to Therapy Progress

Using the PFM, Silberschatz, Fretter, and Curtis (1986) hypothesized that therapist interpretations that are plan compatible would be effective in bringing about patient progress whether or not they were transference related. Judges derived formulations according to the PFM. They subsequently rated therapist interventions as interpretations or noninterpretations, distinguishing transference from nontransference interpretations. Focal adherence was measured using the Plan Compatibility of Interventions Scale.

As predicted, they found a significant positive correlation between suitability of interpretations, that is, those that were along the lines of the patient's plan, and progress as rated on the Experiencing Scale (Klein, Mathieu, Gendlin, & Keisler, 1970). Comparing good versus poor outcome cases, they also found high percentages of suitable interventions in the two good outcome cases but higher percentages of antiplan or ambiguous interpretations in the poor outcome case. Although their data set consisted of only three cases, this study inspired further research in tracking moment-to-moment therapeutic progress following therapist interpretations. Thus, a therapist sticking to a plan or focus helps to move the therapy forward.

Based on an earlier randomized controlled trial of BPT, Joyce and Piper (1996) conducted an exploratory analysis of the relationship between a therapist's focal interpretations and treatment process and outcome. Their interests were twofold: They hoped to categorize how patients respond to interpretations and to look more closely at what features of interpretations predicted certain patient responses.

Joyce and Piper (1996) studied 60 cases of manualized BPT with patients matched on QOR, age, and gender and assigned to either immediate therapy or a delayed-therapy control group. In comparison to studies in which judges derived the formulations posttherapy, therapists derived their own formulations. An interpretation was considered focal if it included references to the triangle of conflict (i.e., wish, anxiety, and defense) or to transference interpretations that corresponded with the patient's central emotional concern. Progress was measured by creating factor clusters of patient responses such as "working involvement," which indicated an increase in the patient's engagement in the therapeutic process.

Joyce and Piper (1996) found that focal correspondence interventions were advantageous to both therapeutic process and outcome. Interpretations highest in focal correspondence were directly associated with increased working involvement. However, as reported previously (Piper et al., 1991), they also found that high frequency of transference interpretations specifically had a negative outcome for patients with high QOR. These

5. FACTORS RELATED TO OUTCOME

results underscore the positive impact of focal interpretations and the necessity of using transference interpretations sparingly.

Employing the PFM, Messer, Tishby, and Spillman (1992) used single-case design to examine how the focal plan compatibility and quality of therapist interventions affected therapy process. To assess patient progress, they divided a 15-session therapy into early, middle, and late phases and developed a scale to gauge patient progress in response to therapist interventions. The relationship between focal adherence and patient progress was strongest in the early (Sessions 4–7) and middle (Sessions 8–12) phases of therapy, which suggested to the authors that the emphasis on focal adherence is most important in the working through process of the early and middle stages of treatment.

Also using single-case design, Tishby and Messer (1995) compared the effects of therapist focal adherence according to two different plans. The question posed was, "Would therapist interventions along the lines of one plan lead to more progress than interventions along the lines of the other?" Each therapist intervention was rated according to its plan compatibility with both the Mt. Zion cognitive-dynamic viewpoint (Weiss et al., 1986) and with the Rutgers object relations based plan (Collins & Messer, 1991). The researchers examined patient turns-at-talk by means of the Rutgers Psychotherapy Progress Scale (Holland, Roberts, & Messer, 1998). Therapist compatibility of intervention with the object relations plan was significantly correlated with progress in the early phase of one case and in the middle phase of both. Focal adherence of intervention along the lines of the Mt. Zion cognitive-dynamic plan, however, showed a negative association with patient progress. Thus, it appears that not just any focal interventions will do; they must resonate with the nature of the patient's problems.

To summarize this line of research, there is a significant association between focal adherence and patient progress. Too high a dose of focal transference interpretations, however, can be detrimental depending on the patient's QOR. Timing of focal adherence also seems to be an important variable, with evidence suggesting that the early to middle phases of therapy are most critical within the course of treatment. Further areas for investigation are discussed later in the chapter.

Diagnostic Criteria that Predict Outcome

In this section, we look at which specific diagnostic groups are correlated with satisfactory outcome (see also Messer, 2001b). It should be noted that there are many studies of mixed diagnostic groups of patients—particularly affective and depressive disorders, adjustment disorders, and mild personality disorders—that are included in the meta-analytic and comparative studies described earlier.

Depression. As reported previously, Shapiro et al. (1994) found that patients with depression profited from BPT, especially the 16-session treatment, although the more severely depressed patients did not maintain their gains as well as those less depressed (Barkham et al., 1996). In an effort to compete with the promotion of medication by different psychiatric groups as the treatment of choice for a variety of psychiatric disorders, the American Psychological Association's Division of Clinical Psychology set up a task force to review psychotherapy outcome studies of specific disorders or problems (Division 12 Task Force, 1996). BPT (in the form of Interpersonal Therapy, or IPT) is included in their list of well-established "Empirically Supported Treatments" for depression (Chambless & Task Force, 1998) and in its more traditional psychoanalytic variety as "probably efficacious." The latter designation suggests that not enough studies have been conducted yet to affirm its status as well established.

Opiate Dependency. BPT (Luborsky's supportive-expressive brief therapy; Luborsky, 1984) is listed by the Division 12 Task Force (1996) as "probably efficacious."

Bulimia. BPT (in the form of Interpersonal Therapy) is listed as probably efficacious.

Panic Disorder. In an effort to determine whether BPT was effective in reducing the relapse rate of panic disorder, Wiborg and Dahl (1996) compared two treatment groups: one received clomipramine alone and the other clomipramine plus 15 simultaneous sessions of manualized BPT based on concepts and techniques from Davanloo, Malan, and Strupp and Binder (see Messer & Warren, 1995). All patients became free of panic attacks within 9 months. However, on removal of medication the relapse rate was significantly higher in the medication-only group. On follow-up, anxiety and panic attacks were again lower for the medication plus BPT group, demonstrating the utility of BPT.

Psychosomatic (Somatoform) and Neurotic Disorders. Junkert-Tress, Schnierda, Hartkamp, Schmitz, and Tress (2001) conducted a naturalistic effectiveness study of 75 patients categorized as having neuroses (affective disorders and mild to moderate anxiety disorders), psychosomatic disorders, or personality disorders. Patients were treated with 25 sessions of BPT, which emphasized "analysis of transference manifestations both in the actual therapist–patient relationship as well as in conflictual relationships outside the therapeutic dyad" (Junkert-Tress et al., 2001, p. 188). Therapists used the Strupp and Binder (1984) relational psychotherapy model as a guide. Across a number of patient and therapist measures including both positive and negative introject and symptom status, the neurotic and psychosomatic patients showed significant improvement at termination of therapy as well as at 6-month and 12-month follow-ups.

Personality Disorders. In the same study, Junkert-Tress et al. (2001) found that patients with personality disorders did much less well than the neurotic or psychosomatic patients, although they too showed some improvement. The authors pointed out that results regarding all three diagnostic groups should be interpreted with caution because there was no control group and the sample sizes were relatively small ($n = 25$ per group). On the other hand, the strength of a naturalistic study is that it reflects actual conditions of practice more so than do controlled clinical trials.

Høglend and others (Høglend, 1993; Høglend, Sørlie, Heyerdahl, Sørbye, & Amlo, 1993) studied the relationship between patient suitability and outcome in a BPT based on the approaches of Malan (1976a) and Sifneos (1972). The presence of a personality disorder was a negative predictor of psychodynamic change at both 2 and 4 years following termination of therapy. Paralleling these results, Hardy et al. (1995) found that depressed patients with comorbid, Cluster C personality disorders (avoidant, obsessive–compulsive or dependent) showed less favorable response to a psychodynamic-interpersonal therapy than clients with a comorbid Axis I diagnosis.

Barber, Morse, Krakauer, Chittams, and Crits-Christoph (1997) compared the improvement of obsessive–compulsive and avoidant personality disorders in Luborsky's supportive-expressive therapy. The *obsessive–compulsive* patients improved fairly rapidly, with 50% losing their diagnosis by 16 sessions. However, it was not until 32 sessions that 50% of the *avoidant* patients were similarly improved. Both groups showed substantial improvement in depression and anxiety by 16 and 32 sessions, but interpersonal problems remained unchanged. In another study of undifferentiated Cluster C personality-disordered patients, groups receiving Davanloo's Short-Term Dynamic Psychotherapy (STDP; Davanloo, 1980) or another form of BPT called *brief adaptive therapy* improved more than a wait-list control (Winston et al., 1994).

It would appear that some personality-disordered patients are helped by BPT, especially the milder ones, but that moderate to longer term therapy may be needed for the more severe cases and to show more substantial improvement.

Relation of Dose Effect (Number of Sessions) to Outcome

In this way of studying factors that correlate with outcome of BPT, the number of sessions (or dose) of therapy is related to the percentage of patients improved for that number (the effect). In the earliest of such studies, Howard, Kopta, Krause, and Orlinsky (1986) found that 55% to 60% of patients had improved by 13 sessions and 75% by 26 sessions in open-ended psychodynamic therapy. Borderline patients made gains more slowly than did the anxiety and depressive patients. Their review of the general psychotherapy literature yielded an even lower estimate of 8 sessions for 50% improvement but the same figure of 26 sessions for 75% improvement. Except for the 8 sessions finding, subsequent studies have tended to support these figures. For example, Kadera, Lambert, and Andrews (1996), employing the more stringent criterion of clinically (vs. statistically) significant change, found that 50% of patients had improved by 16 sessions and 75% by 25 sessions.

Anderson and Lambert (2001) used a larger sample, a more varied group of therapists, and combined the data with those of the previous study. Similar to Howard et al. (1986) they found that 13 sessions were necessary before 50% of outpatients attained clinically significant change. Once again, 25 sessions were required for 75% of patients to show such improvement. (Based on a sample of 10,000 patients collected under much less controlled and reliable conditions, Lambert, Hansen, & Finch, 2001, reported that 21 sessions were required for 50% of patients to achieve clinically significant change.) However, many of these studies lack a focus, goals, and other characteristics of brief therapy, which, if employed, might have made the therapies more time efficient. In sum, it probably takes between 8 and 16 sessions for 50% of patients to improve and about 25 sessions for 75% of patients to show gains. (It should be noted that change often refers to symptom improvement or feeling and functioning better but typically does not include other kinds of outcomes measures valued in particular by experiential and psychodynamic therapists (Messer, 2001a).

The overall results have been refined by examining separately the rate of change for well-being, symptoms, and life functioning. Howard, Lueger, Maling, and Martinovitch (1993) reported that feelings of well-being respond most rapidly, followed by symptoms, and last by changes in interpersonal and social functioning. These findings have been confirmed for therapy in general (Lutz, Lowry, Kopta, Einstein, & Howard, 2001) and BPT in particular (Hilsenroth, Ackerman, & Blagys, 2001) and extended by Lutz et al. to a study of different diagnostic groups. In accordance with predictions, the following was the descending rank order of improvement: adjustment disorder, depressive symptoms, obsessive–compulsive symptoms, bipolar symptoms, and anxiety-related symptoms.

FUTURE DIRECTIONS AND CONCLUSIONS

As just discussed (i.e., dose-effect relationship), patient-focused research involves tracking patients' ongoing progress across the course of therapy (e.g., Lambert & Asay, chap. 15, this volume; Lambert et al., 2001; Lueger et al., 2001). If adherence to a focus tends to enhance treatment progress, a potentially fruitful area for investigation is to monitor therapists' focal accuracy during the course of treatment. In connection with such research, therapists could be given feedback as to how well the current focus is working and could then adjust their interventions accordingly. Supervisors also might be encouraged to tailor supervision to focal adherence.

Research is also needed on diagnostic groups not yet carefully studied as well as on serious conditions such as suicidal ideation and behavior. In a recent example of such research (Guthrie et al., 2001), a brief course of psychodynamic therapy was shown to reduce suicidal ideation and attempts at self-harm to a greater degree than usual care among patients who had attempted suicide. Adult patients presenting to an emergency department after an episode of deliberate self-poisoning were randomly assigned to four sessions of psychodynamic interpersonal therapy provided by nurse therapists once a week in the patient's home or to usual care. Usual care involved referral to a psychiatry outpatient clinic for about a third of the patients, referral to an addiction service for a few, and advice to consult a general practitioner for the rest of the patients.

Eighty percent attended a 6-month follow-up evaluation. Compared with the usual-care group, those who received the intervention scored significantly better on the Beck Scale for Suicidal Ideation (Beck, 1991) and significantly lower on the Beck Depression Inventory (Beck, Steer, & Brown, 1996). During the follow-up period, 28% of those in the control group but only 9% of those in the intervention group had harmed themselves again (Guthrie et al., 2001).

To summarize the overall thrust of the findings reviewed in this chapter, BPT, compared to waiting list controls, is generally well supported for mixed diagnostic and symptom groups and provisionally supported for about half a dozen specific diagnoses. Therapist intervention along the lines of a circumscribed psychodynamic focus is associated with better progress and outcome in BPT. Finally, regarding time as a predictive factor, it takes roughly 8 to 16 sessions for 50% of patients to improve and about 25 sessions for 75% of patients to show gains in psychotherapy.

June, the case study referred to in this book, has received nine sessions of psychotherapy. Therefore, statistically she has a good chance of showing significant improvement. There are a number of issues, however, about what kind of outcome criteria one might wish to consider in trying to distinguish the efficacy of brief treatment in general and its effectiveness specifically with June. The outcome could be assessed using an independent criterion such as blood glucose level because this was the concern of the referring medical practitioner. Indeed, at follow-up, June was found to have a blood glucose reading in the range signifying good control. Other measures of improvement might include her ability to take care of herself and to elicit and receive care from others. June's demonstration of insight about her resistance may also help her sustain the gains. The psychodynamic psychotherapy used in this case was cognitive analytic therapy that emphasizes having a clearly defined focus. The focus, however, could be defined in any number of ways and some of the options will be discussed by Eells and Lombart (chap. 6, this volume). The question for the reader is: How would you work with June along the lines of the focus, such as the one we provided previously, to ensure good progress and a satisfactory outcome?

REFERENCES

Anderson, E. M., & Lambert, M. J. (1995). Short-term dynamically oriented psychotherapy: A review and meta-analysis. *Clinical Psychology Review, 15,* 503–514.

Anderson, E. M., & Lambert, M. J. (2001). A survival analysis of clinically significant change in outpatient psychotherapy. *Journal of Clinical Psychology, 57,* 875–888.

Barber, J., & Crits-Christoph, P. (1993). Advances in measures of psychodynamic formulations. *Journal of Consulting and Clinical Psychology, 61,* 574–585.

Barber, J. P., Morse, J. Q., Krakauer, I. D., Chittams, J., & Crits-Christoph, K. (1997). Change in obsessive–compulsive and avoidant personality disorders following time-limited supportive-expressive therapy. *Psychotherapy, 34,* 133–143.

Barkham, M., Rees, A., Shapiro, D. A., Stiles, W. B., Agnew, R. M., Halstead, J., Culverwell, A., & Harrington, V. M. G. (1996). Outcomes of time-limited psychotherapy in applied settings: Replicating the second Sheffield Psychotherapy Project. *Journal of Consulting and Clinical Psychology, 64,* 1079–1085.

Beck, A. T. (1991). *Beck Scale for Suicide Ideation.* San Antonio, TX: Psychological Corporation.

Beck, A. T., Steer, R. A., Brown, G. K. (1996). *Beck Depression Inventory–II.* San Antonio, TX: Psychological Corporation.

Binder, J. (1977). Modes of focusing in psychoanalytic short-term therapy. *Psychotherapy: Theory, Research and Practice, 14,* 232–241.

Chambless, D. L., & Task Force. (1998). Update on empirically validated therapies, II. *The Clinical Psychologist, 51*(1), 3–16.

Collins, W. D., & Messer, S. B. (1991). Extending the plan formulation method to an object relations perspective: Reliability, stability, and adaptability. *Psychological Assessment: A Journal of Consulting and Clinical Psychology, 13,* 75–81.

Crits-Christoph, P. (1992). The efficacy of brief dynamic psychotherapy: A meta-analysis. *American Journal of Psychiatry, 149,* 151–158.

Crits-Christoph, P., Cooper, A., & Luborsky, L. (1988). The accuracy of therapist interpretations and the outcome of dynamic psychotherapy. *Journal of Consulting and Clinical Psychology, 56,* 490–495.

Curtis, J. T., Silberschatz, G., Weiss, J., Sampson, H., & Rosenberg, S. E. (1988). Developing reliable psychodynamic case formulations: An illustration of the plan diagnosis method. *Psychotherapy, 25,* 256–265.

Davanloo, H. (1980). *Short-term dynamic therapy.* New York: Jason Aronson.

Division 12 Task Force. (1996). Training in and dissemination of empirically validated psychological treatments: Report and recommendations. *The Clinical Psychologist, 49,* 3–23.

Eells, T. D. (Ed.). (1997). *Handbook of psychotherapy case formulation.* New York: Guilford.

Grissom, R. J. (1996). The magic number .7+−.2: Meta-meta-analysis of the probability of superior outcome in comparisons involving therapy, placebo, and control. *Journal of Consulting and Clinical Psychology, 64,* 973–982.

Guthrie, E., Kapur, N., Mackway-Jones, K., Chew-Graham, C., Moorey, J., Mendel, E., Marino-Francis, F., Sanderson, S., Turpin, C., Boddy, G., & Tomenson, B. (2001). Randomised controlled trial for brief psychological intervention after deliberate self poisoning. *British Medical Journal, 323,* 135–138.

Hardy, G. E., Barkham, M., Shapiro, D. A., Stiles, W. B., Rees, A., & Reynolds, S. (1995). Impact of Cluster C personality disorders on outcomes of contrasting brief psychotherapies for depression. *Journal of Consulting and Clinical Psychology, 63,* 997–1004.

Hilsenroth, M. J., Ackerman, S. J., & Blagys, M. D. (2001). Evaluating the phase model of change during short-term psychodynamic psychotherapy. *Psychotherapy Research, 11,* 29–47.

Høglend, P. (1993). Personality disorders and long-term outcome after brief dynamic psychotherapy. *Acta Psychiatrica Scandinavica, 7,* 168–181.

Høglend, P., & Heyerdahl, O. (1994). The circumscribed focus in intensive brief dynamic psychotherapy. *Psychotherapy and Psychosomatics, 61,* 163–170.

Høglend, P., & Piper, W. E. (1995). Focal adherence in brief dynamic psychotherapy: A comparison of findings from two independent studies. *Psychotherapy, 32,* 618–628.

Høglend, P., Sørlie, T., Heyerdahl, O., Sørbye, O., & Amlo, S. (1993). Brief dynamic psychotherapy: Patient suitability, treatment length, and outcome. *Journal of Psychotherapy Practice and Research, 2,* 230–241.

Holland, S. J., Roberts, N. E., & Messer, S. B. (1998). The reliability and validity of the Rutgers Psychotherapy Progress Scale. *Psychotherapy Research, 8,* 104–110.

Horowitz, M., Marmar, C., Weiss, D., DeWitt, K., & Rosenbaum, R. (1984). Brief psychotherapy of bereavement reactions. *Archives of General Psychiatry, 41,* 438–448.

Howard, K. I., Kopta, S. M., Krause, M. S., & Orlinsky, D. E. (1986). The dose-effect relationship in psychotherapy. *American Psychologist, 41,* 159–164.

Howard, K. L., Lueger, R. J., Maling, M., & Martinovich, Z. (1993). A phase model of psychotherapy outcome. *Journal of Consulting and Clinical Psychology, 61,* 678–685.

Joyce, A., & Piper, W. (1996). Dimensions and predictors of patient response to interpretation. *Psychiatry, 59,* 65–81.

Junkert-Tress, B., Schnierda, U., Hartkamp, N., Schmitz, N., & Tress, W. (2001). Effects of short-term dynamic psychotherapy for neurotic, somatoform, and personality disorders: A prospective 1-year follow-up study. *Psychotherapy Research, 11,* 187–200.

Kadera, S. W., Lambert, M. J., & Andrews, A. A. (1996). How much therapy is really enough? *The Journal of Psychotherapy Practice and Research, 5,* 132–151.

Klein, M. H., Mathieu, P. L., Gendlin, E. T., & Keisler, D. J. (1970). *The Experiencing Scale: A research and training manual.* Madison: Wisconsin Psychiatric Institute.

Lambert, M. J., Hansen, N. B., & Finch, A. E. (2001). Patient-focused research: Using patient outcome data to enhance treatment effects. *Journal of Consulting and Clinical Psychology, 69,* 159–172.

Luborsky, L. (1984). *Principles of psychoanalytic psychotherapy: A manual for supportive-expressive treatment.* New York: Basic Books.

Luborsky, L., & Crits-Christoph, P. (1990). *Understanding transference.* New York: Basic Books.

Luborsky, L., Rosenthal, R., Diguer, L., Andrusyna, T. P., Berman, J. S., Levitt, J. T., Seligman, D. A., & Krause, E. D. (2002). The Dodo Bird verdict is alive and well—mostly. *Clinical Psychology: Science and Practice, 9,* 2–12.

Lueger, R., Martinovich, Z., Anderson, E., Howard, K., Lutz, W., & Grissom, G. (2001). Assessing treatment progress of individual patients using expected treatment response models. *Journal of Consulting and Clinical Psychology, 69,* 150–158.

Lutz, W., Lowry, J., Kopta, S. M., Einstein, D. A., & Howard, K. I. (2001). Prediction of dose-response relations based on patient characteristics. *Journal of Clinical Psychology, 57,* 889–900.

Malan, D. H. (1976a). *The frontier of brief psychotherapy.* New York: Plenum.

Malan, D. H. (1976b). *Toward the validation of dynamic psychotherapy: A replication.* New York: Plenum.

Menninger, K. (1958). *Theory of psychoanalytic technique.* New York: Basic Books.
Messer, S. B. (2001a). Empirically supported treatments: What's a non-behaviorist to do? In B. D. Slife, R. N. Williams, & S. H. Barlow (Eds.), *Critical issues in psychotherapy: Translating new ideas into practice* (pp. 3–19). Thousand Oaks, CA: Sage.
Messer, S. B. (2001b). What makes brief psychodynamic therapy time efficient? *Clinical Psychology: Science and Practice, 8,* 5–22.
Messer, S. B., Tishby, O., & Spillman, A. (1992). Taking context seriously in psychotherapy research: Relating therapist interventions to patient progress in brief psychodynamic therapy. *Journal of Consulting and Clinical Psychology, 60,* 678–688.
Messer, S. B., & Wampold, B. E. (2002). Let's face facts: Common factors are more potent than specific therapy ingredients. *Clinical Psychology: Science and Practice, 9,* 21–25.
Messer, S. B., & Warren, C. S. (1995). *Models of brief psychodynamic therapy: A comparative approach.* New York: Guilford.
Piper, W. E, Azim, H., Joyce, A., & McCallum, M. (1991). Transference interpretations, therapeutic alliance and outcome in short-term individual psychotherapy. *Archives of General Psychiatry, 48,* 946–953.
Piper, W. E., Debbane, E. G., Bienvenu, J. P., & Garant, J. (1984). A comparative study of four forms of psychotherapy. *Journal of Consulting and Clinical Psychology, 52,* 268–279.
Piper, W. E., Joyce, A. S., Azim, H. F. A., & McCallum, M. (1998). Interpretive and supportive forms of psychotherapy and patient personality variables. *Journal of Consulting and Clinical Psychology, 66,* 558–567.
Piper, W. E., Joyce, A. S., McCallum, M., & Azim, H. (1993). Concentration and correspondence of transference interpretations in short-term psychotherapy. *Journal of Consulting and Clinical Psychology, 61,* 586–595.
Piper, W. E., McCallum, M., Joyce, A. S., Azim, H. F. A., & Ogrodniczuk, J. S. (1999). Follow-up findings for interpretive and supportive forms of psychotherapy and patient personality variables. *Journal of Consulting and Clinical Psychology, 67,* 267–273.
Shapiro, D. A., Barkham, M., Rees, A., Hardy, G. E., Reynolds, S., & Startup, M. (1994). Effects of treatment duration and severity of depression on the effectiveness of cognitive-behavioral and psychodynamic-interpersonal psychotherapy. *Journal of Consulting and Clinical Psychology, 62,* 522–534.
Shapiro, D. A., Rees, A., Barkham, M., Hardy, G. E., Reynolds, S., & Startup, M. (1995). Effects of treatment duration and severity of depression on the maintenance of gains following cognitive-behavioral and psychodynamic-interpersonal psychotherapy. *Journal of Consulting and Clinical Psychology, 63,* 378–387.
Sifneos, P. E. (1972). *Short-term dynamic psychotherapy and emotional crisis.* Cambridge, MA: Harvard University Press.
Silberschatz, G., Fretter, P., & Curtis, J. (1986). How do interpretations influence the process of psychotherapy? *Journal of Consulting and Clinical Psychology, 54,* 646–652.
Strupp, H. H., & Binder, J. L. (1984). *Psychotherapy in a new key.* New York: Basic Books.
Svartberg, M., & Stiles, T. C. (1991). Comparative effects of short-term psychodynamic psychotherapy: A meta-analysis. *Journal of Consulting and Clinical Psychology, 59,* 704–714.
Tishby, O., & Messer, S. (1995). The relationship between plan compatibility of therapist interventions and patient progress: A comparison of two plan formulations. *Psychotherapy Research, 5,* 76–88.
Weiss, J., Sampson, H., & the Mt. Zion Psychotherapy Research Group. (1986). *The Psychoanalytic Process.* New York: Guilford.
Wiborg, I. M., & Dahl, A. A. (1996). Does brief dynamic psychotherapy reduce the relapse rate of panic disorder? *Archives of General Psychiatry, 53,* 689–694.
Winston, A., Laikin, M., Pollack, J., Samstag, L. W., McCullough, L., & Muran, J. C. (1994). Short-term psychotherapy of personality disorders. *American Journal of Psychiatry, 151,* 190–194.

CHAPTER

6

Case Formulation: Determining the Focus in Brief Dynamic Psychotherapy

Tracy D. Eells
Kenneth G. Lombart
University of Louisville

Our goals in this chapter are to help the reader develop formulations of patients for brief psychodynamic psychotherapy and to do so in an efficient, effective manner that is supported by empirical research. For at least two reasons, psychotherapy case formulation is crucial in today's clinical environment. First, the increasing predominance of brief psychotherapy requires the clinician to formulate a focus and to treat quickly. This trend toward brevity requires the clinician to be active in therapy, to treat while formulating, and to select the most important and timely problems to work on. Second, today's nosology for classifying mental disorders is primarily descriptive in nature rather than explanatory, creating a gap between diagnosis and treatment that a formulation can fill.

Psychodynamic case formulation has been a focus of research in recent years. Several methods have been developed and assessed for reliability and validity. We describe five of these methods and summarize the research supporting them. Although these methods were originally developed for research purposes, the focus of our presentation is on applying them to routine clinical work. We show in step-by-step fashion how each method leads to a formulation. Later, we use one of these methods to formulate "June," then show how the other four methods might add information to the formulation or might reshape it. Before presenting the formulation methods, we define case formulation and discuss four goals when developing a case formulation. We review some practical aspects of case formulation, discuss narrative communication as a wellspring of information for formulation, and present a brief history of psychodynamic case formulation.

DEFINITION OF CASE FORMULATION

Case formulation is a core psychotherapy skill. It is the process by which the clinician posits hypotheses about the personal meanings, causes, precipitants, and maintaining influences of a person's psychological, interpersonal, and behavioral problems. As a hypothesis, the formulation is subject to revision as it is tested and as new information comes forth. Although all patients may not need to understand the causes of their problems to get better, we believe that changing the personal meanings associated with problems is critical to resolving many problems that lead people to seek therapy. The focus on precipitants and maintaining influences of problems is a present-oriented focus and is based on the assumption that an exploration of behavior patterns and their associated meanings and connections to symptom onset and perpetuation is crucial to resolving those problems.

A formulation helps organize information about a person. Patients often present with contradictions in their behaviors, emotions, and thought content. A patient may declare that she or he has given up on love, yet this stance of resignation may belie a wish for love, support, and attention. A formulation should contain structures that permit the therapist to contain the contradictions and to categorize important classes of information within a sufficiently encompassing view of the patient. When this is accomplished, the result is a structure facilitating the therapist's understanding of and empathy for the patient.

A formulation should provide a link to treatment by serving as a marker for change and as a predictor of change. A completed formulation may be viewed as an arrow drawn on a bow; it identifies goals, sets a trajectory, anticipates impediments toward goal achievement, and lists strategies and tactics toward those ends.

Although we typically think of constructing a formulation of a specific individual, one can also formulate situations and disorders. Process-experiential and behavioral therapists share an emphasis on formulating situations, although in different ways. Experiential therapists such as Greenberg (Goldman & Greenberg, 1997), deemphasize global formulations of individual patients, instead focusing on a "moment-by-moment process of identifying the current determinants underlying the client's painful or uncomfortable experience and/or the means by which that experience is being interrupted" (p. 406). Behavior therapists (e.g., Koerner & Linehan, 1997; Nezu, Nezu, Friedman, & Haynes, 1997) view the individual in an environmental context and examine how behavioral chains and contingencies of reinforcement produce and can correct problematic behaviors.

6. CASE FORMULATION

Although every psychopathology is unique, therapists may nevertheless be aided by considering prototypical formulations for specific diagnoses. These are theory and empirically based configurations that may apply to some but not all individuals with a particular disorder and may serve as only partial explanations. For example, one could formulate major depressive disorder as caused by anger turned inward, an inability to elicit positive reinforcement from others, or a core belief of oneself as unlovable and worthless and of the future as hopeless. As another example, several reports indicate that individuals with panic disorder tend to have suffered early relationship losses (Kendler, Neale, Kessler, Heath, & Eaves, 1992; Shear, Copper, Klerman, Busch, & Shapiro, 1993). These prototypical formulations would then be revised and tailored according to the life story of a particular individual in treatment. Although prototypical and situational approaches to formulation are important, our focus in this chapter is on formulating persons.

Case formulation involves aspects of both content and process. *Content* aspects refer to the explanation or hypothesis itself. The content may comprise several components that together paint a picture of the person. Although our focus is on content, the process aspects of formulation are also important because they help produce the information necessary to develop the content. *Process* refers to the clinician's activities aimed at eliciting the information required to develop the formulation content, that is, how the clinical interview is conducted.

Two general categories of information should be kept in mind during a formulation-eliciting interview. The first is *descriptive* information, which includes demographics; the presenting problem as depicted by the patient; coping steps taken by the patient; any history of previous mental health care; medical history; and developmental, social, educational, and work history. The second category is *personal-meaning* information, which refers to how the patient experienced and interprets the events described. If the patient's parents divorced when the patient was 6, it is important to learn the patient's view of how that event affected him or her. How has it affected the patient's thoughts, feelings, and behaviors in relationships? Both descriptive and personal-meaning information are important in a case formulation, but the latter is more crucial. In our experience, beginning therapists are often much better at eliciting descriptive information and struggle to elicit personal-meaning information. It is easier to elicit personal-meaning information when one pays close attention to the narratives the patient tells. What are the roles the patient casts the self and others into? What interpersonal transactions occur? Following the thread of the patient's emotional meaning rather than adhering to a preconceived structure for the interview can help elicit personal-meaning information. By asking about or reflecting on a patient's emotions, one is more likely to elicit the meaning of events described. Personal-meaning information can also be elicited by remaining aware of the categories of information needed for the formulation and basing questions accordingly. For example, several of the formulation methods seek wishes, fears, and transactional information. Therefore, if a patient describes how an important person in his or her life behaved, the therapist could ask how the patient responded to that behavior or to speculate on the motivations of the other person.

Four Goals of Formulation

Ideally, a clinician should aspire to four goals when developing a case formulation. First, the formulation should paint a distinct portrait of a unique individual; it should not describe a person in general. At the same time, it should remain consistent with current scientific knowledge about personality, psychopathology, development, and interpersonal relationships. Second, a formulation should be parsimonious and just comprehensive enough to serve its purpose in the therapy. The formulation should not contain excessive or extraneous information or be so complicated that it fails as a practical guide to treatment. Utility is a key objective. Third, a formulation should strike the right balance between observation and inference. Low-level inferences are usually best for effective therapy and are more reliable (Eells, 1997b). These inferences are tightly linked to readily observable behavior but go beyond those observations to a construction of their meaning and consequences. Inferences that go too deep may lack sufficient empirical foundation and may not be meaningful or helpful to patients. The fourth goal of an ideal formulation is objectivity. A formulation should be about the patient and not the therapist. Researchers have extensively documented many biases in clinical judgment that therapists are prone to committing (e.g., Garb, 1998; Turk & Salovey, 1988). Further, psychoanalysts have long cautioned about the risk of therapists imposing their own psychological needs, characteristics, or problems on patients rather than seeing those patients more objectively.

Some Practical Aspects of Formulation

A formulation should be written down, referred to during treatment, and revised when necessary; otherwise, the therapist is like a builder without the benefit of blueprints. A case formulation should also be systematically constructed early in therapy, typically after the first one or two sessions and certainly within the first five sessions. With practice, a formulation can be constructed within a matter of a few minutes using notes and memories from early sessions. Efficient and high-quality work is facilitated by having an a priori set of formulation categories or "bins" in mind that one "fills in" based on information provided by the patient and others. The formulation systems described later in this chapter provide examples. Research has shown that a formulation is more likely to be reliable and accurate when the therapist is guided by a structured and systematic formulation method (Eells, 1997a).

Some therapists avoid constructing formulations for fear that they may limit the therapist's openness to new experiences of the patient, may lead to a rigid view of the patient, or may place the therapist in an authoritarian role. On the contrary, a well-constructed and well-implemented formulation should facilitate openness to the patient and should help the therapist develop and communicate empathic understanding in the context of a collaborative, mutually respectful relationship. As an expert in interpersonal communication and psychological problem solving, the psychotherapist should avail him or herself of the tools of the trade to facilitate the work.

Therapists sometimes wonder whether and how a formulation should be shared with patients. In a sense, the entire therapy can be viewed as the construction, revision, and imparting of the formulation. Yet the question remains as to how explicitly the written formulation should be shared in a single session or intervention. Opinions are divided on this question. Some (e.g., Ryle & Bennett, 1997) recommend that the entire formulation be shared with the patient and serve as an explicit center point guiding the therapy. Others (e.g., Curtis & Silberschatz, 1997; Luborsky, 1997) believe that sharing the entire formulation in one intervention may be unwise because it could overwhelm a patient, be too much to assimilate at once, be used by the patient in nontherapeutic ways, or be less therapeutic than letting the patient arrive at the formulation on his or her own terms. Instead, these practitioners advise that the therapist select portions of the formulation to be offered in succinct interventions and timed to match the current topic under discussion and the emotional state of the patient. Whichever approach one chooses, the intervention should enhance the therapeutic alliance rather than detract from it. Further, one should not offer the entire formulation until one is reasonably confident of its accuracy.

Narrative Communication: The Wellspring for Case Formulation

Much has been written on the role of narrative in psychology as well as in psychotherapy more specifically (e.g., Bucci, 1995; Polkinghorne, 1988; Spence, 1982). This work ranges from viewing narrative as a root metaphor for science, as a scientific methodology, as a means of organizing information, and as a tool of communication and cultural transmission. We believe that narratives, which are the telling of stories, provide a goldmine of information useful to the therapist in case formulation. Although in this chapter we cannot do justice to the richness of the literature on narrative, we make three key points about the role that narratives play in case formulation.

First, psychotherapy is an attempt to alter the meaning system of suffering individuals, and some researchers have posited that meaning is organized in a narrative form (Bower & Morrow, 1990). Spence (1982) argued that the primary task of psychoanalysis is to repair damaged narratives through the relationship between patient and therapist. If meaning systems are organized in a narrative form, tapping into narratives is the most direct means of understanding the patient's meaning system, a task of both formulation and psychotherapy.

Second, the telling of narratives may be a particularly effective tool of change because narratives tend to bring affect and cognition together and are often interpersonally focused. By their nature, narratives are concretely rooted in space and time, are sequential and episodic, contain an inner logic, and may thus elicit deeper levels of experiencing than other forms of communication. Evidence suggests that this type of cognitive-emotional processing predicts success in therapy (Bucci, 1997).

Third, narrative communication appears particularly apt for eliciting personal-meaning information, as described previously. It is useful for eliciting important elements of formulation in the methods we describe later in this chapter. These elements include a person's wishes and fears, expectations of others' responses to their wishes and fears, how the patient internalizes interpersonal experience, self concepts, concepts of others, and what mechanisms the individual uses to cope or defend against potentially distressing meanings.

HISTORY OF CASE FORMULATION

The modern psychotherapy case formulation can be traced to the medical examination and case history, which are rooted in Hippocratic and Galenic medicine. Hippocratic physicians emphasized viewing the individual as a whole in arriving at a diagnosis and encouraged the patient's active involvement in his or her cure (Nuland, 1988). In contrast to their forebearers' beliefs in polytheism and mythological causes of disease, they based conclusions on observation, reason, and the belief that only natural forces are at play in disease. Hippocratic case reports provided many observable details about physical functioning then drew inferences from these observations before prescribing treatment. Galen's contributions to modern medicine were his emphasis on experimentation and focus on physical structure and function as the foundation of disease.

Consistent with the tradition of Hippocrates and Galen, psychotherapy case formulations depend on close observation as a basis for inference. In accord with the holistic ethos of Hippocrates, a formulation should consider the patient from multiple dimensions, including the biological, psychological, and social. Also consistent with the Hippocratic view, psychotherapists view active patient involvement in treatment as essential for success. Galenic influences are seen in inferences about psychological structure, including concepts such as the id, ego, and superego and more cognitive concepts such as self-representations, faulty reasoning processes, and maladaptive core beliefs about the self, others, and the world.

Within this historical context, the content of a case formulation is influenced by multiple factors. Chief among these is the therapist's worldview, that is, the basic axiomatic tenets that guide the therapist's assumptions about people, the world, and the future. The therapist's worldview in turn influences and is influenced by the therapist's opinions on the nature of psychopathology and his or her approach to psychotherapy and how it works. A further influence is recent case formulation research. It is to these influences that we now turn, with a focus on the influence of psychodynamic theory.

Psychodynamic Contributions to Case Formulation

One's approach to psychotherapy provides a framework for conceptualizing patients. Psychoanalysis has had a pervasive effect on views of personality and psychopathology, as well as on our understanding of the psychiatric interview. Before Freud, the psychiatric interview was viewed simply as an opportunity for the patient to report his or her symptoms. Now we recognize the interview as a vehicle through which the patient's problems express themselves; that is, interpersonal problems outside of therapy may be enacted within the therapy.

Much of the research on case formulations grew from difficulties that psychodynamic investigators identified in achieving consistency among formulations developed by different therapists. The key questions asked are the following: Can case formulations be constructed reliably and validly? To what extent do formulation-based interventions predict psychotherapy outcome and processes? What does the formulation add to outcome? Can a formulation be used to understand psychopathological states?

In 1966, Philip F. Seitz, a Chicago psychoanalyst, reported a 3-year effort to study the extent to which analysts agree in formulating the same clinical material (Seitz, 1966). Six analysts independently reviewed either detailed process notes or a set of dreams from a single case. Each analyst wrote an essay-style narrative addressing the precipitating situation, focal conflict, and defense mechanisms at play in the case. The group distributed the formulations, giving each member the opportunity to revise his work based on the formulation of others, then met weekly to review their findings. The results were largely disappointing in that consensus was reached on relatively few cases.

The primary contribution of Seitz (1966) work is that it alerted the community of psychotherapy researchers to the consensus problem. If psychotherapy research aspired to be a scientific enterprise, progress had to be made in the consistency with which clinicians describe a patient's problems and way of managing them. Another contribution of Seitz was his delineation of why the clinicians failed to agree. One key problem was that group members made inferences at overly deep levels that seemed to stray too far from the clinical material, for example, making references to "phallic-Oedipal rivalry" and "castration fears." Seitz also noted that the group relied too much on intuitive impressions and did not systematically and critically check their interpretations.

Seitz's (1966) paper achieved its stated goal and sparked research efforts to improve methods of case formulation. In the following decades at least 15 formal methods for constructing case formulations have been developed and empirically tested. Most of these methods share several characteristics: They focus on relationship interactions expressed in psychotherapy sessions, they identify core relationship conflicts based on the frequency with which patterns are conveyed in therapy, they rely on clinical judgment rather than rating scales, they include provisions for testing the reliability and validity of the method, they emphasize relatively low-level inferences, they break the formulation task into components, and they reveal a trend toward psychotherapy integration. The following section describes the central psychodynamic methods.

STRUCTURED CASE FORMULATION METHODS: THEORY AND RESEARCH

In this section we describe several of the structured case formulation methods frequently used in dynamic psychotherapy. The methods we describe are the Core Conflictual Relationship Theme (CCRT; Luborsky & Crits-Christoph, 1998), Configurational Analysis (CA; Horowitz, 1997), the Plan Formulation Method (PFM; Curtis & Silberschatz, 1997), Cyclical Maladaptive Patterns (CMP; Schact, Binder, & Strupp, 1984; Levenson & Strupp, 1997), and the Idiographic Conflict Formulation Method (ICF; Perry, 1997). We start the description of each method with basic underlying assumptions including dynamic explanation(s) used. This is followed by a summary of the elements, steps involved in the method, and concludes with a brief summary of the available research.

Core Conflictual Relationship Theme (CCRT)

The first of the structured formulation methods, the CCRT, was introduced by Lester Luborsky in 1977 (Luborsky, 1977). The CCRT is based on Freud's (1958a, 1958b) concept of transference, which states that innate characteristics and early interpersonal experiences predispose a person to initiate and conduct close relationships in particular ways and in repeated fashion later in life. The goal of the CCRT is to reliably and accurately identify a patient's central relationship pattern. The CCRT focuses on narratives a patient tells in therapy, identifying three key components within those narratives: an individual's wishes, expected responses of others, and responses of the self. The CCRT is applicable in everyday clinical use as well as in research. In day-to-day clinical use, therapists may note the relationship components as they arise in therapy and then infer a CCRT later. In the research context, trained judges first extract relationship episodes from therapy transcripts; a second set of judges then identifies each of the three key relationship components. The CCRT is operationally defined as the most frequently observed wish, response of other, and response of self, regardless of whether these components occur sequentially in the separate narratives. Based on a mixed group of patients in multiple studies (Chance, Bakeman, Kaslow, Farber, & Burge-Callaway, 2000; Luborsky & Crits-Christoph, 1998; Okey, McWhirter, & Delaney, 2000), the most frequent CCRT is a wish to be close and accepting; a response from others of rejection and opposition; and a response of the self marked by disappointment, depression, and anger. Luborsky (1997) does not recommend that therapists offer patients the entire CCRT in a single intervention but rather select portions that are most likely to be accepted by patients in the current context of the therapy. He also recommends that therapists link the CCRT to symptoms, focus primarily on wishes and responses from others because these are the most reliably identified components, and focus on negative components of the CCRT but in a manner that enhances the therapeutic alliance.

The CCRT is the most frequently researched of the structured case formulation methods. Crits-Christoph, Luborsky, et al. (1988) and Luborsky, Barber, and Diguer (1992) found adequate to good reliability in identifying the three components. Weighted kappas were .61 and .60 for wish of self, .68 and .70 for response of other, and .61 and .71 for response of self. Other CCRT-related research findings are that approximately four narratives are typically told in a therapy session (Luborsky et al., 1992); interventions based on a patient's CCRT predict psychotherapy outcome (Crits-Christoph, Cooper, & Luborsky, 1988); gaining mastery of the CCRT is associated with successful outcome in therapy (Grenyer & Luborsky, 1996); CCRTs derived from dreams are similar to those derived from waking life (Popp et al., 1996); narratives told outside of a session are similar to those told in sessions (Barber, Luborsky, Crits-Christoph, & Diguer, 1995); greater consistency of relationship patterns as measured by the CCRT is associated with greater psychopathology (Cierpka et al., 1998); and symptom onset seems closely related to central interpersonal conflicts of patients as measured by the CCRT (Luborsky, 1996).

Configurational Analysis (CA)

CA, developed by Mardi J. Horowitz (Horowitz, 1997), is similar to the CCRT in its focus on identifying a central relationship pattern but adds important elements. These elements include inferences about a patient's states of mind, the assumption of multiple rather than single relationship patterns, and defensive control processes. States of mind are recurrent and distinct complexes of affect, cognition, experience, and behavioral propensities. They can be described using simple adjectives such as "depressed and helpless" or "angry and bitter"; in motivational terms (a wished-for or feared state); or according to the degree of affect modulation, or control, characterizing the state. According to Horowitz, states of mind are organized by mental representations, or schemas, about interpersonal relationships and concepts about the self and others. These representations can be depicted in wish–fear–compromise configurations, which Horowitz (Horowitz & Eells, 1977) called role relationship model configurations (RRMC). These describe desired, dreaded, adaptive compromise and maladaptive compromise relationship patterns. We describe RRMCs further in our case formulation of June.

CA also includes a system for formulating an individual's defensive control processes. These are habitual ways an individual controls ideas and affect to maintain a well-modulated state of mind. For example, a patient might control a core belief of himself or herself as cold and unfeeling by any combination of the following processes: becoming somnolent or distracted, accusing others of being cold, being overly and inauthentically nice to others, or avoiding the topic of emotional closeness. A complete list of defensive control processes may be found in Horowitz (1997).

The formulation steps in CA move from description to increasing degrees of inference. They are describe clinically relevant phenomena; identify the patient's repertoire of states of mind; identify self, other, and relationship schemas; and identify defensive control processes. Finally, the therapist plans goals and interventions specific to each category.

Research on CA has shown a similar level of reliability to that shown by the CCRT, although the studies and the number of participants per study are fewer (Eells et al., 1995; Horowitz & Eells, 1993). Convergent validity for CA as well as for CCRT is suggested by the high level similarity between formulations independently constructed with each system (Horowitz, Luborsky, & Popp, 1991). Horowitz and colleagues (Horowitz, Ewert, & Milbrath,

1995; Horowitz, Milbrath, Ewert, Sonneborn, & Stinson, 1994) have also provided evidence that states of mind can be reliably coded using psychotherapy transcripts and a standardized list of states. In a series of quantitative single-case studies of individuals responding to psychosocial trauma, Horowitz and colleagues (Horowitz et al., 1995) found evidence of recurring emotional states, showed that shifts from well-modulated to less well-modulated states of mind are related to whether or not a patient is discussing a conflict-laden topic (Horowitz et al., 1994), and showed that increased signs of defensive control processes occur when conflictual or unresolved themes are being discussed in therapy (Horowitz et al., 1993). A series of single-case studies has also shown convergences between formulations that are clinically derived and independently derived formulations based on ratings of self and significant others provided by patients (Eells, 1995; Eells, Fridhandler, & Horowitz, 1995).

Plan Formulation Method (PFM)

PFM, developed by John Curtis and George Silberschatz (Curtis, Silberschatz, Sampson, & Weiss, 1994), follows earlier formulation work by Joseph Caston (1977, 1986) and is based on Joseph Weiss' (1993) control mastery theory of psychotherapy. Control mastery theory assumes that psychopathology results from pathogenic beliefs stemming from traumatic events that are usually experienced in childhood. Weiss believed that patients develop an unconscious plan to disconfirm these beliefs. The plan may involve testing the therapist through behavioral or verbal challenges or expressions of anger. The therapist must understand the purpose of these events to best help the patient.

The goal of PFM is to identify, categorize, and test the key elements of control mastery theory. Five elements comprise a plan formulation: the patient's goals for therapy, the obstructions (pathogenic beliefs) that may interfere with achieving the goals, the traumas that produced the pathogenic beliefs, insights necessary to help the patient achieve the goals, and tests the therapist might expect from the patient as the patient attempts to disconfirm a set of pathogenic beliefs. For regular clinical use, these components can be inferred from the early sessions of psychotherapy. For research purposes, coders follow a five-step process. First, three or four judges who are versed in control mastery theory review transcripts from early psychotherapy hours and create a list of real and plausible alternative items for each formulation component. Second, a master list of goals, obstructions, traumas, insights, and tests is compiled and randomly ordered within each component. Third, the judges review the master list and rank order each item according to its relevance to the patient. Fourth, mean ratings are obtained and rank ordered; those items ranking below the median are discarded. Fifth, the group meets and consensually finalizes the most relevant items for each formulation category. The final formulation contains a description of the patient and his or her current life circumstance followed by the patient's presenting symptoms and problems. Then the goals, obstructions, tests, insights, and traumas are listed.

The reliability of the PFM is excellent (Curtis et al., 1994), although adherence among the clinical judges to an explicit theory of psychotherapy appears essential. One interesting study (Messer, Tishby, & Spillman, 1992) showed that two independent research teams, one working from the control master perspective and the other working from an object relationship standpoint, independently developed highly reliable plan formulations, but the two formulations correlated poorly with each other. Several studies have been published showing that the degree of a therapist's adherence to the plan formulation predicts patient progress and outcome in psychotherapy (Silberschatz & Curtis, 1993; Silberschatz, Curtis, & Nathans, 1989; Silberschatz, Fretter, & Curtis, 1986). Patients appear to deepen their level of emotional experiencing subsequent to plan-compatible interventions as compared to plan-incompatible interventions. One study (Silberschatz et al., 1989) showed that achieving goals and insights, as listed in the formulation, correlates with standard psychotherapy outcome measures.

Cyclical Maladaptive Patterns (CMP)

CMP (Levenson & Strupp, 1997; Schacht, Binder, & Strupp, 1984) was developed for time-limited dynamic psychotherapy (Strupp & Binder, 1984). The CMP provides a structure for understanding a patient's circular interpersonal behavior patterns that may be inflexible and lead to self-defeating, negative self-appraisals, and dissatisfaction in relationships. The method also addresses goals for therapy and how to stay focused on them.

There are six basic elements to the CMP: acts of the self, expectations of others' reactions, acts of others toward the self, acts of the self toward the self, the therapist's reaction to the patient, and new experiences and new understandings to aim for in therapy. *Acts of the self* are the thoughts, feelings, behaviors, motivations, and perceptions the individual has about relating interpersonally. *Expectations of others' reactions* are how the person expects others to react to him or her interpersonally. *Acts of others* toward the self are the individual's perception of how people actually relate to him or her. *Acts of the self toward the self* are the individual's attitudes and behaviors toward himself or herself. The *therapist's reaction to the patient* is considered important because it likely mirrors what others feel when relating to the patient. This element is based on the TLDP tenet that the therapist will inevitably be drawn into the patient's dysfunctional patterns and that the therapist can be more helpful when the reenactment is anticipated and prepared for. *New experiences and understandings* are different and more effective ways of relating and the emotional appreciation for that different behavior. This element also refers to identifying and appreciating one's maladaptive interpersonal behavior patterns.

Constructing a CMP-based case formulation involves nine steps (Levenson & Strupp, 1997). First, the therapist lets the patient tell his or her own story without attempting to structure it while remaining attuned to how the story is told and to the patient's interpersonal style. Second, one explores symptoms and problems and the interpersonal context in which they arise and are maintained. Third, the therapist probes for information necessary to sort interpersonal information into the categories described previously. Fourth, the therapist searches for common themes in the patient's relationships across people, time, and situations. Fifth, the therapist looks at how he or she is pulled into reenactments of the patient's interpersonal behavior patterns. Sixth, the patient is helped to examine his or her reactions to the relationship that is forming with the therapist. Seventh, from the historical information and the therapist's experience in the room with the person, a short narrative is developed using the first five elements. Next, based on that narrative, the therapist describes the new experience and new understanding goals that will help the person relate more adaptively to others. Finally, the additional information one learns from the individual and from experiences with him or her should be used to revise and refine the CMP throughout therapy.

Although TLDP has been extensively investigated (Strupp, 1993), the CMP method of case formulation has not yet been assessed rigorously for its reliability or validity. However, one study (Johnson, Popp, Schacht, Mellon, & Strupp, 1989) compared a CMP and a CCRT formulation based on the same patient and found considerable similarity. A more recent preliminary analysis (Hartmann & Levenson, 1995) of patients with personality disorder undergoing TLDP in a Veterans Administration setting found better outcomes were achieved when therapy stayed focused on topics relevant to the patients' CMPs. The same study found that independent clinicians could agree on patients' interpersonal problems after reading CMPs prepared by the treating clinicians after one or two sessions, suggesting that the CMP conveys meaningful information.

Idiographic Conflict Formulation (ICF)

Christopher Perry's (1994, 1997) ICF focuses on motivational conflict and how the individual responds to this conflict. An explicit assumption of the method is that behavior is motivated. According to Perry (1997), motives have both psychological and biological bases, may operate unconsciously or consciously, and can be described most simply as wishes and fears. Unlike the CCRT, CA, and CMP, the ICF does not explicitly incorporate a focus on object relations; instead, views about self and other are captured through the concept of wishes and fears. Many of these are about other people and involve the attainment and maintenance of self-esteem. The ICF does not explicitly lay out goals; instead, goals are implied in a person's wishes and fears.

The ICF is embedded in a developmental framework. In ICF, motives are organized according to the eight stages of Erik Erikson's (1963) theory of psychosocial development. When a person experiences positive developmental experiences, motives may adapt or mature.

The chief purpose of the ICF formulation is to "help the clinicians discern the conflicting motives that underlie complaints and symptoms" (Perry, 1997, p. 140). The purpose of ICF-based therapy, in turn, is to help the patient "improve handling of the motives, which requires using more adaptive defense mechanisms" (Perry, 1997, p. 140). In therapy, the clinician can track the individual's adaptation to motives and the developmental maturation of motives as indications of therapeutic progress.

Three components lie at the core of the ICF: wishes, fears, and resultants. Perry (1997) is careful to define dynamic wishes and fears. According to Perry (1997), a wish or fear is dynamic when it plays a causal role in a variety of overtly different behaviors, fantasies, and experiences. For example, a wish for self-esteem may affect a person in multiple spheres, whereas a wish for a particular job may not and thus would not be considered a dynamic wish. Similarly, a fear of intimacy may affect a person in multiple ways, whereas a fear of heights may not.

Procedurally, after conducting up to three psychotherapy assessment interviews and determining a descriptive diagnosis, the therapist infers between two and four centrally important wishes that appear to broadly influence the individual. Perry (1997) prepared a standardized list of these wishes as well as corresponding fears, each categorized according to Erikson's (1963) psychosocial stages of development. For example, wishes based on trust versus mistrust include wishes to survive, to be protected from harm, to be near a significant other, and to be comforted and soothed. Wishes categorized within the Eriksonian identity versus identity confusion stage include wishes for attention from the opposite sex, for a mentor or role model, and for belonging in a social group. For each wish, the therapist should list three to five observations that support its inclusion in the formulation.

A similar process is followed to identify a set of central fears. These represent negative beliefs, expectations, or experiences the individual wants to avoid. The therapist lists the fears that operate in opposition to the person's wishes or to each other; the number of fears need not equal the number of wishes. As in wishes, the therapist lists the observations that support inclusion of each fear.

The next step in ICF is to list the resultants of conflicts among wishes and fears, which Perry (1997) categories as either symptoms and symptomatic behaviors or as avoidant outcomes. Resultants describe how the individual has adapted to conflicts that are either frequent, salient, or appear unresolvable. For example, a depressed mood (symptom), a pattern of frequent arguments (symptomatic behavior) or interpersonal withdrawal (avoidant outcome), may result from a conflict between a wish to communicate needs and a fear of being dependent on others. Symptoms are subjective experiences of distress and may include mood states, recurrent negative experiences, pathological beliefs, negative schemas, and overreactions to events. Symptomatic behaviors may include drug abuse, self-mutilation, arguing, stealing, difficulty maintaining employment, and trouble in intimate relationships. Avoidant outcomes are the characteristic ways the person avoids or mitigates experiencing conflicts, including any character pathology, defense mechanisms, characteristic handling of affect, and limitations in intimacy or achievement the individual uses to deflect awareness of conflicts. As with wishes and fears, the therapist generates a list of resultants then shows which conflict each resultant is related to.

Two additional steps are involved in an ICF formulation. One is identifying the individual's vulnerability to specific stressors, listing those that often trigger the individual's conflicts. At the end of treatment the individual should be able to face these stressors without experiencing negative resultants. The final step is to list the person's best available level of adaptation to conflict. This list serves as a benchmark of the individual's potential healthy functioning.

Research on the ICF has shown adequate reliability for wishes (median weighted kappa = .64) and fair reliability for fears (median weighted kappa = .46; Perry, 1994). Concurrent validity for wishes in ICF was shown by their significant similarity to other formulation methods, including CCRT and plan diagnosis (a precursor to the PFM; Luborsky, Popp, & Barber, 1994; Perry, Luborsky, Silberschatz, & Popp, 1989). Perry (1997) also examined the heuristic value of the Eriksonian (1963) developmental hierarchy. In a sample of patients with personality disorders, many diagnosed with borderline personality disorder, he found that about half of the total wishes and fears were categorized in Erikson's lowest developmental stages (trust versus mistrust and autonomy versus shame and doubt). He also found that the borderline patients scored lower than patients with other personality disorders.

CONFIGURATIONAL ANALYSIS OF JUNE

In this section, we present a case formulation of June using CA. We chose CA because we are most familiar with it and because it is comprehensive, incorporating elements of other methods. After presenting our CA formulation of June, we briefly discuss how the formulation might be changed if she were viewed from the perspective of the other methods. Readers may also compare our formulation with that derived from the standpoint of cognitive analytic therapy, which guided the actual treatment of June.

Step 1: Describe Clinically Relevant Phenomena

We developed a list of the problems discussed by June and her therapist in their third therapy session. Most prominent is her tendency to blank out feelings and numb herself to keep from becoming overwhelmed. Other problems are not feeling "normal," low self-concept, jealousy, resentment, and suicidal ideation. Her low self-concept is supported, among other statements, by her assertions that she does not "matter ninety percent of the time," as well as by her negative body image. Her jealousy and resentment is related to wishing her relationship with her mother was more like that enjoyed by her sister. Her abuse is directed both inwardly (e.g., exercising poor diabetes management) and toward others (e.g., her outbursts of anger).

Step 2: Identify Repertoire of States of Mind

Using CA, we identified four key states of mind, which we organized in a wish-fear-compromise configuration, as shown in Fig. 6.1. June made only a few references to her wishes. Based on what she did say, we first inferred that she "wishes for affection and love." If accurate, this wish should arise later in the therapy. It may be that June does not think she deserves to have wishes or have love and affection. It could also be that her blanked out state is so prominent that it blocks conscious access to more desired states. Second, we inferred a feared state in which she is "jealous, angry, and resentful." June described jealousy of her sister's relationship with her mother and resentment of her sister's expectations for family childcare. Third, a more adaptive state we infer is that of "passively withdrawn and in control," which provides her with a sense of greater self-control and security. The fourth state, which we label "blanked out and numb," is the state that appears to have precipitated the current treatment. She described herself as blanking out feelings and feeling numb to keep from being overwhelmed by emotion.

Step 3: Identify Self, Other, and Relationship Schemas

Figure 6.1 shows the RRMC we developed for June. We infer that she wishes to see herself as strong and normal and experience mutual affection and support with a loved one. However, when she shows affection she feels exploited instead of supported and becomes angry. We infer that she at-

6. CASE FORMULATION

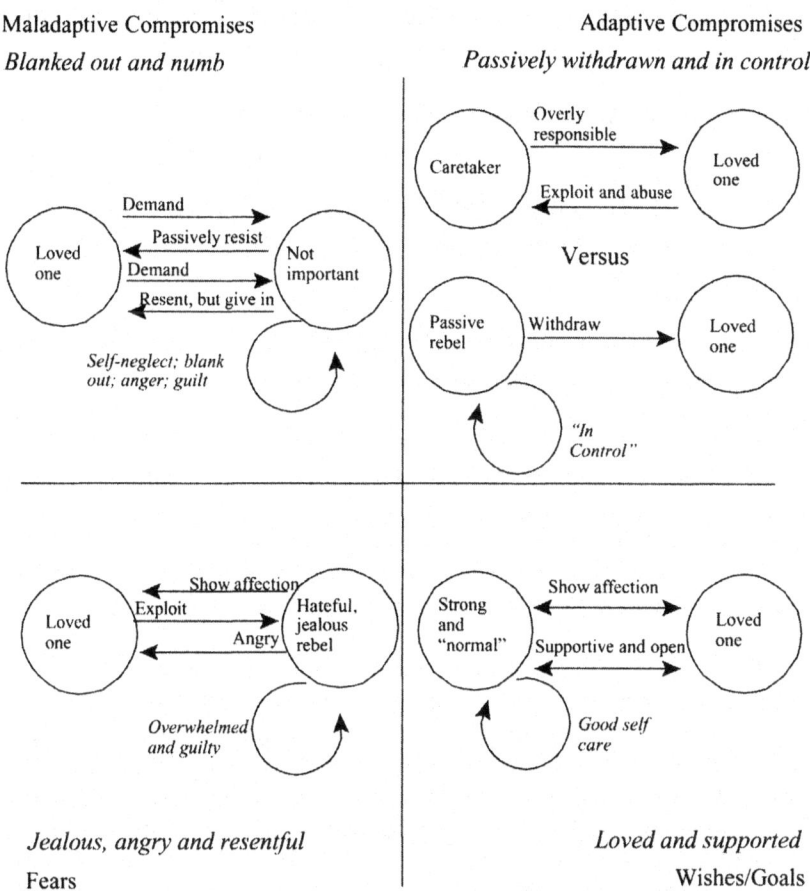

FIG. 6.1. Role relationship models configuration of June.

tempts to resolve this wish-fear dilemma either by assuming a stance of excessive responsibility as a caretaker for others or by withdrawing from them as a passive rebel and maintaining a sense of self-control. Her withdrawal and overresponsibility do not, however, meet her need for affection. She then tries to passively resist demands but eventually gives in. This leads to resentment and guilt, which she blanks out, and to self-neglect.

Identify Defensive Control Processes

June's major defensive process is blanking out her emotions to keep from being overwhelmed. She uses self-numbing to keep from feeling hurt. She also turns anger inward and deals with disappointment passive aggressively. In addition, she may somaticize and identify with her father's passive resistance, lack of perseverance, and abusive temper.

Step 5: Application to Treatment

With the CA case formulation as a focus for therapy, CA-styled interventions would focus on and flow from each of the previous formulation steps. The reader may wish to compare these with the interventions made by the cognitive analytic therapist.

Clinically Relevant Phenomena. In therapy, we would work collaboratively with June to establish a short list of goals for brief therapy. Working from the problem list, one goal would be to eliminate her episodes of blanking out. We would frame blanking out as an attempt to solve a problem, specifically that of her wanting the love and affection of her family, not receiving it, and responding with anger that leads to guilt. We might frame blanking out as her attempt to give herself a time out or vacation from family conflicts, and suggest she seek other, more satisfying ways of vacationing. We would also work on learning more appropriate and effective ways of expressing anger.

A second goal would be to help her take appropriate responsibility for herself and others, rather than being overresponsible. We would gently challenge June to explore how her sense of overresponsibility may reflect a response to the dilemma of wanting affection yet not receiving it and feeling anger and resentment toward her loved ones. We would ask what she imagines would happen if she were less responsible for others, anticipating that she might feel that doing so would harm or destroy a loved one. In particular, being less responsible toward her father might lead to a fear that father could not defend himself against her mother's attacks. Noting that she identifies with her father, we might wonder whether being less responsible toward her father might make her more open to her mother's attacks.

A third goal would be to increase appropriate self-care, certainly with regard to improved management of diabetes but also to grooming. Our hypothesis is that her self-neglect is displaced anger toward loved ones who do not provide her with affection and love.

States of Mind. We would want June to recognize that she enters different states of mind at different times, and we would help her label the most predominant states. We would prefer that she provide her own labels rather than use ours. Because she appears least in touch with desired states, we would hope to identify these better and help her acknowledge them. We might ask whether she feels deserving of love and affection and if not, why not. We would work on enhancing her compassion for herself and encour-

6. CASE FORMULATION 137

aging her to have the courage to wish for good things for herself. In other words, instilling hope that she might gain love and affection, although not necessarily from her family, would be a focus.

Self, Other, and Relationship Schemas. The RRMC summarizes inferences about self, other, and relationship schemas, and serves as the heart of the formulation in CA. We would use the RRMC to help June recognize her interpersonal wishes and fears and how they relate to her symptoms and maladaptive interpersonal behavior patterns. In particular, we would use the RRMC to help her recognize her need for affection and see the role that her anger plays in preventing her from meeting her needs for affection. As more information emerges about her relationship with her parents we might want to help June recognize that she may never gain the love and affection that she wishes from her parents, help her grieve this loss, and begin to work toward finding a relationship where she can gain love and affection. We could also use the RRMC to help June work toward the goal of feeling strong, competent, and normal, as well as to take only appropriate responsibility.

Control Processes. Our chief goal regarding June's control processes would be to address the blanking out, presenting it not only as a maladaptive attempt to solve a problem but also as an impediment to achieving what she wants in life.

JUNE FROM THE PERSPECTIVE OF THE OTHER METHODS

In this section, we discuss what might be added to our formulation of June if we took the perspective of the other methods discussed.

CCRT

The CCRT is contained within CA in the form of role relationship models. If we were to condense the RRMC to one central maladaptive pattern and to use Luborsky's standard categories (Version 3; Barber, Crits-Christoph, & Luborsky, 1998), it would be that June's primary wish of self is to be loved and understood; the response of others is rejecting and opposing; and the response of self is to be disappointed and depressed, although rejecting and opposing also appears to be a response of June's. If using the "tailor-made" approach, we would change only the response of self category, adding three other responses: behaving overresponsibly toward others to avoid guilt, resentfully giving in to the demands of others, and withdrawing to feel in control.

PFM

From the PFM perspective, we would identify June's primary goal for therapy as that of achieving independence from her parents. Pathogenic beliefs may include the following: "My independence will harm my father and possibly destroy him because he is so vulnerable and fragile"; or "If I am healthy and strong, I will lose what little love my parents have for me"; or "I need to be sick and weak in order to hang on to what little love my parents have for me." The transcript of Session 3 does not go into June's developmental history; therefore, we are not able to identify any traumas that may have led to the development of her pathogenic beliefs. We recognize, however, that the source of those beliefs may not be a single traumatic event but could be the accumulated consequence of many disappointments. She alludes to her family as unaffectionate. As a child and adolescent she may have repeatedly sought affection from her parents and been repeatedly disappointed. Insights needed to achieve the stated goal could be that abandoning her excessive responsibility for others and taking better care of herself need not harm her parents or her relationship with them. A test we might expect in treatment is for June to turn passive into active by neglecting the therapist (e.g., being late for treatment or not coming for her appointments). To pass the test, the therapist would need to respond by not becoming angry. Alternatively, a test may be to assert her independence in therapy (e.g., by disagreeing with the therapist or by skipping a session) and seeing whether the therapist appears wounded.

CMP

Like the CCRT, the CMP has much in common with CA. We believe that the RRMC captures the elements of the CMP except for the therapist's reaction to the patient and the goals of new experience and new understanding. Of course, we can only speculate about how the therapist might react to June. Nevertheless, we might expect the therapist to experience frustration at June's blanking out, passivity, continued poor self-care, and dependence; in addition, the therapist may experience an impulse to criticize or to make demands on June or to save June. We identify the following with regard to new knowledge and experiences we would hope for June: to understand how her symptoms are responses to frustrated wishes for love, to experience a stronger need for love and affection, and to experience herself as someone who matters.

ICF

The wishes and fears stated earlier would also be captured by the ICF. What the ICF can uniquely offer is information about the specific stressors that may activate June's conflicts and her best available level of adaptation to conflict. Although June's specific stressors are not readily available to us, we speculate that they involve interpersonal conflict and specifically situations that call for adaptive self-assertion and those involving intimacy. It is also not clear what her best available level of adaptation to conflict is. We speculate that her level of adaptation to conflict in her family changed from blanking out to more adaptive withdrawal. In addition, her account of freely exchanging ideas with an assertive friend suggests that her best level of adaptation could be remaining engaged in stressful interpersonal exchanges and holding her own in them.

CONCLUSIONS AND A RESEARCH PROPOSAL

As we have noted, case formulation is a core psychotherapy skill. Numerous structured formulation methods have been developed in recent years, some of which have shown acceptable levels of reliability and validity. It is important to note, however, that these studies are based on mean ratings of multiple judges. Therefore, a formulation developed by an individual therapist should be viewed as tentative until sufficient data is gathered to support it. The individual practitioner who does not have the benefit of a group to aid in formulation still can benefit from these case formulation methods. Using structured and systematic methods that include a fixed set of components should raise reliability above what it would be otherwise. Using these methods also helps organize clinical information and increases the comprehensiveness and clarity of the formulation. In addition, a focus on low-level inferences should increase reliability and serve to keep interventions focused more closely on what the patient says in therapy. Finally, some argue that it may not be necessary to have an accurate and comprehensive formulation initially. Instead it may be more important to have an explicit working hypothesis that can be tested with the patient then altered and improved as therapy proceeds.

More research is needed on case formulation. First, it has not been shown unequivocally that working from a formulation leads to better outcomes than working without a formulation. Second, reliability and validity might be improved if formulation methods can be developed in an inventory format. Third, more studies are needed showing the effects in therapy of adherence to a formulation as compared to diverging from a formulation.

As an exercise, we encourage the reader to refer to the case description of June and the formulation consistent with cognitive analytic therapy. Note the similarities and differences between the cognitive analytic therapy formulation and each of the structured case formulation methods presented in this chapter. Compare and contrast the types of information each of the case formulation methods yields from the narratives patients tell in therapy. Generate a list of questions you might ask to elicit information necessary to develop each type of case formulation. We also encourage the reader to note the distinction between descriptive and personal-meaning information presented in this chapter. Make a list of each type of information provided by June in the session transcripts and develop a formulation integrating these two forms of information.

REFERENCES

Barber, J. P., Crits-Christoph, P., & Luborsky, L. (1998). A guide to CCRT standard categories and their classification. In L. Luborsky & P. Crits-Christoph (Eds.), *Understanding transference: A guide to the CCRT–The Core Conflictual Relationship Theme method in research and practice* (rev. ed.). Washington, DC: APA Books.

Barber, J. P., Luborsky, L., Crits-Christoph, P., & Diguer, L. (1995). A comparison of core conflictual relationship themes before psychotherapy and during early sessions. *Journal of Consulting and Clinical Psychology, 63,* 145–148.

Bower, G. H., & Morrow, D. G. (1990, January). Mental models in narrative comprehension. *Science, 247,* 44–48.

Bucci, W. (1995). The power of the narrative: A multiple code account. In J. W. Pennebaker (Ed.), *Emotion, disclosure and health* (pp. 71–92). Washington, DC: American Psychological Association.

Bucci, W. (1997). Empirical studies of "good" and troubled hours: A multiple code interpretation. *Journal of the American Psychoanalytic Association, 45,* 1–34.

Caston, J. (1977). Manual on how to diagnose the plan. In J. Weiss, H. Sampson, J. Caston, & G. Silberschatz (Eds.), *Research on the psychoanalytic process: I. A comparison of two theories about analytic neutrality* (Bulletin No. 3, pp. 15–21). San Francisco: The Psychotherapy Research Group, Department of Psychiatry, Mount Zion Hospital and Medical Center.

Caston, J. (1986). The reliability of the diagnosis of the patient's unconscious plan. In J. Weiss, H. Sampson, & the Mount Zion Psychotherapy Research Group (Eds.), *The psychoanalytic process: Theory, clinical observations, and empirical research* (pp. 241–255). New York: Guilford.

Chance, S. E., Bakeman, R., Kaslow, N. J., Farber, E., & Burge-Callaway, K. (2000). Core conflictual relationship themes in patients diagnosed with borderline personality disorder who attempted, or who did not attempt, suicide. *Psychotherapy Research, 10,* 337–355.

Cierpka, M., Strack, M., Benninghoven, D., Staats, H., Dahlbender, R., Pokomy, D., Frevert, G., Blaser, G., Kachele, H., Geyer, M., Korner, A., & Albani, C. (1998). Stereotypical relationship patterns and psychopathology. *Psychotherapy and Psychosomatics, 67,* 241–248.

Crits-Christoph, P., Cooper, A., & Luborsky, L. (1988). The accuracy of therapists' interpretations and the outcome of dynamic psychotherapy. *Journal of Consulting and Clinical Psychology, 56,* 490–495.

Crits-Christoph, P., Luborsky, L., Dahl, L., Popp, C., Mellon, J., & Mark, D. (1988). Clinicians can agree in assessing relationship patterns in psychotherapy: The Core Conflictual Relationship Theme Method. *Archives of General Psychiatry, 45,* 1001–1004.

Curtis, J. T., & Silberschatz, G. (1997). Plan formulation method. In T. D. Eells (Ed.), *Handbook of psychotherapy case formulation.* New York: Guilford Press.

Curtis, J. T., Silberschatz, G., Sampson, H., & Weiss, J. (1994). The plan formulation method. *Psychotherapy Research, 46*, 197–207.

Eells, T. D. (1995). Role reversal: A convergence of clinical and quantitative evidence. *Psychotherapy Research, 5*, 297–312.

Eells, T. D. (Ed.). (1997a). *Handbook of psychotherapy case formulation*. New York: Guilford.

Eells, T. D. (1997b). Psychotherapy case formulation: History and current status. In T. D. Eells (Ed.), *Handbook of psychotherapy case formulation*. New York: Guilford.

Eells, T. D., Fridhandler, B., & Horowitz, M. J. (1995). Self schemas and spousal bereavement: Comparing quantitative and clinical evidence. *Psychotherapy, 32*, 270–282.

Eells, T. D., Horowitz, M. J., Singer, J. L., Salovey, P., Daigle, D., & Turvey, C. (1995). The role-relationship models method: A comparison of independently derived case formulations. *Psychotherapy Research, 5*, 154–168.

Erikson, E. H. (1963). *Childhood and society* (2nd ed.). New York: Norton.

Freud, S. (1958a). The dynamics of the transference. In J. Strachey (Ed.), *The standard edition of the complete psychological works of Sigmund Freud* (Vol. 12, pp. 99–108). London: Hogarth Press. (Original work published 1912)

Freud, S. (1958b). Recommendations to physicians practising psycho-analysis. In J. Strachey (Ed.), *The standard edition of the complete psychological works of Sigmund Freud* (Vol. 12, pp. 111–120). London: Hogarth Press. (Original work published 1912)

Garb, H. N. (1998). *Studying the clinician: Judgment research and psychological assessment*. Washington, DC: American Psychological Association.

Goldman, R., & Greenberg, L. S. (1997). *Case formulation in process-experiential therapy*. New York: Guilford.

Grenyer, B. F. S., & Luborsky, L. (1996). Dynamic change in psychotherapy: Mastery of interpersonal conflict. *Journal of Consulting and Clinical Psychology, 64*, 411–416.

Hartmann, K., & Levenson, L. (1995, June). *Case formulation in time-limited dynamic psychotherapy: Reliability and validity issues*. Paper presented at the Society for Psychotherapy Research, Vancouver, British Columbia, Canada.

Horowitz, M. (1997). *Formulation as a basis for planning psychotherapy treatment*. Washington DC: American Psychiatric Press.

Horowitz, M. J., & Eells, T. D. (1993). Role-relationship model configurations: A method for psychotherapy case formulation. *Psychotherapy Research, 3*, 57–68.

Horowitz, M. J., & Eells, T. D. (1997). Configurational analysis: States of mind, person schemas, and the control of ideas and affect. In T. D. Eells (Ed.), *Handbook of psychotherapy case formulation* (pp. 166–191). New York: Guilford.

Horowitz, M. J., Ewert, M., & Milbrath, C. (1995). States of emotional control during psychotherapy. *The Journal of Psychotherapy Practice and Research, 5*, 20–25.

Horowitz, M. J., Luborsky, L., & Popp, C. (1991). A comparison of the Role-Relationship Models Configuration and the Core Conflictual Relationship Theme. In M. J. Horowitz (Ed.), *Person schemas and maladaptive interpersonal patterns* (pp. 213–220). Chicago: University of Chicago Press.

Horowitz, M. J., Milbrath, C., Ewert, M., Sonneborn, D., & Stinson, C. H. (1994). Cyclical patterns of states of mind in psychotherapy. *American Journal of Psychiatry, 151*, 1767–1770.

Horowitz, M. J., Stinson, C., Curtis, D., Ewert, M., Redington, D., Singer, J., Bucci, W., Mergenthaler, E., Milbrath, C., & Hartley, D. (1993). Topics and signs: Defensive control of emotional expression.

Johnson, M. E., Popp, C., Schacht, T. E., Mellon, J., & Strupp, H. H. (1989, August). Converging evidence for identification of recurrent relationship themes: Comparison of two methods. *Psychiatry, 52*, 275–288.

Kendler, K. S., Neale, M. C., Kessler, R. C., Heath, A. C., & Eaves, L. J. (1992). Childhood parental loss and adult psychopathology in women: A twin study. *Archives of General Psychiatry, 49*, 109–116.

Koerner, K., & Linehan, M. (1997). Case formulation in dialectical behavior therapy for borderline personality disorder. In T. D. Eells (Ed.), *Handbook of psychotherapy case formulation* (pp. 340–368). New York: Guilford.

Levenson, H., & Strupp, H. H. (1997). Cyclical maladaptive patterns: Case formulation in time-limited dynamic psychotherapy. In T. D. Eells (Ed.), *Handbook of psychotherapy case formulation* (pp. 84–115). New York: Guilford.

Luborsky, L. (1977). Measuring a pervasive psychic structure in psychotherapy: The core conflictual relationship theme. In N. Freedman & S. Grand (Eds.), *Communicative structures and psychic structures* (pp. 367–395). New York: Plenum Press.

Luborsky, L. (1996). *The symptom-context method: Symptoms as opportunities in psychotherapy.* Washington, DC: American Psychological Association.

Luborsky, L. (1997). The core conflictual relationship theme: A basic case formulation method. In T. D. Eells (Ed.), *Handbook of psychotherapy case formulation* (pp. 58–83). New York: Guilford.

Luborsky, L., Barber, J. P., & Diguer, L. (1992). The meanings of narratives told during psychotherapy: The fruits of a new observational unit. *Psychotherapy Research, 2,* 277–290.

Luborsky, L., Popp, C., & Barber, J. P. (1994). Common and special factors in different transference-related measures. *Psychotherapy Research, 4,* 277–286.

Messer, S. B., Tishby, O., & Spillman, A. (1992). Taking context seriously in psychotherapy: Relating therapist interventions to patient progress in brief psychodynamic therapy. *Journal of Consulting and Clinical Psychology, 60,* 678–688.

Nezu, A. M., Nezu, C. M., Friedman, S. H., & Haynes, S. N. (1997). Case formulation in behavior therapy: Problem-solving and functional-analytic strategies. In T. D. Eells (Ed.), *Handbook of psychotherapy case formulation* (pp. 368–401). New York: Guilford.

Nuland, S. B. (1995). *Doctors: The biography of medicine.* New York: Vintage Books.

Okey, J. L., McWhirter, J. J., & Delaney, M. K. (2000). The central relationship patterns of male veterans with posttraumatic stress disorder: A descriptive study. *Psychotherapy: Theory, Research, Practice, Training, 37,* 171–179.

Perry, J. C. (1994). Assessing psychodynamic patterns using the Idiographic Conflict Formulation Method. *Psychotherapy Research, 4,* 239–252.

Perry, J. C. (1997). The idiographic conflict formulation method. In T. D. Eells (Ed.), *Handbook of psychotherapy case formulation* (pp. 137–165). New York: Guilford.

Perry, J. C., Luborsky, L., Silberschatz, G., & Popp, C. (1989). An examination of three methods of psychodynamic formulation based on the same videotaped interview. *Psychiatry: Journal for the Study of Interpersonal Processes, 52,* 245–249.

Polkinghorne, D. E. (1988). *Narrative knowing and the human sciences.* Albany: State University of New York Press.

Popp, C. A., Diguer, L., Luborsky, L., Faude, J., Johnson, S., Morris, M., Schaffer, N., Schaffler, P., & Schmidt, K. A. (1996). Repetitive relationship themes in waking narratives and dreams. *Journal of Consulting & Clinical Psychology, 64*(5) 1073–1078.

Ryle, A., & Bennett, D. (1997). Case formulation in cognitive analytic therapy. In T. D. Eells (Ed.), *Handbook of psychotherapy case formulation* (pp. 289–313). New York: Guilford.

Schacht, T. E., Binder, J. L., & Strupp, H. H. (1984). The dynamic focus. In H. H. Strupp & J. L. Binder (Eds.), *Psychotherapy in a new key.* New York: Basic Books.

Seitz, P. F. (1966). The consensus problem in psychoanalytic research. In L. Gottschalk & L. Auerbach (Eds.), *Methods of research and psychotherapy* (pp. 209–225). New York: Appleton, Century, Crofts.

Shear, M. K., Copper, A. M., Klerman, G. L., Busch, F. N., & Shapiro, T. (1993). A psychodynamic model of panic disorder. *American Journal of Psychiatry, 150,* 859–866.

Silberschatz, G., & Curtis, J. T. (1993). Measuring the therapist's impact on the patient's therapeutic progress. *Journal of Consulting and Clinical Psychology, 61,* 403–411.

Silberschatz, G., Curtis, J. T., & Nathans, S. (1989). Using the patient's plan to assess progress in psychotherapy. *Psychotherapy, 26,* 40–46.

Silberschatz, G., Fretter, P. B., & Curtis, J. T. (1986). How do interpretations influence the process of psychotherapy? *Journal of Consulting and Clinical Psychology, 54,* 646–652.

Spence, D. P. (1982). *Historical truth and narrative truth.* New York: Norton.

Strupp, H. H. (1993). The Vanderbilt psychotherapy studies: Synopsis. *Journal of Consulting and Clinical Psychology, 61,* 431–433.

Strupp, H. H., & Binder, J. L. (1984). *Psychotherapy in a new key.* New York: Basic Books.

Turk, D. C., & Salovey, P. (Eds.). (1988). *Reasoning, inference, and judgment in clinical psychology.* New York: Free Press.

Weiss, J. (1993). *How psychotherapy works: Process and technique.* New York: Guilford.

CHAPTER

7

Constructing Interpretations and Assessing Their Accuracy

Mary Beth Connolly Gibbons
Paul Crits-Christoph
Phillip Apostol
University of Pennsylvania Health System

Modern theories of dynamic psychotherapy focus on the interpretation of maladaptive relationship patterns as the primary technique designed to increase self-understanding and relieve psychiatric symptoms. Therapists in training in dynamic psychotherapy are faced with the task of learning to formulate and deliver accurate interpretations. The primary goal of this chapter is to review the research literature on constructing interpretations, with particular attention to studies that evaluate the relation between interpretations and psychotherapy outcome, to enhance the ability of clinicians to develop interpretation skills informed by research. We first consider the definitions of interpretation and review the role of interpretations in the process of change as described in theories of dynamic psychotherapy.

The term *interpretation* is generically used among dynamic theorists to refer to therapeutic interventions that are designed to foster self-understanding. However, the definition of interpretation within dynamic models of psychotherapy has evolved over time. Freud (1912/1958) first described "stereotyped plates" as cognitive structures formed through early childhood relationships that resulted in repetitive maladaptive interpersonal patterns throughout adulthood. Although the initial focus of psychoanalysis was on using interpretation to uncover the repressed memories related to symptom formation, psychoanalysis later evolved to emphasize the interpretation of the products of Freud's stereotyped plates, especially how the repetitive maladaptive patterns played out in the relationship with the analyst.

In 1954, Bibring defined interpretation as interventions that went beyond the patient's awareness in helping the patient to understand how his or her behaviors are determined by wishes and thoughts. Modern theories of dynamic psychotherapy such as Luborsky's (1984) supportive-expressive (SE) psychotherapy and Strupp and Binder's (1984) time-limited dynamic psychotherapy focus interpretations on maladaptive interpersonal themes. Within these models, interpretations can include interventions that help elucidate the components of the pattern, the consistency of the pattern across relationships, the historical development of the pattern, and the relation of the pattern to current symptoms.

The definition of interpretation is further confounded by differential use of the term *transference interpretation*. Although the term *transference* is generally used within modern theories of dynamic psychotherapy to refer to an individual's tendency to repeat maladaptive relationship patterns, we use the term *interpretation* to refer to any therapist statement that has the intent of helping the patient to learn about his or her impairing relationship conflicts. We use the term *transference interpretation* to refer to the subtype of interpretation that helps the patient understand his or her relationship theme within the therapeutic relationship.

Modern theories of dynamic psychotherapy have also provided more precise definitions of the interpersonal components of transference patterns. For instance, Luborsky's (1984) model of SE specifies three main components that comprise a patient's maladaptive interpersonal theme that he terms the *core conflictual relationship theme* (Luborsky & Crits-Christoph, 1990). This core theme consists of the interpersonal wishes experienced by the patient within relationships, the perceived responses of others toward the patient, and the stereotypic and often maladaptive response of the patient toward others. The SE model of treatment focuses on exploring narratives that the patient shares during psychotherapy to gather information needed to accurately formulate interpersonal wish and response patterns. This formulation is used by the therapist to develop accurate interpretations of the impairing relationship conflicts.

The goal of this research review is to inform the use of interpretations by therapists learning to implement dynamic psychotherapy. We first briefly review the literature that provides a descriptive account of the techniques used in dynamic psychotherapy, including a description of the format, content, and frequency of interpretations within dynamic psychotherapy. As therapists learn to implement interpretations within short-term treatments, it is necessary to have an understanding of the frequency with which interpretations should be implemented and an appreciation of the extent to which interpretations in short-term dynamic treatments focus on various other people and time frames.

We then review studies evaluating the consistency of interpersonal themes across the narratives that patient's share during psychotherapy because the therapist uses the material in these narratives to formulate the patient's maladaptive interpersonal patterns and to construct interpretations. The bulk of our research review focuses on studies that examine the relation of interpretation to psychotherapy outcome. These studies include first investigations that examine the frequency and accuracy of interpretations in the prediction of outcome followed by studies that examine the use of transference interpretations in relation to treatment outcome. Each section of this review is followed by a summary of findings that might be translated into clinical practice. Although the research literature might be quite informative, we provide only tentative clinical recommendations. Many more studies with adequate statistical power need to be conducted before we can make definitive recommendations regarding the role of interpretations in the process of dynamic psychotherapy.

We conclude the review with a summary of recommendations for future research. Finally, we provide an exercise designed for beginning therapist to help them begin to learn how to extract relationship patterns from the narratives that are shared during dynamic psychotherapy and to formulate possible interpretations.

FREQUENCY, CONTENT, AND FORMAT OF INTERPRETATIONS IN DYNAMIC PSYCHOTHERAPY

Dynamic psychotherapy is a broad rubric encompassing a variety of therapeutic treatments that have in common the use of interpretations to help alleviate psychiatric symptoms. Studies that have investigated the prevalence of interpretative statements within naturalistic (non-manual guided) dynamically oriented treatments have demonstrated the diversity across dynamic psychotherapies in the definition and use of interpretations. For instance, Hill, Helms, Tichenor, and Spiegel (1988) reported that 8% of therapist utterances within psychoanalytic psychotherapy sessions were classified as interpretations. Stiles (1979) classified a much higher rate of therapist utterances within psychoanalytic psychotherapy sessions as interpretations, with 30% classified as interpretations in terms of form and 49% classified as interpretations in terms of therapist intent.

Manual-guided dynamically oriented treatments have specified more precisely how interpretations should be formulated and implemented within treatment sessions. However, content analyses of manual-guided dynamic psychotherapy sessions are quite rare in the psychotherapy research literature. Stiles, Shapiro, and Firth-Cozens (1988) found that more than 20% of therapist utterances were classified as interpretations in terms of the intent of the therapist in interpersonal dynamic psychotherapy. Piper, Debbane, de Carufel, and Bienvenu (1987) reported that 14% of therapists speaking turns in dynamic psychotherapy sessions were classified as interpretations with an average of five interpretations per session classified as transference interpretations focused on the therapeutic relationship.

We conducted a molecular level process analysis of SE dynamic psychotherapy sessions to provide a more precise guide for practitioners in formulating and implementing dynamic interpretations within our model of dynamic psychotherapy (Connolly, Crits-Christoph, Shappell, Barber, & Luborsky, 1998). We found that therapists on average used about 125 individual speaking turns in an average 50-min sessions. The therapists in these sessions were quite active. It should be noted that 33% of statements did not fit into either the interpretation, clarification, or question categories and were rated by judges as "other" statements. Many of these statements were simple facilitative comments such as "uh-huh." Four percent of therapist statements were classified as interpretations (approximately five statements per session) with less than one statement per session classified as a transference interpretation of the relationship between the patient and the therapist. Further, most therapist interpretations within the SE sessions focused on the patient's relationship patterns with the parents, significant others, and the self. Contrary to some stereotypes of dynamic treatments, the majority of interpretations focused on the current time frame, with only 5% of interpretations focused on the patient's childhood past.

In summary, molecular level assessments of therapist interventions in manual-guided dynamic psychotherapies suggest that interpretations of maladaptive relationship patterns range in frequency from about 4% of therapist speaking turns per session to over 20% of therapist utterances. Dynamic models of treatment also vary regarding the intensity of transference interpretations, with more traditional psychoanalytic models such as Piper's (Piper et al., 1987) providing as many as five transference interpretations per session in short-term psychoanalytic psychotherapy. Models such as SE psychotherapy, which was codified to represent the kind of dynamic psychotherapy often practiced in the community, use more interpretations focused on the current time frame and uses transference interpretations sparingly.

EVIDENCE FOR THE TRANSFERENCE OF MALADAPTIVE INTERPERSONAL THEMES

When formulating interpretations to help patients learn about maladaptive relationship patterns, the therapist uses information provided in patient narratives about their interactions with other people to formulate the patient's core relationship pattern. The research evaluating the consistency of narrative themes and the relation of these themes to the patient's experience with the therapist can be quite informative to therapists who are learning to construct interpretations, including transference interpretations, from the therapeutic material.

Both Luborsky et al. (1985) and Crits-Christoph and Luborsky (1990) reported that core interpersonal themes were pervasive across psychotherapy narratives. Crits-Christoph, Demorest, Muenz, and Baranackie (1994) used the Quantitative Analysis of Interpersonal Themes method to have independent judges rate the wish and response patterns using a standard vocabulary across the psychotherapy narratives of 60 patients. One advantage of this research methodology was that judges rated the patient narratives in random order to prevent judges from perceiving a higher level of similarity between narratives than was actually present. The investigators reported a small but statistically significant level of consistency across narratives in the interpersonal wish and response patterns.

Fried, Crits-Christoph, and Luborsky (1992) examined the similarity between each patient's interpersonal theme and the theme experienced with his/her own therapist. Themes experienced with the therapist were also compared to other patients' interpersonal themes to control for chance similarity. The investigators found that patients' own interpersonal themes were more similar to the themes experienced with their own therapist than the themes expressed by other patients. Connolly et al. (1996) implemented the Quantitative Analysis of Interpersonal Themes method to evaluate the relation between patients' therapeutic narratives about significant others and the narratives told about experiences with the therapist. Across 35 patients, there was usually one predominant theme that was most pervasive across narratives. Most patients also had additional interpersonal themes that were less pervasive across narratives. Overall, about 60% of patients described an interpersonal theme in the narratives told about significant others during treatment that was statistically significantly related to the theme expressed in narratives about the therapist. However, it was not always the most pervasive interpersonal theme. For 34% of patients the most pervasive theme evident in psychotherapy narratives was significantly associated with the therapist theme.

Connolly, Crits-Christoph, Barber, and Luborsky (2000) repeated the methodology implemented by Connolly et al. (1996) with a sample of 18 patients treated with short-term SE psychotherapy for major depression. In this investigation, interpersonal themes extracted from pretreatment interviews about significant others were compared to the themes expressed in narratives about the therapist during treatment. Consistent with the results reported by Connolly et al. (1996), the most pervasive interpersonal theme in the pretreatment narratives was statistically significantly associated with the theme expressed in the treatment narratives about the therapist for 33% of patients. In both the Connolly et al. (1996) study and the Connolly et al. (2000) investigation, only about one third of patients demonstrated a significant transference of their core interpersonal pattern to the relationship with the therapist, at least across the early sessions of the time-limited psychotherapy that we evaluated.

In summary, these investigations suggest that patients' interpersonal themes are consistent across the narratives they tell during psychotherapy. However, therapists in training should be aware that the research shows that there is tremendous variability across patients in the consistency of themes across narratives. Although most patients will express at least one theme that appears to predominate, most patients have multiple maladaptive interpersonal themes that interfere with their current relationships. It is the task of the therapist to extract the predominant themes from the narratives that patients tell and to explore which themes might be causing the patient the most distress in his or her current relationships.

The research studies on transference of interpersonal themes further suggest that although some transference to the therapist is evident in the narratives that patients share during psychotherapy, not all patients early in treatment describe their therapists consistent with their interpersonal relationships outside of treatment. For these patients, it is possible that transference of their maladaptive themes to the therapeutic relationship has not yet developed, or if the patient has begun to experience the therapist consistent with his or her other relationships this material is not evident in the material the patient chooses to share. Thus, for many patients it might be more useful to focus exclusively on the narratives shared about people other than the therapist to understand the impairing relationship conflict.

REVIEW OF STUDIES RELATING INTERPRETATIONS TO PSYCHOTHERAPY OUTCOME

Research investigations have evaluated both the relation of frequency of interpretation and accuracy of interpretation to treatment outcome. Further, studies have focused on both interpretations in general and transference interpretations specifically as predictors of psychotherapy outcome.

Frequency of Interpretation and Psychotherapy Outcome

Although correlational studies do not address the quality or timing of interpretations, studies relating the frequency of interpretation to outcome can inform the clinician in general about whether greater use of interpretation influences the course of treatment. Foreman and Marmar (1985) evaluated the frequency of interpretations for six cases with poor alliances early in treatment. Only three cases improved in terms of the alliance across treatment. There were more interventions that addressed patient defenses in the improved cases compared to the unimproved cases. Piper et al. (1987) used the Therapist Intervention Rating Scale to evaluate the relation between use of interpretations and treatment outcome. In this system, interpretations were defined as therapist statements that address at least one of six possible components, including both dynamic components (impulses, anxiety, defenses, dynamic expressions) and nondynamic components (objects and resultant expressions). The investigators reported that the proportion of interventions that addressed two or three dynamic components was significantly correlated with the therapists' ratings of overall usefulness of therapy.

Contrary to Piper et al. (1987), Hill et al. (1988) did not report a statistically significant relation between the proportion of interpretations and treatment outcome for eight patients who received between 12 and 20 sessions of brief psychotherapy. However, this investigation had low statistical power. There was a moderately large association, although it did not reach statistical significance, between the proportion of interpretations and change in self-concept. Although many more studies with adequate power are needed to address the relation of frequency of interpretation to treatment outcome, these three investigations (Foreman & Marmar, 1985; Hill et al., 1988; Piper et al., 1987) indicate that there is a positive association between the frequency of interpretation provided in psychotherapy and symptom course. These results suggest that it is important for clinicians to formulate the patient's maladaptive interpersonal theme and to provide interpretations designed to help the patient identify and explore the interpersonal patterns that interfere with his or her current relationships.

Frequency of Transference Interpretations and Psychotherapy Outcome

In two early investigations, Malan (1976) evaluated the association between the outcome of treatment and the proportion of interpretations that linked the transference with the therapist to experiences with the parent or a sibling. In both studies, greater frequency of transference interpretations predicted positive treatment outcomes. Piper, Debbane, Bienvenu, de Carufel, and Garant (1986) evaluated therapist response modes across 21 patients treated with short-term psychoanalytic psychotherapy. Contrary to the results presented by Malan (1976), the proportion of interpretations that linked the transference to the parental relationship was not associated with treatment outcome. In fact, the average correlation across 17 outcome measures was only .05.

The inconsistent research results regarding the relation between the frequency of transference interpretations and outcome are clarified somewhat by further studies that included the patient's quality of interpersonal functioning as a moderator of the association between transference interpretations and treatment outcome. Piper, Azim, Joyce, and McCallum (1991) evaluated the relation between the proportion of transference interpretations and therapy outcome separately for patients rated high versus low on the quality of object relations. *Quality of object relations* was defined as the patient's lifelong pattern of relationships. Only for patients with a history of high quality of object relations, high rates of transference interpretation predicted a poor treatment outcome ($r = .58$, $p < .001$). Similarly, Høglend (1993) found a significant inverse relation between frequency of transference interpretation and treatment outcome for the high quality of object relations patients only.

Connolly et al. (1999) also found that quality of interpersonal relationships significantly moderated the relation between proportion of transference interpretations and treatment outcome. Specifically, patients with low quality of interpersonal relationships demonstrated poor treatment outcomes at relatively higher levels of transference interpretations. One might argue that these investigations do not unpack the temporal relation between use of transference interpretations and symptom course. Specifically, it may be that early treatment symptom change prior to the use of transference interpretations predicts both the frequency of transference interpretations used by the therapist and the subsequent symptom course. The investigation by Connolly et al. (1999) unpacked this temporal course of symptom change across treatment, demonstrating that the quality of interpersonal relationships moderated the relation between proportion of transference interpretations symptom change following the use of transference interpretations, controlling for early treatment symptom change.

At first glance, the results presented by Connolly et al. (1999) appear inconsistent with those presented by Piper et al. (1991) and Høglend (1993). Piper et al. (1991) and Høglend (1993) found that high levels of transference interpretations predicted poor treatment outcome for patients with a high quality of object relations, whereas Connolly et al. (1999) found that higher levels of transference interpretations predicted poor outcome for low quality of interpersonal relationship patients. Connolly et al. (1999) presented one possible explanation of how these results might be complementary. The Piper et al. (1991) investigation evaluated a treatment that ranged from moderate to high levels of transference interpretation with an average of five transference interpretations per session. In contrast, Connolly et al. (1999) evaluated a treatment that used very low to moderate levels of transference interpretation often ranging from zero to at most two transference interpretations per session.

In the Piper et al. (1991) investigation, it is possible that patients with low quality of object relations had poor treatment outcomes across the range of moderate to high transference interpretation used in that study. Thus, Piper et al. (1991) found a significant relation only within the high quality of object relations patients, with these patients demonstrating good outcomes at moderate levels and poor outcomes at high levels of transference interpretation.

The results presented by Connolly et al. (1999) could be complimentary in that patients with high quality of interpersonal relationships had good outcomes across the range of low to moderate frequencies of transference interpretation evaluated in the investigation. In contrast, patients with low quality of interpersonal relationships demonstrated good outcomes at the very low levels of transference interpretation implemented in this study and poor outcomes at moderate levels. Taken together, these investigations suggest that patients with high quality of object relationships can benefit from treatments that implement low to moderate levels of transference interpretation. However, at very high levels even patients with high quality of interpersonal relationships have poor outcomes. Although Piper et al. (1991) did not specify the range of transference interpretations evaluated in their investigation, they do report an average of five transference interpretations per session. Therefore, the results might be interpreted to mean that more than five transference interpretations per session, even with patients who experience positive interpersonal relationships, can lead to a poor treatment outcome. These studies also suggest that patients with low quality of interpersonal relationships benefit only from treatments with very low, if any, transference interpretations.

Accuracy of Interpretations and Psychotherapy Outcome

Developing clinicians are trained not only to provide an adequate frequency of interpretations but specifically to construct accurate interpretations of the patient's impairing relationship conflicts. Silberschatz, Fretter, and Curtis (1986) evaluated the plan compatibility of interpretations in three psychotherapy cases. The investigators reported that the patient with the best treatment outcome had a greater number of interpretations that were consistent with the patient's case formulation compared to the patient with the poorest treatment outcome. This study was extended by Norville, Sampson, and Weiss (1996) who evaluated the relation between the average plan compatibility of interpretations and treatment outcome for seven cases, three of which were included in the Silberschatz et al. (1986) investigation just described. The researchers found a significant correlation ($r = .69$, $p = .043$) between the average plan compatibility of interpretations and the patient's plan attainment rating.

Crits-Christoph, Cooper, and Luborsky (1988) assessed the accuracy of dynamic interpretations for 43 patients treated with up to 1 year of dynamically oriented psychotherapy. A composite score representing the average accuracy on the wish and response of other components of the core conflictual relationship theme were significantly associated with treatment outcome.

Although few in number, investigations of the accuracy of interpretation suggest to clinicians in training that the degree to which interpretations accurately address the patient's core maladaptive themes is predictive of a decrease in symptoms across treatment. In addition to learning to provide frequent interpretations, therapists in training should learn to formulate the patient's maladaptive pattern from the narratives that are shared during treatment and learn to construct interpretations that accurately address these themes.

Accuracy of Transference Interpretations and Psychotherapy Outcome

The previous investigations evaluated the relations between interpretation use in general and treatment outcome. One additional investigation specifically evaluated the correspondence of transference interpretations with the therapist's own case formulation in the prediction of treatment outcome (Piper, Joyce, McCallum, & Azim, 1993). Piper et al. (1993) reported that for patients with a low quality of object relations, greater correspondence of transference interpretations was significantly associated with poor 6-month follow-up outcome ($r = .49$, $p < .05$). For patients with a high pretreatment quality of object relations, greater correspondence of transference interpretations was significantly related to a more favorable follow-up outcome at 6 months.

In summary, although greater frequencies of interpretations in general and greater accuracy of interpretations appear to predict a positive symptom course in the studies reported in the research literature to date, the relation between transference interpretations and treatment outcome is more complex. High numbers of transference interpretations appear to be problematic for many patients treated in short-term dynamic psychotherapy. However, patients with good interpersonal functioning may benefit from a few highly accurate transference interpretations provided sparingly across the course of treatment.

The results of this research review on the role of dynamic interpretations in psychotherapy suggest that therapists in training should focus on learning to accurately formulate the patient's core maladaptive interpersonal pattern. Active use of accurate interpretations of this core theme can be useful in teaching patients to identify, understand, and hopefully change the maladaptive themes that lead to unfulfilling relationships and psychiatric symptoms in their current worlds. Therapists implementing short-term dynamic treatments may also, with some patients, experience the transference of the patient's maladaptive theme within the therapeutic relationship. In cases in which the therapist judges the patient to be capable of working within the therapeutic relationship to learn about the interpersonal theme, a few accurate transference interpretations might be quite useful in helping the patient to learn firsthand about the effects of their relationship conflicts.

FUTURE RESEARCH DIRECTIONS

To date, the research literature can be very informative to the beginning clinician learning to formulate interpersonal patterns and learning to construct and deliver accurate interpretations of these maladaptive patterns. However, this review indicates that although clinicians can be informed by the research findings to date, these findings should also be interpreted cautiously. Given the central role of interpretations in dynamic theories of symptom change, relatively little research has evaluated the role of interpretations in the psychotherapeutic process. Many studies published to date were conducted on very small sample sizes, some so small that formal statistical analysis was not possible.

The review of the literature reveals that treatments included within the dynamic camp vary widely in their use of interpretations. Although the few studies done to date suggest that greater numbers of interpretations can be helpful in psychotherapy, much more research is needed to inform the level of interpretation that is optimal with different kinds of patients.

Most important, theories of dynamic psychotherapy are based on the premise that accurate interpretations help patients to understand their interpersonal worlds in a way that allows them to make changes that improve their interpersonal relationships and psychiatric symptoms. Research is needed to demonstrate this change process in psychotherapy. Although a few correlational investigations suggest that accuracy of interpretation predicts treatment outcome, further research is needed to unpack the causal pathway through which accurate interpretations have their impact. Further research is also needed to demonstrate the most effective ways to train therapists to formulate and implement accurate interpersonal interpretations.

TRAINING EXERCISE

Our own experience suggests that the best method for training therapists to competently implement interpretations involves intensive individual supervision of psychotherapy cases by a trained expert. We commonly start by providing therapists with a treatment manual that lays out the theoretical framework for the interventions and provides case examples of the interventions suggested. Therapists usually treat at least three training cases for which they receive 1 hour of individual supervision for every 2 hours of therapy provided.

The supervision focuses on helping the therapist to extract a formulation of the patient's core conflicts from the material that the patient shares during treatment. Therapists are trained in techniques to help the patient expand their narratives so that an accurate formulation can be constructed. The supervisor works with the therapist to role-play possible interventions, including dynamic interpretations, helping the therapist to fine tune wording and learning about appropriate timing of these interpretations.

To supplement training experiences with actual patients, it might be useful to have trainees review transcripts of therapy sessions. We have found that while training judges on the various tasks needed to rate the accuracy of interpretations, judges working from transcripts can be trained to competence on identifying interpretations from session transcripts, identifying the interpersonal patterns in patient narratives and rating the accuracy of dynamic formulations. As these are all skills needed to become a competent therapist, we feel that such training from therapy transcripts might be useful in conjunction with intensive supervision in teaching therapists essential skills that they can fine tune under supervision.

In our experience, judges and therapists in training must rate many transcripts to identify interpretations, interpersonal themes, and accurate interpretations with competence. We have included a training exercise here that is intended to provide only a starting point in this training process.

Training Exercise in Formulating a Core Conflictual Relationship Theme

A patient described in this book's case study told the following narratives during psychotherapy. Each narrative has been edited to conserve space and protect confidentiality. Each narrative can be read to identify the core conflictual relationship theme consisting of the patient's wishes, perceived responses of other, and response of self. The theme can be identified by addressing the questions posed at the end of each narrative.

Narrative 1: Sister Cathy and Mum

Q: Anything else that's happened during the week that's important to you?

A: Um, a bit of an argument with my sister about coming here today, last night. Dad had been in bed all day and I just felt that the argument she was having was basically about somebody looking after Jo rather than being concerned about how Dad was or me having to get up here. And basically what she was saying was, you know, well he's probably willing so don't even ask him whether he wants to come or not, just say that he's going and then has to get out of bed to look after Jo sort of thing. Because she was of the mind that if I came on my own, she'd be leaving Jo with him but Jo would be downstairs on her own all day while he was being ill in bed. I felt that she was saying, that's not good enough. She wanted him to be looking after Jo rather than being ill. And I said, well, hold on a minute, we've all had it, and he's gone through without getting it, for the past . . . well, I've forgotten now how many months I've had it. And he's looked after us you know. I've been there, I was literally in bed for three days solid or something, and he was basically nursemaiding me. And I said, just give him a bit of leeway, after all it was a Sunday, it wasn't as if he had to go to work or anything like that. He wasn't sort of bunking off from anything. Umm, and just basically Cathy and Mum seemed so put out by the fact he was ill, and I just sort of . . . you know, I think give the poor bloke a break . . . the way it sounded was as if he was doing it on purpose. And basically, Jo was not particularly well either, and I sort of said, I basically said to Cathy, well wouldn't it be better for the both of them to stay here in the warm, rather than have to get on buses and trains and things to get up to London, you know. Then neither of them would have to be rushed out of bed in the morning. I said if I just go home, I can get there as easy as anything. No hassles, I haven't got to worry about anyone else.

What does the patient want or need from her sister and Mum? How does the patient see her sister and Mum as responding toward her? How does the patient respond?

Narrative 2: Sister Cathy

A: I was feeling a bit rough. Sat down, had lunch, and it must have got to about half 5 and Jo thumped Cathy and she smacked her and gave her a telling off, and Sally laughed.

A: Jo's got quite a little temper on her. I think that she just got over excited you know, with Christmas and everything. It was all just too much for her.

A: Cathy went mad, smacked her and told her off. But Sally laughed, so Sally got told off. So I said, oh right, so it's all right for you to laugh when Jo thumps me and Sally. So she said, when does she thump you? And I said does it matter when. The fact she did and you laughed. She said oh well, and I said, what are you calling me a liar ... and she went, no when? And me and Sally practically said at the same time, in Safeway's. In the middle of Safeway's with everyone looking at us and you just laughed at us. And this is Sally as well. Cause Sally's been thumped as well. She's been laughed at as well basically. So it wasn't just me.

Q: It's another person who supports your position.

A: Yeah. Well I thought so. Anyway there was a sort of half hearted apology for that, and I just shut up. I thought no I'm not saying another thing. Yi know, I was feeling quiet level headed and fine. I mean not brilliantly happy or anything but probably a lot happier than I'd felt for a lot of the holiday. Oh, and before that Mum had said what does everyone want for tea and everything. Um, Sally and Jo had placed their orders and Cathy had said yeah I'll have the same as them. Then after this happened I just sat there and was staring at the telly. Then Cathy just suddenly says, get your stuff together, to Sally, and Sally just looked at her. Mum said, oh you're not going are you? And she said yeah in a minute. And Mum said, oh why I thought you were having tea. And she said, yeah, well we're going before she goes in to one. And I sat there and I said nothing. Just left it. As far as I was concerned she had given me a very half hearted apology but ...

A: Can I ask, if she said that, and yes I did go in to one, but because she said that. I thought what bloody reason did you have to say that. Anyway I wasn't anywhere near going in to one before she said it ... and of course I did. And basically all the pressure over Christmas came out. A hell of a lot of shouting and swearing and um ...

Q: What you to Cathy, or ...

A: Both ways. And I shut her up by saying if you weren't here then I wouldn't have the bloody problems. I mean she started going on about making out that I was the only one that had problems. And you know, that I was the only one that needed any sympathy.

What does the patient want or need from her sister? How does the patient see her sister as responding towards her? How does the patient respond?

Narrative 3: Doctors, Nurses, Parents

A: Yes. I suppose for 15 years all I've been listening to is, you should be doing this, you should be doing that. It's doctors, nurses, parents or whatever. There's always someone telling you, should you be eating that? And you just think, go away. There's always that someone that is there, it doesn't matter if I switch myself off or not, it still goes in. If someone is telling you something you'll still . . . very halfheartedly, but you do listen.

Q: Then you blank it out.

What does the patient want or need from others? How does the patient see them as responding towards her? How does the patient respond? List the wishes, responses from other, and responses from self that are repeated across the three narratives.

Authors' Ratings of Core Conflictual Relationship Theme

In the first narrative, the patient describes a fight she has with her sister and Mum over whether the father will be able to take care of the sister's daughter and escort the patient to the clinic. The patient describes that she is upset with them for worrying about their own needs rather than "being concerned with how Dad was or me having to get up here." We can infer that the patient's wish is to have others concerned for her. The sister and the mother respond by not being concerned about the patient's need but the patients own response is not described. We can infer from the narrative that her response is to become angry or upset.

In the second narrative, the patient described a fight with her sister is which she points out to the sister that she herself was once hit by the niece and the sister only laughed. In this narrative, the patient describes a wish for the sister to care about the patient and to have sympathy for the patient. The sister responds by not being concerned for the patient, by laughing when the patient was hit, and by providing only a begrudging apology. In this episode, the patient responds by tuning everything out and by then becoming angry.

In the last narrative, the patient describes others telling her what to do. We can infer that she has a wish to be left alone, she sees others as controlling her, and her response is to blank out. Across these three narratives, we can begin to develop a preliminary formulation of her core conflictual relationship theme, including a wish for others to be concerned with her needs, a response of others as not being concerned for her and not providing sympathy for her, and a response of self to become angry and to tune others out.

Training Exercise in Constructing Interventions Based on the Core Conflictual Relationship Theme

So far we have evaluated only three narratives. However, in treatment the therapist is faced with the task of unraveling stories as they are told, looking for similarities across narratives, formulating interventions to help expand one's understanding of the theme, and formulating preliminary interpretations. Based on these narratives, the therapist can develop therapeutic interventions by considering the following questions: What questions might you ask to help expand your understanding of the patient's wishes, responses from other, and responses from self? What clarifications might be useful in helping the patient to deepen her exploration of the pattern? What interpretations might you use to address elements of the patient's theme? What interpretations might you use to address similarities across narratives?

Authors' Suggested Interventions to Address the Core Conflictual Relationship Theme

Based on our preliminary formulation of the patient's core theme, we would recommend both clarifications and questions during the early sessions to help expand our understanding of her wishes and responses. In the first narrative, a therapist might ask questions such as, "What did you want from your sister?" "How did you respond when they didn't seem to be considering your needs?," and "How did you feel" to help both the patient and therapist better understand the components of her theme. In the second narrative, the therapist might provide a clarification regarding the patient's response of self such as, "it sounds like you blanked out when you were feeling angry" to help the patient continue to expand her description of her own response.

Interpretations of specific components as well as interpretations linking the themes across stories can be used throughout the treatment to help the patient understand his or her pattern. After the second narrative, a therapist might say, "You've told multiple stories about your sister in which you wanted her to be concerned with your needs, and you tend to get angry and tune everything out when you feel that she is not concerned about you."

7. CONSTRUCTING INTERPRETATIONS

Training Exercise in Rating the Accuracy of Interpretations

The therapist implemented the following interpretations in the sessions. For each interpretation, the reader can rate the accuracy of the statement in addressing the core wish, response of other, and response of self that you formulated previously.

> Q: I think this thing about you either feel blanked out, i.e., excluding and rejected, or you feel invaded and others are totally involved. And when you get in both those positions as you say, you become abusive to others, shouting, temper, you're more like your Dad and have a temper. So that could be seen as selfish. But generally you are sort of, almost like inappropriately responsible towards others, aren't you? Which is not quite the same as being selfish.
>
> Q: But June, um, lots of very, very different things have happened. You confronted Cathy when, if she hit you and she laughs, it's conformation that you don't matter. Right. You challenged her on that and saying like, I do matter. Actually it does matter. This matters and I matter. Right. I haven't seen you . . . normally you're quite defensive. It's all like, see I'm blank. So you're much more proactive about it. That's another thing. You had some whiskies, but they didn't knock you out, i.e., I wasn't able to blank out my feelings and what happened to me. You were thinking about things. That's a good thing not a bad thing.
>
> Q: They don't have to say it. But your Mum just said it recently. "Is your diabetes sorted out?" Your diabetes is not sorted out because you blank it out, because you treat yourself as if you don't matter, but you complain that they don't treat you like you matter.

Author's Ratings of Accuracy of Interpretation

In the first intervention, the therapist helps the patient to learn about her response of self. This interpretation would be rated as high on accuracy of addressing her response of anger and tuning others out. It does not at all address the wish and response of other. In the second intervention, the therapist is supporting changes that the patient has made in her response of self. Again the therapist accurately addresses her maladaptive tendency to become angry and tune others out. In doing so, the therapist alludes to her wish that others be concerned for her, but doesn't address it directly. We might score the wish for others to be concerned for the patient low on accuracy and the response of other of not providing concern and sympathy as low to moderate. Finally, in the third intervention, the therapist links her response of self of blanking out with her medical problems. The therapist further links June's perceived response of others as not being concerned for the patient to her own behavior toward herself. This interpretation would be rated high on accuracy on the response of other and response of self components.

Our analysis of some of the interventions actually implemented by the therapist suggests that the therapist was highly accurate in helping her to explore her response of self but did not provide much interpretation of the other elements of her theme. Our model of SE psychotherapy, as well as the results reported by Crits-Christoph et al. (1988), suggest that it is important in terms of treatment outcome to accurately interpret for the patient both the wishes and perceived responses of others.

REFERENCES

Bibring, E. (1954). Psychoanalysis and the dynamic psychotherapies. *Journal of the American Psychoanalytic Association, 2,* 745–770.

Connolly, M. B., Crits-Christoph, P., Barber, J. P., & Luborsky, L. (2000). Transference patterns in the therapeutic relationship in supportive-expressive psychotherapy for depression. *Psychotherapy Research, 10,* 356–372.

Connolly, M. B., Crits-Christoph, P., Demorest, A., Azarian, K., Muenz, L., & Chittams, J. (1996). The varieties of transference patterns in psychotherapy. *Journal of Consulting and Clinical Psychology, 64,* 1213–1221.

Connolly, M. B., Crits-Christoph, P., Shappell, S., Barber, J. P., & Luborsky, L. (1998). Therapist interventions in early sessions of brief supportive-expressive psychotherapy for depression. *Journal of Psychotherapy Practice and Research, 7,* 290–300.

Connolly, M. B., Crits-Christoph, P., Shappell, S., Barber, J. P., Luborsky, L., & Shaffer, C. (1999). Relation of transference interpretations to outcome in the early sessions of brief supportive-expressive psychotherapy. *Psychotherapy Research, 9,* 485–495.

Crits-Christoph, P., Cooper, A., & Luborsky, L. (1988). The accuracy of therapists' interpretations and the outcome of dynamic psychotherapy. *Journal of Consulting and Clinical Psychology, 56,* 490–495.

Crits-Christoph, P., Demorest, A., Muenz, L. R., & Baranackie, K. (1994). Consistency of interpersonal themes. *Journal of Personality, 62,* 499–526.

Crits-Christoph, P., & Luborsky, L. (1990). Changes in CCRT pervasiveness during psychotherapy. In L. Luborsky & P. Crits-Christoph (Eds.), *Understanding transference—The CCRT method* (pp. 133–146). New York: Basic Books.

Foreman, S. A., & Marmar, C. R. (1985). Therapist actions that address initially poor therapeutic alliances in psychotherapy. *American Journal of Psychiatry, 142,* 922–926.

Freud, S. (1958). The dynamics of transference. In J. Strachey (Ed. and Trans.), *The standard edition of the complete psychological works of Sigmund Freud* (Vol. 12, pp. 99–108). London: Hogarth Press. (Original work published 1912)

Fried, D., Crits-Christoph, P., & Luborsky, L. (1992). The first empirical demonstration of transference in psychotherapy. *Journal of Nervous and Mental Disease, 180,* 326–331.

Hill, C. E., Helms, J. E., Tichenor, V., & Spiegel, S. B. (1988). Effects of therapist response modes in brief psychotherapy. *Journal of Counseling Psychology, 35,* 222–233.

Høglend, P. (1993). Transference interpretations and long-term change after dynamic psychotherapy of brief to moderate length. *American Journal of Psychotherapy, 47,* 494–507.

Luborsky, L. (1984). *Principles of psychoanalytic psychotherapy: A manual for supportive-expressive treatment.* New York: Basic Books.

Luborsky, L., & Crits-Christoph, P. (1990). *Understanding transference: The core conflictual relationship theme method.* New York: Basic Books.

Luborsky, L., Mellon, J., Alexander, K., van Ravenswaay, P., Childress, A., Levine, F., Cohen, K. D., Hole, A. V., Ming, S., Crits-Christoph, P., Levine, F. J., & Alexander, K. (1985). A verification of Freud's grandest clinical hypothesis: The transference. *Clinical Psychology Review, 5,* 231–246.

Malan, D. H. (1976). *Towards the validation of dynamic psychotherapy: Replication.* New York: Plenum Medical Books.

Norville, R., Sampson, H., & Weiss, J. (1996). Accurate interpretations and brief psychotherapy outcome. *Psychotherapy Research, 6,* 16–29.

Piper, W. E., Azim, H. F., Joyce, A. S., & McCallum, M. (1991). Transference interpretations, therapeutic alliance, and outcome in short-term individual psychotherapy. *Archives of General Psychiatry, 48,* 946–953.

Piper, W. E., Debbane, E. G., Bienvenu, J. P., de Carufel, F., & Garant, J. (1986). Relationships between the object focus of therapist interpretations and outcome in short-term individual psychotherapy. *British Journal of Medical Psychology, 59,* 1–11.

Piper, W. E., Debbane, E. G., de Carufel, F. L., & Bienvenu, J. P. (1987). A system for differentiating therapist interpretations from other interventions. *Bulletin of the Menninger Clinic, 51,* 532–550.

Piper, W. E., Joyce, A. S., McCallum, M., & Azim, H. F. A. (1993). Concentration and correspondence of transference interpretations in short-term psychotherapy. *Journal of Consulting and Clinical Psychology, 61,* 586–595.

Silberschatz, G., Fretter, P. B., & Curtis, J. T. (1986). How do interpretations influence the process of psychotherapy? *Journal of Consulting and Clinical Psychology, 54,* 646–652.

Stiles, W. B. (1979). Verbal response modes and psychotherapeutic technique. *Psychiatry, 42,* 49–62.

Stiles, W. B., Shapiro, D. A., & Firth-Cozens, J. A. (1988). Verbal response mode use in contrasting psychotherapies: A within-subject comparison. *Journal of Consulting and Clinical Psychology, 56,* 727–733.

Strupp, H. H., & Binder, J. L. (1984). *Psychotherapy in a new key: A guide to time-limited dynamic psychotherapy.* New York: Basic Books.

CHAPTER

8

The Evidence: Transference Interpretations and Patient Outcomes— A Comparison of "Types" of Patients

John Ogrodniczuk
William Piper
University of British Columbia

Brief psychodynamic psychotherapies are prominent in many treatment settings. One of their central and defining technical features is the interpretation of transference. Thus, the study of the appropriate use of transference interpretations in brief therapies is an important undertaking. Although various definitions of transference, interpretation, and associated concepts have been proposed, *transference interpretation* is commonly understood to refer to the therapist making reference to the patient's reaction to him or her, which is to some extent determined by the patient's previous relationships (Piper, 1993). There seems to be general agreement that interventions that explicitly address the dynamics of the patient's behavior toward the therapist in the here and now (i.e., transference) have a special impact on outcome. Transference interpretations are affectively immediate and compelling. Thus, analysis of the transference makes it possible for the patient (and therapist) to become directly aware of distinctions between what is real in the therapy situation and what is determined in fantasy by past experience. Transference interpretations set in motion a chain of events that are assumed to bring about insight and dynamic change.

FOCUS OF THIS CHAPTER

This chapter presents a review of the research evidence for the use of transference interpretations in brief psychodynamic psychotherapy. We give particular attention to the consideration of the use of transference interpretations with different types of patients. The rationale for considering different types of patients is provided, as well as the research evidence. Finally, we discuss the clinical implications of the research findings and directions for future research in this area.

TRANSFERENCE INTERPRETATIONS IN BRIEF THERAPY

The question of the appropriate use of transference interpretations in brief therapy is a compelling issue. One of the technical innovations of brief therapies is greater therapist activity than in long-term therapies. Limited time creates pressure on the therapist to make transference interpretations earlier and more frequently. Advocates of transference interpretations in analysis and long-term psychotherapy have warned therapists about their overuse and have even questioned their use at all in brief therapies (Gill, 1982; Strachey, 1934). However, proponents of brief psychodynamic psychotherapy recommend that explicit transference manifestations and also allusions to the transference in the patient's material should be identified and interpreted as soon as they appear (Davanloo, 1978; Malan, 1976a; Mann, 1973; Sifneos, 1976). They hold the view that transference interpretations in brief therapy not only can promote symptom relief but also can cultivate lasting characterological change.

Evidence to support the active use of transference interpretations in brief therapy has relied heavily on case reports. In one of the first studies to examine this issue, Malan (1976b) was unable to demonstrate a significant correlation between the proportion of transference interpretations (relative to all interpretations) and outcome. However, he did find a significant correlation between the proportion of transference/parental linking (T/P) interpretations and outcome. Such interpretations indicate the similarity between the patient's reactions to the therapist and the patient's previous reactions to his or her parents. Malan's (1976b) finding was consistent with Strachey's (1934) emphasis on the importance of the patient making a distinction between the analyst and early influential figures as a step in breaking the patient's neurotic vicious cycle. The finding created considerable excitement in the field and inspired attempts at replication that claimed to support Malan's (1976b) finding (e.g., Marziali & Sullivan, 1980). Two further studies that used independent samples of patients and stronger research methodology were conducted by Marziali (1984) and Piper, Debbane, Bienvenu, de Carufel, and Garant (1986). These investigations provided no evidence of a direct relation between transference interpretations and favorable outcome and only weak evidence of a direct relation between T/P interpretations and favorable outcome.

USE OF TRANSFERENCE INTERPRETATIONS WITH DIFFERENT TYPES OF PATIENTS

Apart from considering the general effects of transference interpretations in brief therapies, it is also important to identify relevant patient characteristics that may affect how these interventions are used. Transference interpretations are considered to be anxiety provoking, particularly within brief therapy. To successfully use this technique, it has been argued that the patients need to be highly suitable (e.g., Høglend, 1993). Unfortunately, suitability for these interventions has not been well defined in the literature.

Although very little has been written on this topic, some authors have made attempts to provide recommendations regarding the use of transference interpretations with certain types of patients. For example, Frances and Perry (1983) suggested that transference interpretations in brief therapy are appropriate when the patient has the psychological mindedness to observe, understand, tolerate, and apply transference interpretations. Luborsky (1984) suggested that patients vary in how much supportive or expressive (interpretive) technique they require. He argued that interpretive features (including transference interpretations) should receive greater emphasis for patients with "adequate ego strength and anxiety tolerance, along with the capacity for reflection about their interpersonal relationships" (Luborsky, 1984, p. 90). Meissner (1988), writing on the treatment of borderline patients, used the notion of a borderline spectrum as a guide to therapy. He suggested that the therapist tailor the use of transference interpretations to the severity of pathology in the patient. With patients at the upper end of the spectrum (i.e., those less disturbed), therapy with an intense focus on the transference can be used effectively. For more disturbed patients who use projective mechanisms extensively or who have vulnerable self-esteem, Meissner cautioned that use of transference interpretations, at least early in treatment, can be experienced as a critical attack. For these patients, he suggested a more supportive approach with a holding–soothing function. Some authors (Gabbard et al., 1994; Winston, McCullough, & Laikin, 1993) have also alluded to the importance that the patient's level of object relations may have in moderating the effect of transference interpretations. *Object relations* refers to an individual's pattern of relating to others. They have argued that patients with less mature object relations will be less able to tolerate the frustration and anxiety caused by an intense examination of the therapeutic relationship.

RESEARCH ADDRESSING THE USE OF TRANSFERENCE INTERPRETATIONS WITH DIFFERENT TYPES OF PATIENTS

Relatively little empirical attention has been paid to considering whether transference interpretations are better suited for certain types of patients. This is, in part, a reflection of the minimal attention this topic has received in the theoretical and clinical literature. In the past 10 years, however, there has been a growing interest in examining the issue of patient suitability for transference interpretations. A small number of studies have provided evidence that patient characteristics do interact with transference interpretations in affecting therapy process and outcome. We provide descriptions of seven published studies following.

Study 1

In-session interactions for five patients with personality disorders were examined by Winston et al. (1993). Their study focused on transference interpretations and patient responses as change episodes. They considered how the patients' level of object relations influences the relation between patient responses to transference interpretations and treatment outcome. Short-term dynamic psychotherapy and brief adaptation-oriented psychotherapy were employed. Brief adaptation-oriented psychotherapy focuses on the patient's maladaptive interpersonal patterns, emphasizing their presence in the transference relation. Short-term dynamic psychotherapy places greater emphasis on confronting defenses and resistances and eliciting affect. Treatment length ranged from 27 to 53 sessions. Four complete sessions per case were rated.

Winston et al. (1993) found that patients who had more meaningful recent relationships and less social isolation, that is, more mature object relations, responded positively to active work on the transference. Patients who lacked truly close relationships, that is, less mature object relations, responded to transference interpretations with hurt, anger, and withdrawal. For these patients, the authors suggested that supportive interventions could be used to focus on the needs specific to a primitive level of relatedness (e.g., anxiety over the therapist's perceived disapproval or low self-esteem).

Study 2

Piper, Azim, Joyce, and McCallum (1991) examined the relations between the proportion of transference interpretations provided by therapists and both the therapeutic alliance and treatment outcome for patients with a history of low or high quality of object relations (QOR). These relations were investigated for a sample of 64 patients who had received approximately 20 sessions of short-term, individual, psychodynamic psychotherapy within a controlled, clinical trial investigation (Piper, Azim, McCallum, & Joyce, 1990).

Therapist interventions were categorized using the Therapist Intervention Rating System (TIRS; Piper, Debbane, de Carufel, & Bienvenu, 1987) for eight of the sessions (4, 7, 9, 11, 14, 16, 18, and 20). All therapist statements from each session were assigned to one of nine categories that range from simple utterances (e.g., "MmHmm") to complex interpretations. An intervention was defined as an interpretation if it contained a reference to one or more dynamic components. A *dynamic component* is one part of a patient's conflict that exerts an internal force on some other part of the patient, for example, a wish, an anxiety, or a defense. The TIRS also assessed the type of object (person) included in the intervention. A *transference interpretation* was operationally defined as an interpretation that included a reference to the therapist. Qualitatively, it addresses a dynamic conflict involving the therapist. The TIRS was used to calculate the proportion of transference interpretations provided relative to all interventions provided. The per session mean number of interventions, interpretations, and transference interpretations were 44 (range 16–94), 11 (range 3–23), and 5 (range 0–14). This indicated that the therapists were active, interpretive, and transference oriented.

QOR was defined as a person's enduring tendency to establish certain kinds of relationships with others. Scores range along a dimension ranging from 1 (*primitive*) to 9 (*mature;* Azim, Piper, Segal, Nixon, & Duncan, 1991; Piper & Duncan, 1999). At the primitive end of the 9-point scale, the person tends to react to perceived separation or loss of the object, or to disapproval or rejection by the object, with intense anxiety and affect. There is inordinate dependence on the object, who provides a sense of identity. At the mature end of the scale, the person tends to enjoy equitable relationships characterized by love, tenderness, and concern for objects of both sexes. There is a capacity to mourn and tolerate unobtainable relationships. The sample of 64 patients was divided into high-QOR (≥ 5.0) and low-QOR (< 5.0) groups. There were 32 patients in each group.

Piper et al. (1991) found that a greater proportion of transference interpretations were related to a weaker therapeutic alliance and less favorable outcome for high-QOR patients. Similar associations were found for low-QOR patients; however, they were not statistically significant. Because the study was naturalistic rather than experimental in design, more than one causal explanation of the significant findings was offered by Piper et al. (1991). With regard to the alliance, a high proportion of transference interpretations could have weakened the alliance with subsequent negative effects on outcome, a weak alliance could have prompted a high use of transference interpretations from the therapist, or both could have occurred. Further examination of session material in the study provided evidence that was consistent with both explanations. It was also clear that continuation of a high use of transference interpretations either within or across sessions did not serve to strengthen a weak alliance. As an additional step, they plotted dose-response relations for the proportion of transference interpretations and outcome. An *effective response* was defined as traversing a clinically significant cutoff level for each of several outcome measures for which considerable normative data were available. An effective response occurred for 50% or more of the patients when the proportion was equal to or less than one transference interpretation in every 12 interventions. Piper et al. (1991) believed that the results of the study were sufficiently strong to warrant alerting clinicians to the possibility of negative treatment effects when high proportions of transference interpretations are used with certain types of patients who receive brief therapy.

Study 3

Høglend et al. (1993) conducted a study that examined the relation between transference interpretations and outcome for 43 patients who were classified as either being highly suitable or not suitable for treatment that included transference interpretations. *Suitability* was defined as having a circumscribed conflict and motivation for self-understanding. It was assessed by a group of clinicians who independently rated patients on ten 8-point scales. Highly suitable patients received treatment that encouraged early and persistent focus on transference interpretations, whereas less suitable patients received few, if any, transference interpretations. The therapies for the two groups did not differ on other aspects. All patients received dynamic psychotherapy of brief to moderate length. The total number of sessions varied from 9 to 53.

Høglend et al. (1993) found that persistent analysis of the patient–therapist relationship (i.e., a high frequency of transference interpretations) had a negative effect on long-term dynamic change (assessed at 4-year follow-up) for patients who were deemed to be highly suitable to receive transference interpretations. Patients who received few or no transference interpretations evidenced better long-term dynamic change. The authors concluded that their findings support the traditional position within psychoanalysis that a careful and very moderate use of transference interpretations is more appropriate than use of a high number of transference interpretations from early on in treatment. They recommended that transference interpretations be used sparingly, with great care, and only with the particular needs of the individual patient as the primary determinant. Unfortunately, these conclusions are limited by the fact that patient type and therapist technique were confounded in this study. That is, only highly suitable patients received therapy that provided a high number of transference interpretations and only unsuitable patients received therapy that minimized the use of transference interpretations. Thus, it is not known how unsuitable patients would have responded to the transference-oriented therapy and how suitable patients would have responded to the therapy that abstained from transference interpretations.

Study 4

Høglend (1993) further examined the data from the study just described, this time looking at the relation between transference interpretations and outcome for patients with high or low QOR. He found that for high-QOR patients, a frequent use of transference interpretations was associated with less favorable outcome. For the low-QOR patients, however, there was not a statistically significant association between transference interpretations and outcome. Høglend's (1993) findings, as with the findings of Piper et al. (1991), are counterintuitive and somewhat difficult to explain. Høglend (1993) offered the following explanation. He suggested that the early spontaneous transferences of patients with low QOR might take on a dependent or pathological form that is more evident and, therefore, is more suitable to interpretation. In contrast, patients with high QOR who habitually establish mutual relationships to others, may present more subtle transference cues, thus forcing the therapist to base early transference interpretations more on inference than concrete evidence. A high level of transference interpretations in the absence of concrete evidence may result in a high level of resistance. Piper et al. (1991) also suggested that high-QOR patients might be prone to perceive transference interpretations as criticism.

Study 5

Connolly et al. (1999) examined the use of transference interpretations early in therapy and their subsequent effect on treatment outcome for 29 patients who received short-term, time-limited, supportive-expressive psychotherapy for depression. They were interested in determining whether transference interpretations had a differential effect on outcome for patients with either good or poor interpersonal functioning. Therapist interventions from Sessions 2, 3, and 4 (when available) were classified to determine the proportion of transference interpretations provided. The quality of the patient's current interpersonal relationships was assessed during a clinical interview using a global rating in the Health Sickness Rating Scale (Luborsky & Bachrach, 1974). Patients who scored below 50 on this 100-point scale were classified as having poor interpersonal relationships.

Connolly et al. (1999) found that the association between proportion of transference interpretations and outcome varied as a function of the level of quality of interpersonal relationships. Patients with a low level of current interpersonal functioning showed less favorable improvement in depressive symptomatology with greater proportions of transference interpretations. This finding held even when early symptomatic change was factored into the analysis, thus indicating that high levels of transference interpretations may be causally related to poor treatment outcome for some patients.

These findings are interesting if one considers the proportion of transference interpretations provided in Connolly et al.'s (1999) study. The authors revealed that across all sessions sampled, the average percentage of transference interpretations per session was only .27. This indicates that about one fourth of 1% of all therapist interventions were transference interpretations, meaning that less than one transference interpretation per session was provided. Additionally, 48% of the 29 cases examined had no transference interpretations provided in any session sampled. Yet, despite these very low levels of transference interpretations, the authors found a significant association between their use and treatment outcome. Their findings may be interpreted as providing evidence of the extremely powerful negative effect that these interventions have for some patients.

One obvious difference in the findings of this study compared to the studies of Piper et al. (1991) and Høglend (1993) is that they found that the negative effect of transference interpretations was more pronounced for those patients with high levels of interpersonal functioning, whereas Connolly et al. (1999) found that the negative effect of transference interpretations was more pronounced for those with low levels of interpersonal functioning. This contrast in findings may be partly the result of differences in how the patient's interpersonal functioning was characterized. Piper et al. (1991) and Høglend (1993) regarded the patient's level of interpersonal functioning as a personality characteristic and evaluated the patient's life-long history of interpersonal relationships. Connolly et al. evaluated only the patient's current level of interpersonal functioning. Another distinction between the studies concerns time. Piper et al. (1991) and Høglend (1993) examined aggregated transference scores from across the entire treatment period. Connolly et al. used averaged transference scores from early treatment sessions. A third difference concerns the technical activity of the therapists in the studies. Connolly et al. indicated that only 4.3% of the therapists' average of 125 interventions per session was interpretations. Piper et al. (1991) indicated that 25% of the therapists' average of 44 interventions per session was interpretations. Clearly, the therapists in Connolly et al.'s study were much more active and less interpretive than the therapists in Piper et al.'s (1991) study. Despite these differences, each study highlighted the importance of the patient's level of interpersonal functioning when providing transference interpretations in brief dynamic therapies.

Study 6

The most recent study to explore the potentially differential effect of transference interpretations for different types of patients was conducted by Ogrodniczuk, Piper, Joyce, and McCallum (1999). This study attempted to validate (replicate) the findings of the Piper et al. (1991) study. Ogrodniczuk et al. (1999) examined the relations between the frequency and proportion of transference interpretations provided by therapists and both the therapeutic alliance and treatment outcome for patients with a history of low or high QOR. These relations were investigated for a sample of 40 patients who had received approximately 20 sessions of short-term, individual, interpretive psychotherapy within a comparative clinical trial investigation (Piper, Joyce, McCallum, & Azim, 1998). As in the Piper et al. (1991) study, therapist interventions were classified using the TIRS. The mean number of interventions, interpretations, and transference interpretations per session were 74.3, 14.4, and 3.7, respectively. The patient's QOR was assessed using the QOR Scale (Azim et al., 1991), the same assessment instrument used in the Piper et al. (1991) study. Again, the sample was divided into high-QOR ($\geq$ 5) and low-QOR (< 5.0) groups. There were 10 high-QOR cases and 30 low-QOR cases.

Ogrodniczuk et al. (1999) found significant inverse relations between the frequency of transference interpretations and both patient-rated therapeutic alliance and favorable outcome for low-QOR patients. For high-QOR patients, however, increased use of transference interpretations was associated with more positive ratings of the alliance by both patients and therapists, although these relations were not statistically significant (due to the small sample of high-QOR patients). There was minimal association between transference interpretations and outcome for high-QOR patients.

The findings of this study (Ogrodniczuk et al., 1999) are consistent with the findings of Connolly et al. (1999) and with recommendations from Luborsky (1984) and Gabbard et al. (1994) who have suggested that transference interpretations should be reserved for patients who have the capacity to reflect on their interpersonal relationships (e.g., high-QOR patients). Conceptually, transference interpretations serve the purpose of helping patients understand their interpersonal difficulties as they are currently enacted within the therapeutic relationship. Thus, it is likely that patients with poor interpersonal functioning outside of therapy would have difficulty making use of the therapeutic relationship as a means of understanding their problems. The findings may reflect the negative effect of providing transference interpretations to these patients. When patients are encouraged to work directly with transference reactions, conflictual issues are identified and patient anxiety is heightened. The patient may perceive the therapist's behavior as critical. Unable to tolerate strain in the relationship, an interpersonally immature patient may become more anxious and frustrated. This could lead to the patient becoming disengaged from the working relationship, as well as regressing to a more maladaptive defensive style. Also, because the conflictual issues are interpersonal (between patient and therapist), it is possible that other interpersonal relationships (familial relationships) of the patient may suffer as a result of the patient's negative reaction.

Alternatively, the findings may reflect the therapist's transference interpretation response to a weak alliance, resistance, negative transference, or some other indicator of potential poor outcome among low-QOR patients. Therapists may be especially prone to focus on the transference with patients who do not progress well through therapy. In other words, the therapist could be reacting to the patient's lack of progress with an increased examination of the transference as a way to resolve the impasse and facilitate improvement. Such increased examination could make the situation worse.

The findings of Ogrodniczuk et al.'s (1999) study are clearly different from those of Piper et al.'s 1991 investigation that found an inverse relation between transference interpretations and both alliance and favorable outcome for high-QOR patients but not low-QOR patients. Despite their different conclusions, the two studies may actually complement each other. As indicated earlier, although Piper et al.'s (1991) study highlighted significant inverse relations between transference interpretations, alliance, and favorable outcome for high-QOR patients, a number of similar but statistically nonsignificant associations were found for the low-QOR patients. This was particularly true for the relation between transference interpretations and alliance. In Piper et al.'s (1991) investigation, transference interpretations were inversely associated with alliance and to some extent with outcome for all patients. However, the relations were more pronounced for the high-QOR patients.

It is also important to consider the technical activity of the therapists in the two studies when comparing their findings. Therapists in Ogrodniczuk et al.'s (1999) study were considerably more active yet focused significantly less on the transference. Approximately 6% of the therapist interventions in that study were transference interpretations, compared to 12% in Piper et al.'s 1991 investigation. As Connolly et al. (1999) cleverly suggested, and as illustrated in Fig. 8.1, low-QOR and high-QOR patients may respond differently to different levels of transference interpretations. In Piper et al.'s (1991) investigation, moderate-to-high levels of transference interpretations

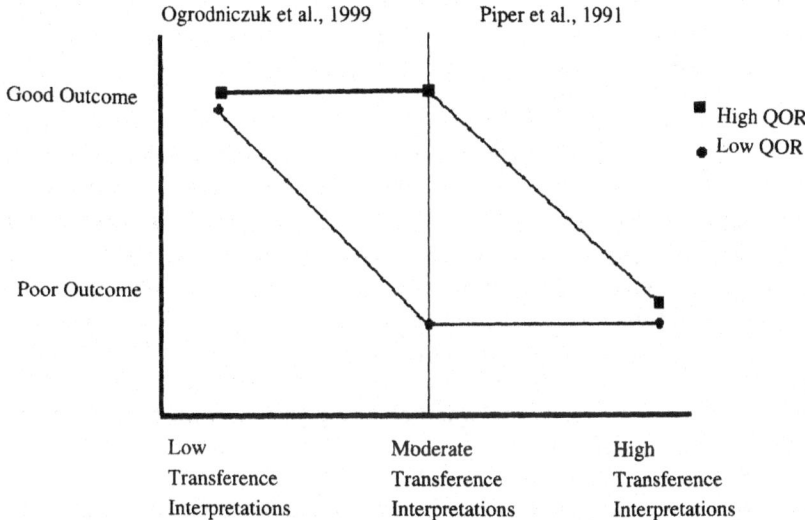

FIG. 8.1. Comparison of the findings of Ogrodniczuk, Piper, Joyce, and McCallum (1999) and Piper, Azim, Joyce, and McCallum (1991).

were provided. Low-QOR patients showed less improvement than the high-QOR patients throughout this moderate-to-high range. With limited variation in outcome scores for the different levels of transference interpretations for the low-QOR patients, no significant associations were found. High-QOR patients benefited from moderate levels of transference interpretations but experienced difficulty with high levels, thus producing the inverse relation for this group of patients. In contrast, Ogrodniczuk et al.'s study examined comparatively low-to-moderate levels of transference interpretations. High-QOR patients benefited from these levels. Low-QOR patients benefited from treatment at low levels of transference interpretations but had less favorable outcome at moderate levels. To summarize, the findings of Ogrodniczuk et al.'s study and Piper et al.'s (1991) investigation suggest that high-QOR patients may benefit from low-to-moderate levels of transference interpretations and only have difficulty with high levels. The benefit of transference interpretations to low-QOR patients may be limited to only low levels at most. Thus, the relation between transference interpretations, alliance, and outcome might not only be a function of the patient's QOR but also of the level of transference interpretations provided.

The following clinical illustration demonstrates the difficulty that low-QOR patients may have when the therapy includes an exploration of the transference. The patient was a 44-year-old woman that was self-referred to the psychiatric outpatient clinic that was the site for Piper et al.'s (1990,

1998) clinical trials. She reported feeling a loss of control over her life and "being in trouble emotionally." The patient received a QOR rating of 3.2, which is on the low end of the continuum. A major theme of the therapy was the patient's history of abandonment and rejection. Throughout the therapy, the patient lamented the many losses in her life and agonized over her inability to find a man to love and take care of her. Between Sessions 14 and 15, her therapist had planned a 5-week interruption. The patient "forgot" to attend Sessions 11 and 13. She was 25 min late for the (prehiatus) 14th session. Given the importance of abandonment in the patient's life and the suspected acting out in reaction to the therapist's imminent departure, her therapist attempted to explore the patient's feelings with respect to the break. The following section presents a segment of Session 14. The patient spent the first 10 min of the shortened session talking about her fear of losing a close woman friend who was becoming serious with a man. She had picked a fight with her friend.

Patient: ... So maybe I'm sabotaging the friendship because I'm losing it.

Therapist: Well, interesting choice of words "sabotaging because I'm losing it." Because of course, I'm going to be away for 5 weeks and is it again a coincidence that you short-changed yourself today by being about half an hour late?

Patient: Yeah.

Therapist: Well, maybe there are some feelings about this relationship ending.

Patient: I don't know. I'm angry with myself again for doing this to myself today and I don't understand why.

Therapist: What about some feelings about me?

Patient: About you?

Therapist: About me or about this situation.

Patient: Again, I don't feel anything negative. I feel I have a lot more work to do in developing the relationship. I don't know, there's still a certain amount of it that feels forced. Like I'm supposed to feel all these things and sometimes I'm at a loss. Well what do I say? And yes, insecurity or being unsure. But it's not enough for me to be aware of ... I tend to forget because I get involved—once I'm involved in a project my memory just goes. I seem to have problems with my memory right now. I attribute it to doing too many things.

Therapist: So maybe there's a feeling of relief that you'll have one less thing to do. You won't have to come and feel like you're on the spot having to give to me what you think I might want.

Patient:	Maybe 1%—but for the most part I know I'm here to help me; not to please you and not to feel uncomfortable. Because basically, why should I be uncomfortable with myself when I'm talking about me? I don't know. I just know I was really upset again 'cause I looked up at the clock and it was 4:05. So I threw everything in my desk and ran out and then I got stuck in traffic longer than I anticipated. My only conscious feeling was one of remorse.
Therapist:	And remorse because I might punish you? Or because you short-changed yourself?—and you really wanted to talk about stuff. Remorse that I might think differently of you? What do you think the remorse is about?
Patient:	Mostly the remorse is short changing myself. That's what I would think it is. Because I'm not seeing you for a few weeks and I know you're going to be away. And again to me subconsciously, this is important to me and it's out of character for me to forget like this but . . .
Therapist:	Well maybe there's also a part of you that doesn't want to open yourself up to the pain and the anger knowing that we can't continue it.
Patient:	I don't know. I could explore it on my own.
Therapist:	Well, maybe the feelings become overwhelming.
Patient:	Well, definitely the anger is so far down there still and I know it has to come up. I know that because it seems like—well, everyone negates my anger so why talk about it? I'd like to call [my friend] and tell her how I feel.
Therapist:	What would you say?
Patient:	That I feel really wronged . . .

In this segment, the therapist explored whether the patient was harboring any feelings regarding the 5-week hiatus. The patient's insight that she may be sabotaging her friendship because she was losing it may have enboldened the therapist that the time was right for this exploration. She wondered if the patient was relieved about the break. She also wondered if there was some reluctance to open up the painful feelings right before the break because there may not be any closure for several weeks. The therapist also explored many possible reasons for the remorse that the patient acknowledged feeling. Despite the seemingly nonthreatening threads of exploration offered by the therapist, the patient could only admit that "1%" of her was anything but remorseful that she had short changed herself of her therapy time. She returned to the safer target of her friend and her anger with her. The therapist relented and allowed the patient to move on.

In the segment, the therapist was exploring the transference. The segment depicted the patient's inability to work with the therapist's transference interventions. It appears that the patient's low QOR interfered with her ability to benefit from the session. The therapist was inviting the patient to see her as yet another person who abandoned her. The patient resisted this association. Initially, she had difficulty with the idea that she might have any feelings about the therapist, asking "about you?" Then, she stated that the whole idea "seemed forced." It is possible that the patient needed to see the therapist as a benign figure toward whom she had no feelings or at least only positive ones. Exploring negative feelings toward the therapist may have been too frightening for the patient.

Study 7

Piper et al. (1999) conducted a study that examined the contribution of different process variables to dropping out of brief psychodynamic psychotherapy. Of particular interest was the effect of transference interpretations. Although the study was not conducted with the intention of determining for which patients transference interpretations were most suitable, it provided important information concerning the use of these interventions in particular situations, that is, when the patient threatens to drop out of therapy prematurely.

To achieve a better clinical understanding of the patient-therapist interactions during the dropout's last session, Piper et al. (1999) listened to audiotapes of each of the last sessions of 22 patients who dropped out of short-term therapy. For the dropouts in the study, the pattern that was observed over the course of the last session was consistent and striking. The pattern was represented by a sequence of nine features. The nine features:

1. The patient made his or her thoughts about dropping out clear, usually early in the session.
2. The patient expressed frustration about the therapy sessions. This often involved expectations that were not met and the therapist's repeated focus on painful feelings.
3. The therapist quickly addressed the difficulty by focusing on the patient-therapist relationship and the transference. Links were made to other relationships.
4. The patient resisted the focus on transference and engaged in little dynamic exploration (work). Resistance was often active, for example, verbal disagreement, and sometimes passive, for example, silence.
5. The therapist persisted with transference interpretations.
6. The patient and therapist argued with each other. They seemed to be engaged in a power struggle. At times the therapist was drawn into being sharp, blunt, sarcastic, insistent, impatient, or condescending.

7. Although most of the interpretations were plausible, the patient responded to the persistence of the therapist with continued resistance.
8. The session ended with encouragement by the therapist to continue with therapy and a seemingly forced agreement by the patient to do so.
9. The patient never returned.

This pattern is illustrated in the following excerpt from the last attended session of a male patient who dropped out of therapy after only six sessions.

Therapist: Let's stick to the feelings 'cause this is what we need to keep working on. Wanting to fire yourself from me or fire me is about being angry.
Patient: Not so much angry as not wanting to waste my time.
Therapist: It's about being angry 'though, with me, we need to be clear.
Patient: I admit, angry at first, maybe but more disappointed that—
Therapist: It's about feelings, let's say that. Let's be clear too that I was saying last week that the fear you have is that I would be like your father.
Patient: No, no, not at all! If I have to work with you, you're a human being first—but I don't see that, maybe that's one of your techniques, you don't show your human side but I can't operate like that. I need to know you're a human being first.
Therapist: What are you feeling right now?
Patient: Oh, so you come back to that (sigh).

The session continued in much the same vein. Finally, the patient announced that he wanted to terminate therapy. The therapist continued to insist that the patient was angry with him and that this was a reenactment of his relationship with his father. Conversely, the patient talked about not trusting the therapist. Eventually, he became quite subdued, no longer initiating any disclosures. The patient's final statement was, "I'll do some hard thinking about it." He did not return. The excerpt illustrates the nonproductive pattern in the last session of many dropouts, characterized by resistance and transference interpretation.

SUMMARY OF FINDINGS

The studies we reviewed focused on a key aspect of therapist technique: the use of transference interpretations in brief therapy. Theoretically, analysis of transference reactions makes it possible for the patient to become directly aware of distinctions between what is real in the therapy situation and what is determined in fantasy based on past experiences. It is regarded as a central process in helping the patient achieve insight and change.

Research has indicated that in the context of certain patient characteristics, higher levels of transference interpretations are associated with negative effects. Piper et al. (1991) and Høglend (1993) found that the associations were stronger among patients with a high level of QOR. In contrast, Connolly et al. (1999) and Ogrodniczuk et al. (1999) found that the associations were stronger among patients with low levels of object relations or interpersonal functioning. Winston et al. (1993) also provided clinical evidence that suggested that transference work was more appropriate for patients with higher levels of object relations. Although the findings of Piper et al. (1991) and Høglend (1993) differ from those of Connolly et al. and Ogrodniczuk et al., they are consistent in highlighting the importance of the patient's level of interpersonal functioning in understanding the correlates of transference interpretations. A fifth study, that of Høglend et al. (1993), examined the use of transference interpretations with patients suitable for such interpretive work. *Suitability* was defined as having a circumscribed conflict and motivation for self-understanding. Despite the apparent suitability of these patients, high levels of transference work were associated with poor long-term outcome. The findings from these studies form a small but growing body of evidence that indicates that there may be limitations in the use of transference interpretations with certain types of patients.

In addition, the study by Piper et al. (1999) suggested that transference interpretations should be used carefully in certain situations, for example, when a patient threatens to terminate therapy prematurely. Clinical observations of last sessions revealed a consistent pattern for many of the dropouts in their study. The patient and therapist appeared to be caught up in an unproductive power struggle that increased the frustration of both. Persistent use of transference interpretations on the therapist's part was not successful in resolving the impasse. Despite considerable clinical experience and success in treating many other patients in brief psychodynamic therapy, the therapist was often unable to avoid countertransferential reactions. After the difficult session, the patient never returned.

CLINICAL IMPLICATIONS

Few studies have examined the use of transference interpretations with different types of patients, and as we have indicated, there are different possibilities for the nature of the causal sequences. Nevertheless, tentative recommendations can be entertained. First, in brief psychodynamic psychotherapy, the therapist should consider avoiding a focus on the transference with patients who have a low QOR, even when the patient may seem highly motivated for self-understanding. Persistent use of transference interpretations may contribute to a weak alliance, poor outcome, and possibly dropping out of therapy prematurely. In the interest of enhancing favorable outcome in brief therapy, therapists should consider providing a low number of transference interpretations to low-QOR patients. For high-QOR patients, low to moderate numbers of transference interpretations appear to be appropriate. High numbers may be counterproductive. It has been suggested that exploration of the transference with all patients (with low-QOR patients especially) be integrated with supportive interventions. As Gabbard et al. (1994) argued, "expressive and supportive approaches are often artificially juxtaposed or polarized when, in fact, elements of both may work synergistically" (p. 66).

Supportive techniques are often considered important tools for the development of a strong working relationship with the patient. It is recommended that a strong alliance be present for the effective use of transference interpretations. As Bond, Banon, and Grenier (1998) described, when the alliance is weak, transference interpretations not only fail to help repair the alliance, but also they increase patient defensiveness and further weaken the alliance. They suggested that a strong alliance is necessary for work in the transference to provide a safe environment for the patient to experience the strong affect that is typically aroused by such work. This sentiment is echoed by Gabbard et al. (1994) who advised therapists to "carefully cultivate and weigh the state of the therapeutic alliance before attempting transference interpretation" (p. 66). They pointed out that effective transference interpretations often follow a series of supportive interventions, which build the alliance and thus pave the way for interpretive work. This is particularly important in the treatment of patients with low QOR who appear to be highly sensitive to transference interpretations.

DIRECTIONS FOR FUTURE RESEARCH

There are several limitations to the studies that we have reviewed, for example, small sample sizes, confounding of patient variables, and therapist technique, which should be avoided in future research. Sample sizes need to be increased to allow the investigator enough power to be able to detect significant relations within the data. Furthermore, because the studies reviewed in this chapter examined only a few patient characteristics, it is important to consider other patient variables that interact with the use of transference interpretations. The field also needs to achieve consistency in the definition and operationalization of transference interpretation. Without this, it is difficult to synthesize the findings from research and make recommendations for clinical practice. Other important considerations include addressing patient behaviors that precede transference interpretations to further examine causal processes involved in patient change. Another issue concerns the use of aggregated data across treatment phases. Use of such data may obscure significant time-dependent associations. For example, the use of transference interpretations early in therapy may have a different relation to outcome compared to their use during a later phase of treatment. There is a need, then, to examine therapist technique at different stages of therapy. Another potential pitfall is artificially isolating transference interpretations when they should be considered as a series of interventions. Thus, it is important to investigate whether different sequences of interventions affect outcome differentially. Finally, as discussed in chapter 7, the accuracy or correspondence, as well as the timing of transference interpretations should be considered. The few studies that have examined these complex issues, which are related to therapist skill, have provided significant findings that have important clinical implications. This work should be encouraged in future studies.

SUMMARY

Transference interpretations are an important feature of brief psychodynamic psychotherapies. Despite their importance, the clinical and theoretical literature provide little guidance regarding the use of these powerful interventions in the treatment of different types of patients. Research, however, has contributed to our knowledge of the appropriate use of transference interpretations. Thus, some tentative conclusions have emerged. These include ensuring technical flexibility in the use of transference interpretations, with the particular needs of patients as the primary determinant. The needs and tolerances of high- and low-QOR patients, for example, may be different and require different technical approaches in their treatment. Only careful exploration of the multiple factors operating simultaneously in treatment, however, will yield information to guide clinicians more effectively in the future.

REFERENCES

Azim, H. F. A., Piper, W. E., Segal, P. M., Nixon, G. W. H., & Duncan, S. (1991). The Quality of Objects Relation Scale. *Bulletin of the Menninger Clinic, 55,* 323–343.
Bond, M., Banon, E., & Grenier, M. (1998). Differential effects of interventions on the therapeutic alliance with patients with personality disorders. *Journal of Psychotherapy Practice and Research, 7,* 301–318.

Connolly, M. B., Crits-Christoph, P., Shappell, S., Barber, J. P., Luborsky, L., & Shaffer, C. (1999). Relation of transference interpretations to outcome in the early sessions of brief supportive-expressive psychotherapy. *Psychotherapy Research, 9,* 485–495.

Davanloo, H. (1978). *Basic principles and techniques in short-term dynamic psychotherapy.* New York: Spectrum.

Frances, A., & Perry, S. (1983). Transference interpretations in focal therapy. *American Journal of Psychiatry, 140,* 405–409.

Gabbard, G. O., Horowitz, L., Allen, J. G., Frieswyk, S., Newsom, G., Colson, D. B., & Coyne, L. (1994). Transference interpretation in the psychotherapy of borderline patients: A high-risk, high-gain phenomenon. *Harvard Review of Psychiatry, 2,* 59–69.

Gill, M. M. (1982). *Analysis of transference: Volume I: Theory and technique.* New York: International Universities Press.

Høglend, P. (1993). Transference interpretations and long-term change after dynamic psychotherapy of brief to moderate length. *American Journal of Psychotherapy, 47,* 494–507.

Høglend, P., Heyerdahl, O., Amlo, S., Engelstad, V., Fossum, A., Sorbye, O., & Sorlie, T. (1993). Interpretations of the patient–therapist relationship in brief dynamic psychotherapy. *Journal of Psychotherapy Practice and Research, 2,* 296–306.

Luborsky, L. (1984). *Principles of psychoanalytic psychotherapy: A manual for supportive-expressive treatment.* New York: Basic Books.

Luborsky, L., & Bachrach, H. M. (1974). Factors influencing clinicians' judgments of mental health: Experiences with the health–sickness rating scale. *Archives of General Psychiatry, 31,* 292–299.

Malan, D. H. (1976a). *The frontier of brief psychotherapy.* New York: Plenum.

Malan, D. H. (1976b). *Toward validation of dynamic psychotherapy.* New York: Plenum.

Mann, J. (1973). *Time-limited psychotherapy.* Cambridge, MA: Harvard University Press.

Marziali, E. A. (1984). Prediction of outcome of brief psychotherapy from therapist interpretive interventions. *Archives of General Psychiatry, 41,* 301–304.

Marziali, E. A., & Sullivan, J. M. (1980). Methodological issues in the content analysis of brief psychotherapy. *British Journal of Medical Psychology, 53,* 19–27.

Meissner, W. W. (1988). *Treatment of patients in the borderline spectrum.* Northvale, NJ: Aronson.

Ogrodniczuk, J. S., Piper, W. E., Joyce, A. S., & McCallum, M. (1999). Transference interpretations in short-term dynamic psychotherapy. *Journal of Nervous and Mental Disease, 187,* 572–579.

Piper, W. E. (1993). The use of transference interpretations. *American Journal of Psychotherapy, 47,* 477–478.

Piper, W. E., Azim, H. F. A., Joyce, A. S., & McCallum, M. (1991). Transference interpretations, therapeutic alliance, and outcome in short-term individual psychotherapy. *Archives of General Psychiatry, 48,* 946–953.

Piper, W. E., Azim, H. F. A., McCallum, M., & Joyce, A. S. (1990). Patient suitability and outcome in short-term individual psychotherapy. *Journal of Consulting and Clinical Psychology, 58,* 475–481.

Piper, W. E., Debbane, E. G., Bienvenu, J. P., de Carufel, F., & Garant, J. (1986). Relationships between the object focus of therapist interpretations and outcome in short-term individual psychotherapy. *British Journal of Medical Psychology, 59,* 1–11.

Piper, W. E., Debbane, E. G., de Carufel, F. L., & Bienvenu, J. P. (1987). A system for differentiating therapist interpretations and other interventions. *Bulletin of the Menninger Clinic, 51,* 532–550.

Piper, W. E., & Duncan, S. C. (1999). Object relations theory and short-term dynamic psychotherapy: Findings from the Quality of Object Relations Scale. *Clinical Psychology Review, 19,* 669–685.

Piper, W. E., Joyce, A. S., McCallum, M., & Azim, H. F. (1998). Interpretive and supportive forms of psychotherapy and patient personality variables. *Journal of Consulting and Clinical Psychology, 66,* 558–567.

Piper, W. E., Ogrodniczuk, J. S., Joyce, A. S., McCallum, M., Rosie, J. S., O'Kelly, J. G., & Steinberg, P. I. (1999). Prediction of dropping out in time-limited, interpretive individual psychotherapy. *Psychotherapy, 36,* 114–122.

Sifneos, P. E. (1976). *Short-term dynamic psychotherapy evaluation and technique.* New York: Plenum.

Strachey, J. (1934). The nature of therapeutic action of psychoanalysis. *International Journal of Psychoanalysis, 15,* 127–159.

Winston, A., McCullough, L., & Laikin, M. (1993). Clinical and research implications of patient–therapist interaction in brief psychotherapy. *American Journal of Psychotherapy, 47,* 527–539.

PART
III

KEEPING AN EYE ON THE RELATIONSHIP

CHAPTER

9

Defining and Identifying Alliance Ruptures

Lisa Wallner Samstag
Long Island University

J. Christopher Muran
Beth Israel Medical Center

Jeremy D. Safran
New School University

A compelling body of empirical evidence has established the therapeutic alliance as a core psychotherapy process that directly contributes to overall patient change across a range of theoretically diverse treatments (Horvath & Symonds, 1991; Martin, Garske, & Davis, 2000). There are numerous theoretical conceptualizations of the therapeutic alliance and several instruments have been developed to measure it. A common feature among them is a description of the general affective quality of the patient–therapist relationship, including the interaction of patient and therapist interpersonal characteristics (e.g., therapist's capacity for empathy, patient's degree of involvement in treatment) in their moment-to-moment collaboration toward agreed on treatment goals (Horvath & Greenberg, 1994).

Over the course of treatment, the alliance is formed as a dynamic interpersonal process. In this process, specific technical treatment interventions (e.g., therapist interpretations or empathic reflections) are integrated and take on meaning within each unique patient–therapist relationship (Butler & Strupp, 1986; Safran & Muran, 2000). The alliance functions both as an early treatment predictor of patient change and as a focus of therapeutic intervention, such as when a breakdown occurs or an impasse is reached between patient and therapist (Horvath & Greenberg, 1994). For instance, an impasse may occur when a therapist is unaware that a patient is dissatisfied with treatment or felt criticized by something the therapist said.

Working through impasses in the therapeutic relationship is considered to be a critical part of the change process, particularly within contemporary, relationally focused perspectives (e.g., Davies, 1994; Ehrenberg, 2000; Safran & Muran, 2000; Stolorow, Brandchaft, & Atwood, 1994). The term *impasse* is used in the clinical literature as a general description of "stuckness" in treatment, although many other overlapping concepts are also applied to this experience. Such overlapping terms include *alliance rupture* or *breach, misalliance, false self, defensiveness, resistance, difficult patient, transference, countertransference, misattunement,* and *empathic failure.* We have adopted the term *alliance rupture* to represent a particular type of therapeutic impasse, the definition and identification of which is the focus of this chapter.

A *therapeutic alliance rupture* is broadly defined as a negative shift in the quality of the existing alliance or as difficulty establishing one. It is thought to be an inevitable event in treatment that is contributed to by both patient and therapist (Safran, Crocker, McMain, & Murray, 1990). The interpersonal nature of alliance ruptures distinguishes the term from other definitions of impasse that emphasize either patient characteristics (e.g., resistance, negative transference) or therapist characteristics (e.g., empathic failure, countertransference reaction). In other words, a rupture is not a phenomenon that is located exclusively within the patient or caused exclusively by the therapist. Rather, a rupture is an interactive process that includes these kinds of defensive experiences as they play out within the context of each particular therapeutic relationship. The difference between intrapsychic and interpersonal conceptualizations of impasse has important implications for the way in which a therapist will intervene toward resolving one.

Aspects of an alliance rupture (e.g., unacknowledged patient or therapist hostility) may not be fully in a participant's awareness, making it a challenge to describe by self-report. To create a comprehensive picture of a rupture episode, we found it important to capture patient and therapist subjective experiences as well as an objective assessment from trained third-party observers using videotaped recordings of sessions. This makes conducting research on ruptures a laborious, expensive, and time-consuming enterprise.

Elsewhere, we (Muran, 2001; Muran & Safran, 2002; Safran, 1993a, 1993b; Safran & Muran, 2000; Safran, Muran, Samstag, & Stevens, 2002; Safran & Segal, 1990) have identified how therapeutic alliance ruptures provide a clinical opportunity to explore and restructure a patient's maladaptive relational schemas and thereby function as an important mechanism of psychological transformation. *Relational schemas* are mental representations of an individual's experience of self in relationships that develop from repeated interactions with caregivers and serve as a guide to what to expect from others in new relationships (e.g., "Others are generally warm and accepting of me," or "Others are often hostile and rejecting of me"). Interpersonal behaviors are expressed in accordance with these expectations in a way that balances the conflicting human needs for both individuation and relatedness (e.g., "I will need to protect myself and not let myself be too vulnerable with others whom I expect to be critical of me"). According to Sullivan (1953), relational schemas or "introjects" develop as individuals treat themselves in a manner that is consistent with the way they were treated by their caregivers and other important authority figures. In the therapeutic relationship, a clinician's behavior should be sufficiently different and not confirm a patient's negative introject and allow for introject change. Research has found patient introject change in brief dynamic psychotherapy to be directly linked to the way in which therapists behaved toward them and that therapists with negative introjects engaged in countertherapeutic interactions (Henry, Schacht, & Strupp, 1986, 1990).

Alliance ruptures also provide an opportunity for therapists to make critical adjustments in technique, as where an impasse is precipitated by the therapist's empathic failure or misattunement to a patient's relational needs. Beginning therapists will often repeat an intervention when a patient responds by shutting down emotionally or by objecting rather than shifting the clinical task to an exploration of how the patient understood that intervention. Here, a kind of "vicious circle" (Horney, 1950; Wachtel, 1982) ensues in which a therapist unwittingly acts in a manner that reconfirms and entrenches a patient's negative introject.

This chapter is an effort to outline, in greater detail and from our perspective, what a rupture is and what it is not. We begin with a brief history of the alliance concept and a discussion of the importance of working with treatment impasses and ruptures. Next, the interpersonal components of alliance ruptures as we currently define them are provided. There are two main components of rupture episodes: misunderstanding events and patient rupture marker behaviors. Descriptions of these components as well as different rupture types are illustrated with clinical examples. There is an overview of therapist facilitative interventions called *metacommunications* that are suggested as a way for therapists to disentangle themselves from vicious circles with their patients and resolve alliance ruptures. Finally, we end with a summary of some research findings from our Brief Psychotherapy Research Program at Beth Israel Medical Center in New York.

ALLIANCE VERSUS TRANSFERENCE VERSUS THE REAL RELATIONSHIP

To understand what alliance ruptures are, it is important to be grounded in the history of concept of the alliance itself. Certain definitions of the alliance emphasize patient or therapist contributions, whereas others support an interactive model of the relationship with both patient and therapist behaviors included in its development and breakdown.

Historically, broad distinctions have been made in the evolution of the alliance between rational and irrational, mature and primitive, neurotic and nonneurotic, and real and transferential aspects of the therapeutic relationship and a patient's ability to cooperate with the analyst in the tasks of treatment. The articulation of a "therapeutic split" in the ego emphasized the importance of the patient's ability to move back and forth between an experiencing and an observing ego in the process of identifying with the analyst and engaging in self-reflection. The term *therapeutic alliance* (Zetzel, 1956) embodied the affective bond or emotional rapport the patient developed with the person of the analyst, and it was thought to be a prerequisite for successful treatment. Zetzel (1956) defined the therapeutic alliance as reflecting positive aspects of the mother–child relationship in which the therapist worked with a patient's capacity to develop an attachment to a primary caregiver.

Luborsky (1976), using the general term "helping alliance" to describe the quality of the therapeutic relationship, labeled this kind of alliance *Type 1*. In a Type 1 alliance, the patient experiences and is able to accept the therapist as warm, helpful, and supportive. Definitions of the alliance that emphasize patient contributions, such as the patient's particular experience of the therapeutic relationship and his or her early relationship history, are most consistent with the definition of transference (e.g., Frieswyk et al., 1986).

The therapist's early relationship history has also been demonstrated to impact on treatment process and overall patient change at termination. Hilliard, Henry, and Strupp (2000) evaluated patient, therapist, and observer ratings of interpersonal behaviors in Session 3 using Structural Analysis of Social Behavior assessments (SASB; Benjamin, 1974), as well as self-report introject assessments from the patient and therapist in their early parental relationships and in the therapeutic relationship. Hilliard et al. (2000) found that both patient and therapist early parental relationships had an indirect impact on overall patient outcome (i.e., change in symptomatology and introject), which was mediated by the therapeutic process (i.e., what the patient and therapist actually did to foster or impede the alliance).

In comparison to the therapeutic alliance and transference, the term *working alliance* (Greenson, 1967) was intended to capture the active, explicit collaboration between patient and analyst who shared in negotiating the treatment tasks in a process that was distinct from transference or unconscious distortion (i.e., the patient's reasonable ego allied with the analyst's analyzing ego). This is consistent with Luborsky's (1976) *Type 2* alliance, based on the joint effort between patient and therapist in overcoming the patient's difficulties and includes the patient's ability to eventually work independently on the tasks that had been engaged in with the therapist.

Finally, the working alliance was also distinguished from the "real" relationship that was forged between the patient and person of the analyst (Greenson, 1967), although this aspect of the therapeutic relationship has not been addressed as fully in the literature (see Gelso, 2002 for an exception). Greenson (1967) considered therapist behaviors that helped forge the alliance, such as degree of openness and genuineness, to be components of the real relationship. However, the real relationship sounds similar to Luborsky's (1976) Type 1 alliance if we include how the patient perceives these therapist qualities and experiences being helped by the therapist. This highlights the limitations of a concept of the alliance that does not consider the interaction of patient and therapist behaviors.

There remains confusion and disagreement regarding the definition of and types of alliance, transference, and real components of the relationship that have important implications for clinical intervention. Some criticisms of the alliance construct include the degree to which the transferential and real interactions between patient and therapist play a role in the overall conceptualization of the relationship. There are implications for how impasses should be handled technically, for example, if the relationship is considered to be based primarily on patient distortion, defense, and transference, or alternatively, as including actual responses of the individuals in the consulting room. For instance, the therapist may deal with an impasse by providing an interpretation of the transference or intrapsychic conflict. However, as Langs (chap. 10, this volume) points out, when a therapist commits a technical error, the patient's response and resulting impasse cannot simply be interpreted as a transference reaction. Ultimately, a model of the therapeutic relationship that does not incorporate both patient and therapist ongoing reactions to each other is inadequate.

AN INTEGRATED VIEW OF THE ALLIANCE AND THE IMPORTANCE OF IMPASSES

The view of impasses or ruptures as manifestations of patients' defenses can be contrasted with a conception of the therapeutic alliance as an ongoing negotiation and collaborative process between a specific patient and a specific therapist. This conception acknowledges the role of therapist "failure." Such a position is rooted theoretically in object relations, interpersonal, self-psychological, attachment, and intersubjective movements that emerged largely in opposition to what was identified as Freud's overly restrictive emphasis on the physiological drives of the individual and inadequate explanation of what occurred in the two-person analytic experience (e.g., Greenberg & Mitchell, 1983).

Indeed, one of the fundamental mechanisms of psychological change, according to Kohut (1984), came via the exploration of the inevitable ruptures between patient and analyst. These experiences were considered to be inevitable because no analyst could always be perfectly empathic or available to a patient. Kohut defined a *rupture* as a break in the therapeutic relationship resulting from the empathic failure of the analyst, which may contribute to the patient's resistance in treatment. Hopefully, the analyst can recognize when this failure occurs and understand the patient's experience of that rupture. Having been understood, then, the patient has the opportunity to increase his or her capacity for self-regulation.

Strikingly, Strupp and his colleagues have shown in their research on brief psychodynamic therapy that impasses reflect hostile exchange sequences between a patient and therapist (e.g., Henry, Schacht, & Strupp, 1986, 1990). These researchers demonstrated in studies beginning in the 1940s that therapist hostile communication, such as even subtle criticism of the patient, is particularly destructive and contributes to poor overall outcome (see Strupp, 1993). Binder and Strupp (1997) emphasized "that negative process is a major obstacle to successful treatment, and its pervasiveness has been underestimated" (p. 121) in the psychotherapy research literature. Bordin (1979, 1994) suggested that severe alliance ruptures could result in premature and unilateral termination by the patient.

To date, a few empirical studies have demonstrated that therapists can address poor alliances in ways that promote improvement in the quality of the relationship (Foreman & Marmar, 1985; Kivlighan & Schmitz, 1992; Lansford, 1986; Safran & Muran, 1996; Safran, Muran, & Samstag, 1994). Incorporating aspects of this literature on impasses and alliance ruptures into a comprehensive description of the therapeutic relationship contributes to an expanded understanding of clinical mechanisms of change and allows for a wider range of responsive and effective interventions.

An integrated view of the alliance also emphasizes the interactive relationship between patient and therapist rather than independent patient and therapist contributions. For example, Gaston (1990) considered the definitions of therapeutic alliance (the affective bond between patient and therapist) and working alliance (the patient's ability to work purposefully in the treatment) to be complementary rather than existing in opposition to each other. This is consistent with Bordin's (1979) conceptualization of the alliance as a dynamic interrelationship of three components that operate across theoretical models of change: the quality of the emotional bond between patient and therapist and how that bond mediates the explicit agreement on the tasks and goals of treatment. The alliance involves both patient and therapist attitudes and behaviors toward the other and expectations of each other in the relationship.

In an overview of such an integrated conceptualization of the alliance, Safran and Muran (2000) highlighted how technical interventions (e.g., interpretation, homework assignment, etc.) take on particular meanings within the context of each patient–therapist relationship matrix: "Any intervention may have a positive or a negative impact on the quality of the bond between the patient and the therapist depending on its idiosyncratic meaning to the patient, and conversely any intervention may be experienced as more or less facilitative depending on the preexisting bond" (p. 14). As such, it is erroneous to consider transference, alliance, and real relationship components of the patient–therapist dyad existing independently. Butler and Strupp (1986) also argued that it is problematic for psychotherapy researchers to consider the relative contributions of specific technique factors (i.e., therapist interventions) separate from the context of common relationship factors (i.e., the alliance). The importance of this ongoing negotiation between the patient and therapist in terms of tasks, goals, needs, and desires is emphasized in Safran and Muran's relational treatment approach (Muran & Safran, 2002; Safran & Muran, 2000).

OPERATIONALIZING ALLIANCE RUPTURES

We define an alliance rupture as being many things. Broadly speaking, a rupture is a complex interpersonal process between a patient and therapist that is often subjectively experienced as a kind of tension within the therapeutic relationship. This tension can range in intensity from subtle to extreme and can take on qualitatively different forms. A rupture is an emotional disconnection between patient and therapist creating a negative shift in the quality of the alliance. This disconnection may be caused by a misunderstanding between patient and therapist regarding the tasks, goals, or frame of treatment (e.g., a patient questioning the usefulness of a task or a therapist pushing his or her own treatment agenda on the patient). It can be related to emotional or relational bond factors (e.g., a patient's mistrust of the therapist or a therapist's dislike of a patient). In addition, it can involve an interaction of technique and relationship factors (e.g., therapist rigidity in the use of interventions can lead to patient frustration and increasingly hostile exchanges). As stated earlier, ruptures are considered to be an inevitable part of treatment and their successful resolution is theorized to be a critical mechanism of psychological change. Ruptures can occur at any time in a therapy, such as at the very beginning of a treatment when the patient and therapist first meet or later within the context of an established and strong alliance. They may emerge as single events or as repeated themes across many sessions. It is important to underscore here that the development of a rupture is always a bidirectional process in which the patient and therapist each play a role.

A rupture is characterized by movement and emotional shifting in the session, typically occurring as a patient begins to feel more vulnerable with the therapist or when a patient is working on something he or she considers particularly meaningful and is thereby experiencing increased emotional investment in that task. A therapist who is insensitive to the patient's increased emotional needs or vulnerabilities may unwittingly cause a rupture. For example, a patient who is beginning to feel more emotionally connected to the therapist and simultaneously vulnerable to rejection due to this increased intimacy might all of a sudden have an angry reaction to the therapist answering the telephone during session, whereas this same behavior was not previously an issue for the patient. At that moment, the therapist was unaware that the patient required his or her undivided attention.

This type of negative therapeutic process in which the therapist is actively participating can be difficult for therapists to identify and manage (Binder & Strupp, 1997). A therapist who is unaware of the occurrence of a rupture in the treatment (e.g., perhaps due to his or her own feelings of helplessness or incompetence) will likely respond in ways that intensify the patient's negative experience, increasing tension in the relationship and prompting subsequent rupture episodes. For instance, if the therapist who answered the telephone in the previous example interpreted the patient's anger as an intrapsychic event or as part of the patient's general relationship pattern rather than understanding the patient's experience of his behavior as rejecting at that moment, he or she would likely come across as critical and dismissing of the patient, who in turn might feel even more misunderstood. If a therapist is aware of a patient's negative reactions and can facilitate the direct expression and exploration of them, an improvement in the alliance will occur: Unresolved ruptures become the vicious circles that may lead to protracted treatment impasses and premature patient termination.

Although a rupture is a particular type of negative therapeutic process, it also marks the beginning of a potential change process or change event in therapy (Rice & Greenberg, 1984; Safran, Greenberg, & Rice, 1988). We define *rupture episodes* as such a change event and have been influenced in our work by the task analytic research model. The task analytic research model identifies observable patient behaviors or markers of some distress (e.g., anxiety reflecting internal conflict) and therapist operations (e.g., specific response to the patient's distress) as two components of a clinical change event.

Our own research on the alliance and rupture-repair cycles in treatment has forced an increasing precision in our understanding of this important clinical phenomenon. The definition and assessment of alliance ruptures has been elaborated from Safran's early work establishing the alliance rupture as a clinical event for empirical study (Safran, Crocker, McMain, & Murray, 1990). Initially, seven themes emerged from the analysis by observers of sessions in which both patients and therapists identified problems in the alliance. These rupture themes included patient (a) overt expressions of negative sentiments, (b) indirect communication of negative sentiments or hostility, (c) disagreement about the goals or tasks of therapy, (d) compliance, (e) avoidance maneuvers, (f) self-esteem-enhancing operations, and (g) nonresponsiveness to interventions (Safran et al., 1990, pp. 157–159). Here, the beginning of a rupture episode was identified as the patient's expression of dissatisfaction with the therapist or some aspect of the treatment, regardless of whether the impasse was initiated by the patient or the therapist. We call this the patient *rupture marker*. A consequence of our ongoing research was the realization of the importance of clearly defining the precipitating rupture experience, as well as explicitly including the therapist's participation in the impasse.

COMPONENTS OF A RUPTURE EPISODE: MISUNDERSTANDING EVENTS AND RUPTURE MARKERS

A *rupture episode* is defined as a constellation of two primary components involving both patient and therapist contributions: a misunderstanding event and patient rupture markers.

Misunderstanding Events

Consistent with the work of Rhodes, Hill, Thompson, and Elliott (1994), we found that identifying a specific misunderstanding event is an important component of the rupture episode and its eventual resolution.[1] A misunderstanding event includes the immediate background (e.g., the therapeutic task in which the dyad was engaged at the moment) and the precipitant or way in which the therapist did something the patient did not need or else failed to provide what the patient needed (Rhodes et al., 1994).

We also found it useful to include as an aspect of the misunderstanding event experiences that occurred outside of the session (e.g., a trauma or loss that leaves the patient feeling emotionally raw) and the impact of accumulated and fluctuating experiences with the therapist (e.g., reaching a

---

[1] We are grateful to Dalia Spektor and Anthea Paterniti for their efforts in clarifying components of the misunderstanding event and rupture episode.

threshold of frustration and expressing anger). These experiences contribute to the patient undergoing a shift in his or her sense of self and requiring something specific or different from the therapist. They are referred to as "patient expectations of therapist" and form a kind of prerupture interpersonal pattern. The way in which a patient interprets treatment events will be a function of his or her expectations of the relationship with the therapist, based in part on early relational experiences with important caregivers. This aspect of the misunderstanding event is consistent with the Core Conflictual Relationship Theme (CCRT) method of case formulation and the components called "expected response of other" and "actual response of other" (Luborsky, 1977; Luborsky & Crits-Christoph, 1998). However, we do not incorporate a patient's general relational history into this part of the misunderstanding event but rather develop a description of the patient's current expectations of the relationship with the therapist based on what is observed and articulated in each session. There can be subtle (and not so subtle) changes in a patient's relationship expectations with the therapist over time and we find that using an abstract and static case formulation as a guide to understanding moment-to-moment interpersonal behaviors often serves to minimize the importance of these fluctuations. Therapists who remain wedded to an initial case formulation of a patient, unable to amend or abandon it in the face of new and specific interpersonal experiences with that patient, run the risk of causing a misunderstanding event.

The following example illustrates the multifaceted, dynamic nature of a misunderstanding event in a rupture episode and how a lack of awareness by the therapist about the significance of the specific event led to the patient terminating treatment.

Ms. D. Ms. D, a bright and successful single woman in her mid-20s, had been in weekly treatment with an older male therapist for about 3 months at the time of the misunderstanding event. She sought therapy for symptoms of mild depression due to generally unsatisfying romantic relationships. The patient was currently involved with a man but was beginning to have doubts about the relationship, and she feared it was going to end unhappily the way most of the others had. Ms. D described the first 2 months of therapy as "ok" but was aware of a nagging sense that the sessions were becoming a chore.

Ms. D came to her session one day after finally ending the relationship with her boyfriend (they had been working on how hard this was for her in the therapy for the last several weeks). She said she looked forward to this session with her therapist, having experienced a shift in her emotions (i.e., she felt "raw" after the break-up) and was aware of "needing" him more than usual. However, the therapist was unexpectedly delayed in returning from an out-of-town trip that day; he was not in his office for the scheduled appointment, nor did he call Ms. D to let her know he was going to be late. The patient finally left the office waiting room after 20 min feeling angry, confused, and upset.

In the next session, the patient was angry about the missed session and the therapist responded to his absence by commenting on how Ms. D "must have felt frustrated." Ms. D reported feeling "pathologized" by him and came away seeing this therapist to be just as disappointing as other men in her life had been. At that point, she made the decision to terminate treatment.

There are actually two examples of misunderstanding events in this vignette. The first occurred when the patient waited alone in an emotionally vulnerable state (the immediate context or background) for the therapist who neglected to inform her of his absence, failing to provide her with something she needed in that moment (the precipitant). The patient was feeling particularly sensitive to loss and rejection because of the recent breakup of her relationship with her boyfriend (patient expectation of rejection by the therapist based on recent experiences with her boyfriend). The patient was angry and considered the therapist to have disregarded her the same way that other men had done in the past (misunderstanding event). Although this kind of situation is sometimes unavoidable in therapy, it could have been utilized to restructure the patient's relational schemes regarding how a particular man (e.g., the therapist) responded to her needs.

The second misunderstanding event in the example occurred in the session following the missed appointment. Here the therapist attempted to empathize with the feelings of frustration he assumed she had (feelings that were consistent with her relationships with other men), but he did not take into consideration specifically how he had contributed to her frustration by not calling her about his lateness. The patient had previous experiences being rejected and disappointed by men, but this man, the therapist, also behaved in a way that was felt by the patient to be rejecting. In the second occurrence, the immediate context was the patient expressing her negative feelings about the missed session. The precipitant was the therapist's inaccurate interpretation about her feelings of frustration (i.e., that she always felt disappointed and frustrated by men). He failed to take responsibility for his role in the first misunderstanding event (the missed appointment) due to his own feelings of guilt for having neglected her and as a result, he created a second misunderstanding event (an unempathic analysis of her pathology). The therapist missed an opportunity here to validate her feelings and to help her begin to disentangle her reactions to men based on previous experiences from those based on her current disappointment in him.

Rupture Markers

The second component of a rupture episode is the patient rupture marker. On the basis of empirical evidence, we identified a number of patient behaviors as rupture markers (see Table 9.1).[2] These are expressions or indications of a patient's distress resulting from an emotional disconnection from the therapist. Patient markers of distress may also serve to push a therapist further away. The rupture marker is a behavioral reflection of the patient's cognitive construal of, and emotional reactions to, a specific event or experience with the therapist that is generally described by patients as an experience of not benefiting from therapy and feeling fundamentally misperceived and misunderstood by the therapist. This experience may be the intensification of a pattern that had begun between the patient and therapist whereby a particular aspect of the patient's self that had previously been inhibited or unrecognized emerges in the treatment (e.g., a increased vulnerability and need for closeness with the therapist or a growing capacity for self-assertion and need for autonomy). In the previous vignette, the rupture markers in the second example were identified as the patient's indirect expression of her anger toward the therapist for not calling her about the missed session. She spoke in a vague and limited way about feeling "upset" that she "traveled all the way uptown for nothing" without addressing explicitly that she was angry at the therapist. In that moment, the patient experienced a conflict between wanting to express her dissatisfaction and fearing retribution in the way of continued rejection by the therapist if she did.

To identify a taxonomy of rupture marker behaviors, therapy sessions from the Brief Psychotherapy Research Program's database at Beth Israel Medical Center (Muran, 2002) were selected for observation based on patient and therapist subjective descriptions of rupture episodes that had occurred. On the postsession questionnaires completed after every meeting (Samstag, Batchelder, Muran, Safran, & Winston, 1998), patients and therapists independently rated whether or not they had experienced "tension" in the relationship at any point during that session and if so the degree and nature of that tension. Additional questions included the extent to which the problem in the relationship was discussed and the degree to which the tension was resolved. We chose sessions for observation that were indicated by patients or therapists or both as evidencing high tension, as these were usually the sessions with the clearest examples of ruptures. Sessions in which the tension was rated as "low" provided ambiguous data.

The rupture marker behaviors listed in Table 9.1 were observed in these patient- and therapist-identified high tension sessions (although it is not

---

[2]We thank Christopher L. Stevens for his suggestion of the rupture behavior checklist used in our coding of rupture-repair cycles.

TABLE 9.1
Three Categories of Patient Rupture Marker Behaviors Found
in Withdrawal and Control Rupture Episodes

Physical behaviors or appearance
  Averting gaze or looking down
  Turning body away
  Crossing arms
  Slumping in chair
  Face falling
  Raised eyebrows
  Furrowed brow
  Wearing overcoat or keeping bag on lap during session
  Restlessness, such as shifting in chair or fiddling with object
  Self-soothing or self-regulating behaviors (e.g., playing with hair)
  Stiffness in body
  Clenching fists or gripping arms of chair
  Wringing hands
  Wearing revealing clothing, removing clothing in suggestive way
  Sexually suggestive sitting positions
  Flipping hair or objects of clothing (e.g., scarf).
  Overly casual sitting positions (e.g., putting feet up on table)
  Touching therapist
  Changing aspects of the physical space (e.g., pulling chairs closer together)
  Eating food
  Glaring
  Refusal to end the session
  Leaving the session early
Narrative manner or tone
  Long silence
  Minimal response
  Refusal to respond
  Changing topic
  Quiet voice
  Loud voice
  Demanding, emphatic tone
  Whining tone
  Use of sarcasm or mocking tone
  Coy or flirtatious manner (e.g., teasing)
  Heavy sighs
  Hisses through teeth
  Interrupts and talks over therapist
  Disregards or dismisses therapist
  Directs therapist (e.g., "you should," "you must," or asks pointed questions)
  Mimics therapist
  Talks directly to recording device
  Laughing at therapist
  Nervous laughter

(Continued)

TABLE 9.1
(Continued)

Narrative content
  Intellectualization
  Denial
  Tangential, vague, or abstract narrative
  Storytelling
  Talking about other people
  Content of narrative mismatched with affective expression
  Overly ingratiating comments
  "Yes-ing" therapist but then responding in contradictory way
  Self-critical statements
  Self-justifying statements
  Helpless, manipulative behavior (e.g., request that therapist call patient to remind about session)
  Passive–aggressive or threatening behavior (e.g., patient making suicidal threats)
  Name dropping, use of obscure references or unusually sophisticated vocabulary
  Criticizes therapist as a person
  Criticizes therapist's competence
  Questions relevance of therapist's interventions or treatment tasks
  Doubts about being in therapy
  Complains about parameters of therapy (e.g., inconvenient session time)
  Complains about lack of progress

---

meant to be an exhaustive list); we then inferred from these behaviors that a patient was in a *rupture state* (i.e., an experience of being misunderstood by the therapist and feeling demoralized and alone). The rupture state is a construct that is not directly observable. The observed patient rupture markers fell into three general categories: behavior or appearance, narrative manner, and narrative content. Typically, there was a clustering of behaviors from two or more of these categories during rupture episodes. For example, a patient who criticized the therapist (narrative content) was also noted to be speaking in a mocking tone (narrative manner) and observed to be wringing his or her hands (physical behavior); a patient responded to the therapist's interpretation with a long silence (narrative manner) during which time the patient looked away from the therapist at the floor and tapped his or her foot nervously (physical behavior).

TWO CATEGORIES OF RUPTURE EPISODES: WITHDRAWAL AND CONTROL RUPTURES

Early on in our research, we adopted the names "withdrawal rupture" and "confrontation rupture" from work conducted by Harper (1989a, 1989b) as part of the Sheffield Psychotherapy Research Studies, describing two distinct types of challenges in therapy. Later, we struggled to distinguish confrontation ruptures, in which patients expressed anger in an indirect and hostile manner (i.e., negative therapeutic process), from a patient's direct expression of negative feelings toward the therapist and open exploration about their impact on themselves and on the work (i.e., positive therapeutic process). Furthermore, we found evidence of patient behavior that was not overtly hostile in nature but was often described by therapists as an experience of feeling pressured or manipulated by the patient to respond in a certain way.

Three subcategories of rupture states were found in our recent observations of rupture sessions (Samstag, Safran, & Muran, 2000): withdrawal ruptures and two subcategories of what we now call *control ruptures,* identified as attacking and blaming the therapist (the former confrontation rupture) and manipulating the therapist. Examples of patient rupture marker behaviors are outlined following. To differentiate ruptures from patient expressions of anger as evidence of good therapy, we used the SASB (Benjamin, 1974). The SASB is a circumplex model of behavior and a system of assessment instruments used for rating interpersonal behaviors on two general intersecting dimensions of affiliation (e.g., ranging from warmth and friendliness to coldness and hostility) and interdependence (e.g., ranging from domineering to submissive). Benjamin made an important distinction in her model between assessment of narrative content (i.e., what the patient and therapist talked about) and therapy process (i.e., the impact of patient and therapists verbalizations on each other).

What seemed to distinguish different patient expressions of anger for us, and emerge as a common element in hostile patient confrontations and manipulative behavior, was the degree of interpersonal control exerted by the patient onto the therapist. This was measured on the SASB with items such as, "Subject (S) takes charge of everything and makes Object (O) follow his/her rules," and "S puts O down, blames him/her, punishes him/her" (Grawe-Gerber & Benjamin, 1989). The SASB was also used to operationalize withdrawal rupture states. Items identifying a withdrawal rupture include "S thinks, does, becomes whatever O wants," or "S defers to O and conforms to O's wishes." Many features of rupture episodes and stages of subsequent resolution processes were operationalized using SASB, and we refer the reader to Safran and Muran (1996), and Safran et al. (1994) for specific findings using this system.

In addition to ratings using these kinds of items to distinguish rupture types, the SASB was used to assess interpersonal complementarity. *Complementarity* is defined as an interpersonal context in which two individuals engage in a back and forth cycle in which each elicits or pulls for certain predictable behaviors from one another. Reciprocity and correspondence are two components of complementarity: Reciprocity occurs on the control axis (dominance elicits submission, and submission elicits dominance) and correspondence occurs on the affiliation dimension (friendliness elicits friendliness, and hostility elicits hostility). Combining the two axes, an example of a complementary transaction would include friendly dominance followed by friendly submission. Ratings on these dimensions reflect ongoing negotiations between patients and therapists in terms of how friendly or hostile they want to be with each other and who will be in control of the interactions. Such moment-to-moment interpersonal negotiations are considered to occur at an automatic level, outside of the awareness of both patient and therapist. The theory of interpersonal complementarity thus provides an explanation for why therapists may sometimes respond to their angry patients with counter hostility or to their passive, withdrawn patients with controlling behavior. This theory has been validated, in part, by studies demonstrating a significant relation between hostile correspondence, or negative complementarity, with both alliance and treatment outcome (Henry et al., 1986; Keisler & Watkins, 1989; Samstag et al., 1999).

Withdrawal Rupture Markers

Withdrawal markers include patient behaviors such as physically moving away from the therapist (e.g., averting gaze, turning body away), verbal disengagement (e.g., changing the topic, long silences, or use of vague, abstract language), and displaying a mismatch between affective expression and narrative content (e.g., patient is obviously tearful but denies feeling anything). Withdrawal rupture behaviors are passive in nature and they can be very subtle and fleeting moments in a session, making them a challenge for therapists to attend to. A slight decrease in the patient's speaking volume or a deep sigh after a therapist's intervention, for instance, can be a clue to a patient feeling misunderstood by the therapist. A therapist who is unaware of his or her patient's dissatisfaction and the meaning of the self-protective stance in the moment may unconsciously repeat the same type of intervention that was not previously responded to by the patient and initiate another withdrawal rupture. According to the interpersonal theory of complementarity, a therapist will be pulled to respond to a patient's withdrawal marker behaviors in a controlling fashion.

In the process of a patient withdrawing from the therapist and the task at hand, the patient may express negative emotions about himself or herself. Drawing a patient's attention to markers of disengaging behaviors is facilitative in resolving withdrawal ruptures (e.g., "I noticed you frowned just now, were you aware of that?"). Insightful patients sometimes notice these behaviors themselves and reflect on their feelings and experiences, often successfully initiating their own resolution processes (e.g., "As I left here last week, I realized I was annoyed that you were not more flexible in trying to reschedule our missed appointment. You must have been some kind of inhibiting force because I was suddenly aware of how I felt when I was outside on the street"). These examples of withdrawal rupture markers are consistent with our original definition of this category (see the description of our rupture research following).

Attacking and Blaming Rupture Markers

Examples of attacking and blaming rupture markers are most evident in the patient's verbal criticisms of the therapist either as a person or in terms of his or her training, qualifications, and technique. A constellation of attacking and blaming rupture behaviors also typically includes physical evidence of the patient's hostility or aggressive state (e.g., gripping the chair arms, clenching fists, or crossing arms) and a hostile, dismissive, or sarcastic manner of communication.

Compared to subtle withdrawal rupture markers, the attacking and blaming rupture marker behaviors are challenging in their power to pull therapists into complementary and reciprocal interpersonal positions. When a patient acts in a hostile manner, for example, it is extremely difficult for a therapist to respond to criticisms and demands in an accepting and nondefensive manner. In other words, it is extremely difficult for a therapist not to respond automatically to a hostile patient with counter hostility. Disembedding or unhooking from this kind of cycle of hostility and control by focusing on the process of communication becomes the therapist's first priority in working through this type of rupture (e.g., "I have the feeling that what I just said seemed to rub you the wrong way"). Interventions that facilitate a disembedding and mark the beginning of the repair cycle are elaborated later in the chapter.

Manipulative Rupture Markers

The effect of manipulative rupture behavior seems to be that therapists feel pulled to shift the role relationship with the patient in some way. For example, a female patient who wears revealing clothing or sits in a sexually suggestive position may be provoking her male therapist to respond in a complementary sexual fashion outside of his clinical role. Patients may act in an overly casual fashion (e.g., calling the therapist by his or her given name in their first meeting) in a manner that pressures therapists to treat them more like friends or colleagues.

Markers of manipulative rupture episodes are also identified as patients acting in a helpless or passive–aggressive fashion. For instance, a patient who indicated he or she might have difficulty getting to an early morning session on time and indirectly hinted that the therapist should do something to ensure the patient gets there, was experienced to be pushing the therapist into occupying a more nurturing role. Similarly, a patient who is overly ingratiating and idealizes the therapist is not allowing the therapist an autonomous, individuated position in the relationship.

A challenge for the therapist in identifying manipulation markers is confronting the gratification the therapist may feel in occupying a particular role with a patient. A therapist may enjoy the experience of a patient being attracted to him, for instance, or may feel relieved to offer some concrete caretaking behavior that temporarily satisfies a needy patient. This is consistent with what Langs (1975) defined as a therapeutic misalliance in which he illustrated how certain patient–therapist dyads paradoxically sought to create misalliances as a method of "symptom relief." He conceived of misalliance as a collusion between patient and therapist to avoid areas that were anxiety provoking for both members of the dyad, including feelings of closeness and intimacy, a denial of separateness through unconscious fantasies of omnipotence and inappropriate gratification, and circumvention of the potentially painful change process through repetition and justification of unsatisfying relationships. Langs considered such an avoidance to reflect major or minor disruption in the alliance and therapeutic work, but the experience was always mutually reinforcing in that it resulted in a temporary feeling of relief or "cure" through shared defenses of the dyad.

The rupture marker behaviors listed in Table 9.1 were not organized by rupture categories because the same behavior might be observed in both withdrawal and control rupture episodes. For example, a patient gripping the arms of his chair may do so to control his anger within the context of an attacking and blaming rupture or as a result of anxiety about how the therapist might respond in the context of a withdrawal rupture. However, a number of rupture marker behaviors do also seem to be characteristic of separate rupture categories. Compliance and passive disengagement through physical and verbal disconnection are common features of withdrawal ruptures, indirect expression of hostility and direct criticisms of the therapist or the treatment are specific to attacking and blaming ruptures, and flirtatious and helpless behavior reflect manipulative ruptures.

Patient–therapist dyads may consistently evidence only one type of rupture (e.g., withdrawal ruptures) or they may demonstrate combinations and patterns of more than one type. It is not uncommon, for instance, to find cycles of rupture episodes occurring in which there is first an attacking and blaming rupture followed by a withdrawal rupture. Patients who express hostility may become anxious about their aggressive impulses and then disengage from the therapist, fearing retribution. Conversely, a series of withdrawal ruptures may contribute to a patient feeling increasingly frustrated, and such an emotional shift may result in the patient expressing hostility toward the therapist in an attacking and blaming rupture or trying to manipulate the therapist through increased helplessness.

The examples of rupture episode components provided to this point primarily reflect experiences in ongoing treatments. The following example illustrates how rupture episodes can also occur at the beginning of a treatment prior to an alliance being established.

Mr. R. Mr. R was a man in his mid-50s who had grown up the eldest of six children. He had undergone a long-term treatment in his early adulthood that he described as helping him gain insight into how his painful experiences of neglectful parents contributed to a general mistrust of others. His therapist became pregnant 4 years into the treatment and she was forced to terminate due to extensive health problems. Years later, the patient responded to an advertisement in a local newspaper describing an innovative, time-limited therapy. Mr. R was accepted into the program, presenting with symptoms of anxiety and stress about a number of changes in his life (e.g., his daughter had recently left for university resulting in a greater focus on his unsatisfying marriage). Mr. R reported feeling hopeful about this new treatment in spite of the lingering resentment he still felt toward his last therapist for abandoning him. The clinic assistant had scheduled the appointment for the initial consultation with the therapist.

On the day of the first session, Mr. R met his new therapist in the waiting room offering her a wane smile and extending a limp hand in greeting. He wrote on the postsession questionnaire that he was aware of a sense of disappointment in response to how young and inexperienced she looked as she approached him in the waiting room. The clinic assistant had told the therapist that this man was very cooperative in completing the paperwork and she thought that he was going to be "a great patient." The therapist was aware of the lukewarm reception she received from Mr. R and focused on working hard to understand his presenting problems in the context of his early relational experiences. The patient called to cancel the next session and did not respond to the therapist's subsequent attempts to contact him.

This patient, as in the example of Ms. D, also presents with a need for something specific from the therapist that for the moment is not being met. The therapist may play less of an active role in this rupture episode, with patient expectations of the relationship with the therapist in the foreground of the rupture episode, but the pattern is similar. Here, the misunderstanding event is defined as the patient and therapist engaged in the task of an initial contact and treatment negotiation (immediate background), how the therapist looked on first impression (precipitant), and an assumption the patient made about the therapist's ability to be helpful and meet his needs based on physical appearance (patient expectation of therapist). The patient was in a highly motivated state at the initiation of the treatment, which reflects the emotional investment component of the misunderstanding event. The patient rupture markers included his weak smile and limp handshake (this was not captured on videotape because the meeting took place in the waiting room, but it was noted by the therapist). This withdrawal rupture episode provided a window of opportunity for the therapist to make the features of their initial interaction explicit and help the patient to voice his feelings of resentment and expectations that she too would leave him.

THERAPIST FACILITATIVE INTERVENTIONS: PRINCIPALS OF METACOMMUNICATION

One of the key principles outlined in the resolution model for disentangling from the vicious cycle that defines the quality of patient and therapist engagement in an alliance rupture and treatment impasse is the process of therapeutic metacommunication. *Metacommunication* was a term first used by Keisler (1988) in the context of psychotherapy and "is synonymous with impact disclosure" (p. 1). It is employed in "an attempt to step outside of the relational cycle that is currently being enacted by treating it as the focus of collaborative exploration: that is, communicating *about* the transaction or implicit communication that is taking place" (Safran & Muran, 2000, p. 108). This approach represents a particular clinical sensibility that emphasizes an ongoing experiential awareness of the therapeutic process as it is created and evolves in a moment-to-moment fashion. The skill of mindfulness (e.g., Epstein, 1995) is cultivated in the tracking of disconnections and fluctuations in relatedness, concentrating on therapist's subjectivity as a way to facilitate the process of metacommunication (Muran & Safran, 2002; Safran & Muran, 2000).

Safran and Muran (2000) outlined three general principals of metacommunication referring to the quality of the therapist's participation with the patient and orientation toward the rupture experience, the focus of the therapist's attention in the context of a treatment impasse, and the therapist's experience of working through an impasse.

First, the therapist should approach the experience with a genuine curiosity, tentativeness, and exploratory attitude, encouraging the patient to collaborate in coming to an understanding of the treatment impasse. Metacommunications are inspired by a subjective experience in the moment and any theme or patterns that emerge in the context of the therapeutic relationship should not be treated as a parallel to outside relationships. For example, a therapist may use her immediate reactions to a patient's presentation as a starting point for exploration of the patient's experience: "I am aware of my attention wandering just now and I wonder if it might have something to do with the way you are speaking. Are you aware of how you are talking at this moment?" Another type of metacommunication may be in the form of a descriptive image the therapist has of the way in which he or she experiences being with the patient that has not been fully articulated: "I am trying to put into words my sense of what is going on between us right now but I feel like it would be easy to say something that would irritate you further." The purpose of these interventions is to initiate exploration of an aspect of the relationship that is not yet fully articulated or explicit. Clarification of the therapist's contribution and acceptance of responsibility for his or her role in the misunderstanding event and ensuing impasse is a particularly powerful aspect of this principle.

Second, the therapist maintains a here-and-now focus on the therapeutic relationship, offering concrete and specific observations about his or her subjective experience of the interaction. Evaluations are made of how patients are experiencing therapist interventions, and degree of emotional closeness between the patient and therapist is continuously assessed. A shift in relatedness toward greater emotional distance may indicate that a particular intervention by the therapist came across as critical, dismissive, or otherwise hindering.

Third, therapists should be aware that their initial attempts to resolve an impasse will often instigate additional rupture episodes. For example, a metacommunication motivated by frustration will serve to intensify the treatment impasse (e.g., a therapist describing the "wall" felt between him or her and the patient may leave the patient with the sense that the wall shouldn't be there). As such, therapists may find themselves reexperiencing the same type of rupture over and over again. This can result in a feeling of hopelessness about the prospects of change, especially during prolonged impasses. The experience of hopelessness is considered to be a part of the process of working through ruptures. The reader is referred to Safran and Muran (2000) for detailed features of these general metacommunication principles, as well as several specific principals regarding the practice of mindfulness in communication using extensive clinical vignettes for illustration.

AN OVERVIEW OF OUR RESEARCH ON ALLIANCE RUPTURES

Our research efforts involve detailed qualitative and quantitative analysis of session process in time-limited relational therapies, describing distinct rupture types and the processes by which these negative shifts or problems in the alliance are resolved by the therapist. In our research program, examples of ruptures were collected from a number of corresponding sources. We use videotaped recordings of therapy sessions for observer assessment, patient and therapist self-report of alliance quality and descriptions of tension in the relationship in the form of postsession questionnaires (Samstag et al., 1998), information from in-depth interpersonal process recall interviews (Elliott, 1984), and descriptions from members of our research group in their roles as patients and therapists.

Videotapes are critical in the assessment of ruptures due to the importance of tracking nonverbal behaviors and the interaction between patient and therapist. Without videotapes of the four sessions with the patient, June, the transcripts of which many of the other contributors to this book analyzed, it was impossible to identify complete rupture episodes. For instance, in Session 8 the patient embarks on a lengthy description of conflicts with her sister, brother, and father, starting out with the patient going to London and ending with the issue of her own happiness. This section is incoherent and difficult to follow. There is a sense that the patient is not giving the therapist any openings, but it is unclear from the narrative alone if the patient is evidencing a kind of defensive avoidance or if this, in fact, was the agreed on therapeutic task. The therapist began the session with a number of directive interventions (e.g., questions such as "Have you changed much since Monday?" and "So were you passive and bottled things up?") that perhaps the patient experienced as controlling. To identify this as part of a rupture episode, we would need to evaluate the nonverbal behavior of the patient (rupture markers) and the quality of interactions between patient and therapist.

Empirically derived models of rupture resolution that have evolved over the past decade are described in three stages of "rational-empirical" validation research (Safran & Muran, 1996; Safran et al., 1994). Different types of ruptures capture distinct conflicts occurring in the ongoing negotiation of the alliance, for example, the tension and conflict experienced in negotiating the fundamental human needs for relatedness versus individuation or agency in both the patient and the therapist (Safran & Muran, 2000).

Two rupture resolution models emerged from this task analytic research: one model for passive withdrawal ruptures and another for active confrontation ruptures, which is a subtype of what we now define as a control rupture (described previously). In both models, patients initially respond to therapists in a defensive way (i.e., the rupture marker). A patient rupture marker reflects a breakdown in the collaboration between the patient and therapist and is manifested as a patient emotionally withdrawing from the therapist or, conversely, as critically attacking the therapist. This is directly followed by the therapist's focus on that moment through friendly and supportive inquiry, empathic reflection, or self-disclosure (e.g., "I noticed that you just sighed ... what is your experience right now?" or "I have a sense of us playing cat and mouse. Are you aware of that?") and then encouragement of the patient's exploration of his or her own experience, expression of any negative feelings toward the therapist, and fears that serve to block or interfere with the exploration of the rupture experience. Finally, in the full resolution model, the therapist encourages direct expression of the underlying relational need or wish (e.g., "I feel so sad and alone and I don't know where to turn"). In the context of withdrawal ruptures, the therapist facilitated a patient's direct assertion of an underlying or unconscious relational wish (e.g., a need for nurturance) in a series of five stages. In the context of confrontation ruptures, a six-stage model outlined the process of encouraging a patient's expression of vulnerability (e.g., a fear of abandonment; Muran & Safran, 2002; Safran & Muran, 2000). Therapists who responded to patient rupture markers with any expressed hostility or criticism did not evidence later components of the resolution models. Instead, repeated ruptures were evidenced in these sessions, provoked by the therapist's misattunement to patient's relational needs and confirmation of negative relational schemas.

A number of reliable and valid observer-rated measures of therapeutic process and content were used in this intensive, single-case research. In addition to the observer-rated SASB and CCRT previously mentioned, we used the Patient and Therapist Experiencing scales (Klein, Mathieu-Coughlan, Keisler, & Gendlin, 1986) and the Client Vocal Quality Scale (Rice & Kerr, 1986) to identify clinically meaningful, moment-to-moment shifts in the sequential analysis of patient and therapist interpersonal behaviors leading to either confirmation or disconfirmation of patients' maladaptive relational schemas. Patient- and therapist-rated alliance and session evaluation measures were also completed after each therapy session.

Two comparatively large-sample studies (Muran, Samstag, Jilton, Batchelder, & Winston, 1997; Samstag et al., 1998) we conducted examined the relationship between evaluations of interpersonal process using an interpersonal adjective scale and overall outcome in cases of time-limited psychotherapy. First, we found that repeated observer ratings of patient and therapist hostile behavior (e.g., the degree to which a participant was "coldhearted" or "impolite") across treatment were significantly negatively related to overall patient outcome (Muran et al., 1997). Degree of friendly behavior in sessions did not have any relation to outcome.

In the second study, we separated patient–therapist dyads in outcome categories (i.e., good outcome, poor outcome, or premature termination) and found that the link between interpersonal process and overall outcome was different depending on the rating perspective (Samstag et al., 1998). From the therapist perspective, and consistent with the previous findings, ratings of patient hostility significantly differentiated the groups (i.e., levels of patient hostility were highest in the dropout condition and lowest in the good outcome group, and no relation between patient friendliness and outcome was found). From the patient perspective, however, the reverse was true: Ratings of therapist friendliness significantly differentiated the three outcome conditions (i.e., levels of friendly therapist behavior were highest in the good outcome condition and lowest in the dropout group), whereas therapist hostility had no relation to outcome.

These studies highlight the often demonstrated relation between interpersonal process and outcome and the importance of assessing multiple rating perspectives. Patients, therapists, and observers experience or view process differently and thereby contribute unique information to an overall understanding of the alliance and alliance ruptures.

Our students have also conducted a number of preliminary studies on patient and therapist reported impasses across different types of treatment. We use the more general term of *impasse* in this type of exploratory research to capture a wide range of difficulties experienced in the therapeutic relationship. For instance, Nagy, Safran, Muran, and Winston (1998) found that therapists consistently reported a greater frequency of impasses (25% to 53%) compared to patients (11% to 38%) in a sample of 75 patient–therapist dyads across three types of manualized, time-limited therapies. They also found that patients and therapists in cognitive behavioral therapy reported fewer instances of impasses compared to ego-psychological and relational treatments.

Other student projects examined the content of impasses reported. Two separate hierarchical cluster analyses were conducted on a sample of 15 patient–therapist dyads in a time-limited, ego-psychological treatment: One evaluated patient-reported ruptures (Jilton et al., 1994), and the other evaluated ruptures reported by their therapists (Paterniti, Samstag, Gorman, & Muran, 2002). The categories of patient-reported impasses (using 100 raters) captured patients' experiences of feeling misunderstood by their therapist (e.g., "feeling judged and incompetent" and "feeling pressured to accept therapist's agenda"), experiencing the therapist as hostile or unempathic (e.g., "feeling attacked and defensive" and "difficulty trusting therapist"), and behaving in an angry or challenging manner with their therapists (e.g., "feeling frustrated and angry" and "being assertive"). Therapist-reported impasses, using a smaller sample of 30 raters, were consistent with aspects of the treatment model, such as therapists most commonly experiencing their patients as "resistant" and "defensive."

Our current research efforts focused on the development of an observer-rated scale of the expanded conceptualization of ruptures and the resolution processes in withdrawal and control types (Samstag, Safran, & Muran, 2000). Preliminary coding with this scale revealed acceptable levels of interrater reliability (Samstag, Safran, Muran, & Stevens, 2002). We are also in the process of testing a procedure in which patients who are demonstrating difficulties developing alliances with their therapists are offered the possibility of switching to a new therapist who has expertise in resolving alliance ruptures.

SUMMARY AND CONCLUSIONS

In general, an alliance rupture is a particular conceptualization of a treatment impasse or misalliance involving both patient and therapist contributions in a complex interpersonal process. It includes features that are outside of subjective awareness but visible to observers, and features that are exclusively the internal experiences of the patients and therapists in the room and only accessible by their self-descriptions. A rupture is also a pattern of relating and disengaging within the ebb and flow of the therapeutic relationship that captures the ways in which the participants negotiate the dialectically opposing, essential human needs they both have for relatedness and individuation.

More specifically, ruptures are experienced as a kind of tension in the therapeutic relationship and are described by patients as a sense of feeling misunderstood, alone, and demoralized: They range in intensity from subtle to severe, in duration from isolated to protracted, and in frequency from few to several; they take on qualitatively different forms with different clusters of patient interpersonal behaviors marking different internal conflicts and experiences of distress; and they can occur within the context of an ongoing treatment and strong alliance or at the beginning of a therapy when the patient and therapist meet for the first time. Clinically, ruptures provide a unique opportunity to explore and reconfigure a patient's relational schemas and maladaptive interpersonal experiences. A rupture is all of these things and as such, it is a challenge to define comprehensively yet succinctly.

Our conceptualization of this important change event has been enhanced by assessment methods that incorporate patient and therapist descriptions of their own rupture experiences and observer ratings of videotaped recordings: Patient and therapist subjective experiences provide information that cannot be witnessed by objective observers, but observers pick up on behavior that is outside of the participants' subjective awareness. Videotaped sessions are a critical part of the assessment process because many of the rupture marker behaviors are nonverbal and could not be rated by audiotape or transcript alone. Increasing specificity regarding the components of a rupture episode—the misunderstanding event and rupture marker behaviors—have helped to further distinguish the breakdown in the alliance from stages of the resolution process. Additional features of withdrawal ruptures and two types of control ruptures (attacking and blaming and manipulative) have been identified through intensive observation and analysis of rupture episodes, deepening our understanding of these distinct clinical phenomena.

The observer-rated Rupture Resolution Scale (Samstag et al., 2000) emerged out of our observational analyses and is in an early stage of development. Future research efforts will focus on the reliable assessment of cycling rupture episodes and effective repair processes, validating our new way of thinking about confrontation and manipulation as control ruptures, and the role these processes play in the evolving therapeutic relationship as a mechanism of psychological change.

REFERENCES

Benjamin, L. S. (1974). Structural analysis of social behavior. *Psychological Review, 81,* 392–425.

Binder, J. L., & Strupp, H. H. (1997). "Negative process": A recurrently discovered and underestimated facet of the therapeutic process and outcome in individual psychotherapy of adults. *Clinical Psychology: Science and Practice, 4,* 121–139.

Bordin, E. (1979). The generalizability of the psychoanalytic concept of the working alliance. *Psychotherapy: Theory, Research, and Practice, 16,* 252–260.

Bordin, E. (1994). Theory and research on the therapeutic working alliance: New directions. In A. O. Horvath & L. S. Greenberg (Eds.), *The working alliance: Theory, research, and practice* (pp. 13–37). New York: Wiley.

Butler, S. F., & Strupp, H. H. (1986). Specific and nonspecific factors in psychotherapy: A problematic paradigm for psychotherapy research. *Psychotherapy, 23,* 30–40.

Davies, J. M. (1994). Love in the afternoon: A relational reconsideration of desire and dread in the countertransference. *Psychoanalytic Dialogues, 4,* 153–170.

Ehrenberg, D. B. (2000). Potential impasse as an analytic opportunity: Interactive considerations. *Contemporary Psychoanalysis, 36,* 573–586.

Elliott, R. (1984). A discovery-oriented approach to significant change events in psychotherapy: Interpersonal process recall and comprehensive process analysis. In L. N. Rice & L. S. Greenberg (Eds.), *Patterns of change: Intensive analysis of psychotherapeutic process.* New York: Guilford.

Epstein, M. (1995). *Thoughts without a thinker.* New York: Basic Books.

Foreman, S. A., & Marmar, C. R. (1985). Therapist actions that address initially poor therapeutic alliances in psychotherapy. *American Journal of Psychiatry, 142,* 922–926.

Frieswyk, S. H., Allen, J. G., Colson, D. B., Coyne, L., Gabbard, G. O., Horowitz, L., & Newsom, G. (1986). Therapeutic alliance: Its place as a process and outcome variable in dynamic psychotherapy research. *Journal of Consulting and Clinical Psychology, 54,* 32–38.

Gaston, L. (1990). The concept of the alliance and its role in psychotherapy: Theoretical and empirical considerations. *Psychotherapy: Theory, Research, and Practice, 27,* 143–153.

Gelso, C. J. (2002). Real relationship: The "something more" of psychotherapy. *Journal of Contemporary Psychotherapy, 32,* 35–40.

Grawe-Gerber, M., & Benjamin, L. S. (1989). *Structural Analysis of Social Behavior (SASB): Coding manual for psychotherapy research.* Unpublished manuscript, University of Bern, Switzerland.

Greenberg, J. R., & Mitchell, S. A. (1983). *Object relations in psychoanalytic theory.* Cambridge, MA: Harvard University Press.

Greenson, R. (1967). *The technique and practice of psychoanalysis.* New York: International Universities Press.

Harper, H. (1989a). *Coding Guide I: Identification of confrontation challenges in exploratory therapy.* Unpublished manuscript, University of Sheffield, Sheffield, England.

Harper, H. (1989b). *Coding Guide II: Identification and classification of therapist markers and withdrawal challenges.* Unpublished manuscript, University of Sheffield, Sheffield, England.

Henry, W. P., Schacht, T. E., & Strupp, H. H. (1986). Structural analysis of social behavior: Application to a study of interpersonal process in differential psychotherapeutic outcome. *Journal of Consulting and Clinical Psychology, 54,* 27–31.

Henry, W. P., Schacht, T. E., & Strupp, H. H. (1990). Patient and therapist introject, interpersonal process, and differential psychotherapy outcome. *Journal of Consulting and Clinical Psychology, 58,* 768–774.

Hilliard, R. B., Henry, W. P., & Strupp, H. H. (2000). An interpersonal model of psychotherapy: Linking patient and therapist developmental history, therapeutic process, and types of outcome. *Journal of Consulting and Clinical Psychology, 68,* 125–133.

Horney, K. (1950). *Neurosis and human growth.* New York: Norton.

Horvath, A. O., & Greenberg, L. S. (1994). Introduction. In A. O. Horvath & L. S. Greenberg (Eds.), *The working alliance: Theory, research, and practice.* New York: Wiley.

Horvath, A. O., & Symonds, B. D. (1991). Relation between working alliance and outcome in psychotherapy: A meta-analysis. *Journal of Counseling Psychology, 36,* 223–233.

Jilton, R., Batchelder, S. T., Muran, J. C., Gorman, B. S., Safran, J. D., Samstag, L. W., & Winston, A. (1994, June). *Content analysis of therapeutic alliance rupture events.* Paper presented at the annual meeting of the Society for Psychotherapy Research, York, England.

Keisler, D. J. (1988). *Therapeutic metacommunication: Therapist impact disclosure as feedback in psychotherapy.* Palo Alto, CA: Consulting Psychologists Press.

Keisler, D. J., & Watkins, L. M. (1989). Interpersonal complementarity and the therapeutic alliance: A study of relationship in psychotherapy. *Psychotherapy, 26,* 183–194.

Kivlighan, D. M., & Schmitz, P. J. (1992). Counselor technical activity in cases with improving working alliances and continuing poor working alliances. *Journal of Counseling Psychology, 39,* 32–38.

Klein, M. H., Mathieu-Coughlan, P. L., Gendlin, E. T., & Keisler, D. J. (1986). The experiencing scales. In L. S. Greenberg & W. M. Pinsoff (Eds.), *The psychotherapeutic process: A research handbook* (pp. 21–71). New York: Guilford.

Kohut, H. (1984). *How does analysis cure?* Chicago: University of Chicago Press.

Langs, R. J. (1975). Therapeutic misalliances. *International Journal of Psychoanalytic Psychotherapies, 4,* 77–105.

Lansford, E. (1986). Weakenings and repairs of the working alliance in short-term psychotherapy. *Professional Psychology: Research and Practice, 17,* 364–366.

Luborsky, L. (1976). Helping alliances in psychotherapy: The groundwork for a study of their relationship to its outcome. In J. L. Claghorn (Ed.), *Successful psychotherapy* (pp. 92–116). New York: Brunner/Mazel.

Luborsky, L. (1977). Measuring a pervasive psychic structure in psychotherapy: The Core Conflictual Relationship Theme. In N. Freedman & S. Grand (Eds.), *Communicative structures and psychic structures* (pp. 367–395). New York: Plenum.

Luborsky, L., & Crits-Christoph, P. (Eds.). (1998). *Understanding transference: The Core Conflictual Relationship Theme method* (2nd ed.). Washington, DC: American Psychological Association.

Martin, D. J., Garske, J. P., & Davis, M. K. (2000). Relation of the therapeutic alliance with outcome and other variables: A meta-analytic review. *Journal of Consulting and Clinical Psychology, 68,* 438–450.

Muran, J. C. (Ed.). (2001). *Self-relations in the psychotherapy process.* Washington, DC: American Psychological Association.

Muran, J. C. (2002). A relational approach to understanding change: Plurality and contextualism in a psychotherapy research program. *Psychotherapy Research, 12,* 113–138.

Muran, J. C., & Safran, J. D. (2002). A relational approach to psychotherapy: Resolving ruptures in the therapeutic alliance. In F. W. Kaslow (Ed.), *Comprehensive handbook of psychotherapy* (pp. 253–281). New York: Wiley.

Muran, J. C., Samstag, L. W., Jilton, R., Batchelder, S., & Winston, A. (1997). Development of a suboutcome strategy to measure interpersonal process in psychotherapy from an observer perspective. *Journal of Clinical Psychology, 53,* 405–420.

Nagy, J., Safran, J. D., Muran, J. C., & Winston, A. (1998, June). *A comparative analysis of treatment process and therapeutic ruptures.* Paper presented at the annual meeting of the Society for Psychotherapy Research, Snowbird, UT.

Paterniti, A., Samstag, L. W., Gorman, B. S., & Muran, J. C. (2002, June). *A typology of therapist reported alliance ruptures.* Poster session presented at the annual meeting of the Society for Psychotherapy Research, Santa Barbara, CA.

Rhodes, R. H., Hill, C. E., Thompson, B. J., & Elliott, R. (1994). Client retrospective recall of resolved and unresolved misunderstanding events. *Journal of Counseling Psychology, 41,* 473–483.

Rice, L. N., & Greenberg, L. S. (Eds.). (1984). *Patterns of change: Intensive analysis of psychotherapeutic process.* New York: Guilford.

Rice, L. N., & Kerr, G. P. (1986). Measures of client and therapist voice quality. In L. S. Greenberg & W. M. Pinsoff (Eds.), *The psychotherapeutic process: A research handbook* (pp. 73–105). New York: Guilford.

Safran, J. D. (1993a). Breaches in the therapeutic alliance: An arena for negotiating authentic relatedness. *Psychotherapy: Theory, Research, and Practice, 30,* 11–24.

Safran, J. D. (1993b). The therapeutic alliance ruptures as a transtheoretical phenomenon: Definitional and conceptual issues. *Journal of Psychotherapy Integration, 3,* 33–49.

Safran, J. D., Crocker, P., McMain, S., & Murray, P. (1990). The therapeutic alliance rupture as a therapy event for empirical investigation. *Psychotherapy, 27,* 154–165.

Safran J. D., Greenberg, L. S., & Rice, L. N.(1988). Integrating psychotherapy research and practice: Modeling the change process. *Psychotherapy, 25,* 1–17.

Safran, J. D., & Muran, J. C. (1996). The resolution of ruptures in the therapeutic alliance. *Journal of Consulting and Clinical Psychology, 64,* 447–458.

Safran, J. D., & Muran, J. C. (Eds.). (1998). *The therapeutic alliance in brief psychotherapy.* Washington, DC: American Psychological Association.

Safran, J. D., & Muran, J. C. (2000). *Negotiating the therapeutic alliance: A relational treatment guide.* New York: Guilford.

Safran, J. D., Muran, J. C., & Samstag, L. W. (1994). Resolving therapeutic alliance ruptures: A task analytic investigation. In A. O. Horvath & L. S. Greenberg (Eds.), *The working alliance: Theory, research and practice* (pp. 225–255). New York: Wiley.

Safran, J. D., Muran, J. C., Samstag, L. W., & Stevens, C. (2002). Repairing alliance ruptures. In J. C. Norcross (Ed.), *Psychotherapy relationships that work: Therapist contributions and responsiveness to patients* (pp. 235–254). New York: Oxford University Press.

Safran, J. D., & Segal, Z. V. (1990). *Interpersonal process in cognitive therapy.* New York: Basic Books.

Samstag, L. W., Batchelder, S. T., Muran, J. C., Safran, J. D., & Winston, A. (1998). Early identification of treatment failures in short-term psychotherapy: An assessment of therapeutic alliance and interpersonal behavior. *Journal of Psychotherapy Practice and Research, 7,* 126–143.

Samstag, L. W., Muran, J. C., Wachtel, P. L., Slade, A., Safran, J. D., & Winston, A. (1999, June). *Interpersonal and attachment perspectives on developing therapeutic alliances.* Paper presented at the annual meeting of the Society for Psychotherapy Research, Braga, Portugal.

Samstag, L. W., Safran, J. D., & Muran, J. C. (2000). *The Rupture Resolution Scale and coding manual.* Unpublished manuscript.

Samstag, L. W., Safran, J. D., Muran, J. C., & Stevens, C. L. (2002, June). *Development of the Rupture Resolution Scale.* Paper presented at the annual meeting of the Society for Psychotherapy Research, Santa Barbara, CA.

Stolorow, R., Brandchaft, B., & Atwood, G. (1994). *Psychoanalytic treatment: An intersubjective approach.* Hillsdale, NJ: Analytic.

Strupp, H. H. (1993). The Vanderbilt psychotherapy studies: Synopsis. *Journal of Consulting and Clinical Psychology, 61,* 431–433.

Sullivan, H. H. (1953). *The interpersonal theory of psychiatry.* New York: Norton.

Wachtel, P. L. (1982). Vicious circles: The self and the rhetoric of emerging and unfolding. *Contemporary Psychoanalysis, 18,* 273–295.

Zetzel, E. (1956). Current concepts of transference. *International Journal of Psychoanalysis, 37,* 369–375.

CHAPTER

10

The Power of Ground Rules

Robert Langs
Mount Sinai School of Medicine

This chapter, devoted to the ground rules of brief or time-limited psychotherapy, is written in circular fashion. That is, the very introduction that you are now reading was developed only after the completion of the working draft of this contribution. The writing, which seemed to have a life of its own, turned out to be an exploration into uncharted lands and brought out a series of unexpected realizations that called for a fresh set of introductory comments. I must say that while I was quite surprised by where it took me, I suspect that what follows will surprise my readers even more, especially those who are unfamiliar with the communicative-adaptive approach on which it is based.

I began to write without preconceived ideas about time-limited treatments. I soon saw that because I have not, in recent years, engaged in this type of practice, I could not write a chapter based on direct observations of this treatment form. Instead, I realized that I would have to fashion a theoretical essay, but it would be one that had an empirical base of its own. It would be developed in light of years of clinical research into the nature, functions, and effects of ground-rule conditions and management of the framework of the usual types of dynamic psychotherapy available today (Langs, 1998).

COMMUNICATIVE-ADAPTIVE APPROACH

The communicative-adaptive approach on which this discussion of the ground rules is based is a relatively new paradigm of dynamic psychotherapy or psychoanalysis (Kuhn, 1962; Raney, 1984). The following are the distinctive features of this approach (Langs, 1993):

1. The human mind has evolved a special set of functions with which to adapt to emotionally charged events (triggers) and their meanings (Langs, 1996). The special set of functions essentially comprise an *emotion-processing mind,* which is a two-system entity, with a *conscious system* whose contents and processes are accessible to awareness and a *deep unconscious system* whose contents and processes are not directly accessible to awareness but reach consciousness through encoded narratives.

2. Many of the most vital and influential aspects of emotional life and psychotherapy are experienced and processed in the deep unconscious system. This is the case largely because many emotionally charged events are too anxiety provoking to be tolerated in awareness.

3. Both the conscious and deep unconscious systems have capabilities for perception, processing (intelligence), assessments of ethical and moral issues, and other adaptive activities. Each system's operations are, however, relatively independent of the other and differ in respect to what is perceived, how it is processed, and the values and standards with which thoughts and actions are judged.

4. An adaptive framework—the study of what patients are coping with—is utilized for listening to and formulating of the patient's material. With this framework, it has been discovered that deep unconscious processes are reflected in narrative communications evident in stories about life experiences and other events, as well as dreams and daydreams.

5. These narrative communications have manifest (directly stated) and encoded (disguised) meanings. Manifest meanings tend to be responses to triggering events outside of therapy, whereas encoded meanings almost always are reactions to triggers that take place in therapy, largely in the form of therapists' interventions. The encoded level of expression deals mainly with the most recent and immediate comments of and ground rule management by therapists. These triggers are a source of considerable anxiety in psychotherapy, which accounts for patients' disguised (encoded) responses to them.

6. To properly decode the encoded or disguised meanings of narratives, a therapist needs to identifying the activating, triggering events that have occurred in therapy. This process is called *trigger decoding.*

The importance of this communicative approach is that it considers that not all patient communications are related to their own presenting problems and the formulation of their maladaptive repetitive interpersonal patterns. Instead, the patient is credited with accurately perceiving the effective and ineffective efforts of the therapist, including the therapist's management or mismanagement of the conditions and rules of the psychotherapy. In short, a therapist can manifest, often repetitive, maladaptive therapy management including maladaptive interpersonal patterns in their work. Patients perceive and process these patterns and make sense of them in the light of their own patterns. It becomes important that therapists engage in trigger decoding to understand the patient's response to the therapist's own frame-related interventions. None of the ideas that I present here can be directly experienced or truly appreciated for their soundness and import unless trigger decoding is undertaken.

Background to the Development of Communicative Approach

Present-day dynamic theories of psychotherapy appear to see the ground rules of psychotherapy as relatively inconsequential in respect to understanding the nature of the treatment process and its outcome. Management of the ground rules or framework of therapy is seldom observed in detail, or linked in any way with the contents of patients' material, or given much serious consideration. The effects of the conditions of treatment and their changes on the dynamics of a therapeutic interaction are afforded little, if any, attention. In addition, manifest or direct observations of issues related to ground rules and their management tend to be thought of as quite unrevealing in terms of understanding the patient's dynamics.

This restricted theoretical vision is seen in the attention or lack thereof given to boundary conditions of therapy. Throughout nature—animate and inanimate, physical and mental—boundary conditions create frameworks for interactions that are a critical determinant of the nature, meanings, and outcomes of the transactions so contained. Indeed, in most circumstances, knowing the status of the boundary conditions tells you almost everything you need to know about what's happening in the interior (Langs, 1999). In most theories of psychotherapy, there is a relative lack of theoretical understanding among psychotherapists regarding the effects of the conditions in which therapy takes place—the rules, frames, and boundaries of treatment interactions (Langs, 1998, 1999)—even though psychotherapy practice may address these issues somewhat pragmatically and unsystematically.

A shift of paradigm is required to move away from formulating patients' material and therapists' interventions based entirely around interpersonal phenomena. It is only with such a shift in paradigm and with it a new way of observing and formulating the transactions between the parties in therapy that the significance of the framework of psychotherapy and a therapist's management of the ground-rule conditions come to the fore and reveal their enormous power and consequences. The shift involves moving to accepting the idea that the parameters of psychotherapy itself and the therapist's management of them consistently impacts on patients and the outcome of their therapies (Langs, 1993, 1998).

Communicative Approach and Ground Rules, Frames, and Boundaries

The two systems of the emotion-processing mind have dramatically different responses to events and interventions in psychotherapy that involve rules, frames, and boundaries. For its part, the conscious mind has a rather casual attitude toward these dimensions of treatment. Consciously, both patients and therapists pay relatively little attention to this area and there is considerable individual variation in conscious attitudes and behaviors in this respect. Thus, to the conscious mind, discussions that claim that ground-rule conditions are critical to the therapeutic experience seem strange and difficult to comprehend.

The picture is very different when one explores the responses of the deep unconscious mind to transactions involving rules, frames, and boundaries. In contrast to the conscious system, this deeper system is almost entirely focused on this dimension of treatment. If therapists examine patient encoded narratives generated in response to frame-related interventions, these narratives will reveal deep meaning in relation to those interventions. In addition, these deep unconscious responses are consistent across individuals and cultures.

From experience in being alert to therapist-created triggers and decoding patient narratives around those triggers, my theoretical position is that there is a single set of ground rules that apply for all patients, that is, that there is a definable, ideal, unconsciously validated framework for all forms of psychotherapy. The empirical evidence for these ground rules is based on the narratives from patients. These narratives can be decoded to determine what impact the ground rules and deviations to the ground rules have on the patient's perception of the process of therapy and of the therapist.

Specifically, patient narratives validate a specific set of rules that constitute an ideal or secured frame for all forms of therapy. Adherence to these rules and conditions evokes encoded images of helpful, wise, caring, and otherwise healing therapists, and adherence is actively healing in its impact. Departures from these rules and conditions evoke images of inappropriate harm, seductiveness, and insensitivity and are actively harmful in their effects. Clinically, whenever a ground-rule issue arises, the patient's subsequent narrative storied material will indicate if the frame change is being experienced unconsciously as constructive and healing (positive and affirming stories will appear) or as harmful and antitherapeutic (negative and harm-related stories will appear).

When the therapist decodes these narratives accurately and consistent with the patient's unconscious processes and conveys his or her decoding or interpretations to the patient, the patient will, with utmost consistency, subsequently provide positively toned narratives that indicate that the intervention—the decoding—is validated unconsciously. If instead the patient subsequently provides narratives that are negatively toned after the intervention, themes are taken to indicate that the therapist's interpretation is inaccurate and the effort at decoding is considered to be invalid.

The method may seem indirect to those not trained in this tradition. However, it is clear that conscious views and experiences of ground-rule interventions vary greatly and deep unconscious views and experiences do not. For example, if a patient needs to change the appointment time, and the therapist complies, the conscious experience is one of compassion and accommodation. Nevertheless, the encoded themes will allude to inappropriate seductions and a lack of stability—and the unconscious experience is quite negative.

Secure-Frame Therapy

The ideal validated framework comprises a set frequency and length of sessions; a set fee; total privacy and confidentiality; the relative anonymity of the therapist with no self-revelations, directives, personal opinions, and the like; the patient saying whatever comes to mind (the absence of censorship); the absence of physical contact; and a group of additional, implied rules such as a soundproofed, private office in a professional building. One final rule is pertinent here: The therapy continues until the patient is relieved of his or her symptoms or chooses to terminate the therapy for that or any other reason.

A therapeutic situation that meets all of these unconsciously sought for conditions is called a *secured-frame therapy* and it has a basic set of features and effects that are common to all such therapies. Secure frame therapy inherently provides sound holding, safety, security, healing, ego reenforcement, psychological strength, and support. It is a frame that is applicable to all therapy forms and situations, and with minor variations, to all types of relationships and interactions. A psychotherapy situation that departs from one or more of these ideal conditions is called a *deviant-frame* or *frame-modified therapy* and it too shares a group of features and effects in common, which are of course quite different from those seen in secured frame treatment settings.

When a Therapist Changes the Ideal Ground Rules

In this context, it is well to be aware that rules, frames, and boundaries allude to what therapists—and patients—actually do in respect to the framework and conditions of a therapy. Frame-related activities are real actions that create real conditions of interacting with real effects in and of themselves. Whenever a therapist or patient moves to alter an aspect of the frame, for example, come late, miss a session, alter the appointment time, go on holidays, change the frequency or duration of sessions, then these serve as triggers. At the level of conscious mind, the therapist or the patient may have unavoidable reasons for altering the frame in some way. However, the effects of these triggers need to be understood at the level of deep unconscious experience where the impact is uniformly negative and harmful. If the therapist is the source of the change, words of apology or regret do not diminish these deep unconscious effects. Indeed, therapists' reassuring verbal communications often contradict their harmful frame-related actions and thereby produce very disturbing mixed inputs for patients. This is seen, for example, when a patient accepts a therapist's explanation for a unilateral change in the time of a session but then alludes to hurtful, manipulative people in his narratives. To compound the problem, if the therapist ignores this unconscious accusation or interprets it as encoded transference distortion—when it actually is an accurate unconscious perception—much harm is done to the patient. Whenever the ideal and universal frame is deviated from, the therapist should be alert to the patient's encoded or unconscious perceptions. The deviations serve as triggers for the encoded, unconscious material and its accurate view of the departure from the secured frame of therapy.

To reiterate, the deep unconscious system of the emotion-processing mind validates and supports only those interventions that have frame-securing qualities. In addition, therapist's values that are consistent with deep unconscious values are far more healing and healthier guides to successful patient adaptations than those that are only consciously wrought. Similarly, unconscious wisdom is far wiser and healing than is conscious wisdom.

What Do Deviations Provoke in the Patient and Therapist?

One needs to understand why the conscious mind accepts a wide range of unconsciously objectionable frame deviations and tends to accept, if not prefer, changes to frames rather than those that are secure. The key to understanding this discrepancy lies with an appreciation of the nature of human death anxieties. There are three forms of death anxiety (Langs, 1997).

Predatory Death Anxiety. Humans experience a full range of physical threats to their immediate survival, including dangers that arise from other humans and other types of living organisms, as well as natural dangers such as earthquakes and tornadoes. They also experience psychological forms of predatory threat. Direct or manifest threats prompt the rapid mobilization of physical and mental resources in preparation for fight or flight. On the other hand, the situation is very different for unconsciously perceived predatory threats, which are mostly psychological in nature. In these situations, there is an absence of a conscious appreciation of the danger and thus no possible fight or flight response—and largely for reasons of unconscious guilt, the unconsciously perceived harm is unwittingly accepted by the patient.

We see then that all departures from the ideal ground rules, frames, and boundaries are experienced deep unconsciously as predatory acts—as psychological forms of harm. Thus, when a therapist establishes a modified framework for a treatment experience as is done for time-limited therapies, he or she activates strong predatory death anxieties in the patient, although the deviating therapist experiences strong predator (causing harm to others) death anxiety as well.

There are two major reasons why patients so often accept deviant frames for their psychotherapies. The first is that these predatory frames satisfy their guilt ridden and rather pervasive needs for punishment; the second is that they are spared much-dreaded secured frame anxieties.

Predator Death Anxiety. This form of death anxiety is distinctly human and the unconscious response to the conscious and unconscious self-perception of damaging others that creates pressures on the conscious system to make choices and engage in actions that are self-punitive and self-harmful. This deep unconscious mechanism appears to have evolved as a way of enhancing survival by helping to curtail the strong, natural human tendency to do harm to others when frustrated, harmed, deprived of food and shelter, in a state of jealously or envy, and the like. As noted, this type of death anxiety can come into play whenever an individual modifies a ground rule, be it therapist or patient.

Existential Death Anxiety. Language has fostered a clear sense of personal identity and the ability to anticipate the future, including the eventual death of all humans and including, of course, oneself. In this way, existential death anxiety became a feature of the human condition and a potentially disruptive force that needed to be mollified lest it interfere with activities needed for survival. The selected solution to this problem was to turn to the use of denial and obliteration in its myriad of mental and behavioral forms.

Perhaps the most prevalent and least appreciated means of denying the inevitability of personal death is the violation of the ideal, unconsciously validated ground rules of relationships and interactions, including, of course, those that are psychotherapeutic. Although as noted, secured frames are optimally and inherently supportive, ego-enhancing, safe, and healing, they also evoke severe and dreaded existential death anxieties. This arises because strict—and I must add eminently sound and unconsciously validated—adherence to the ideal ground rules is limiting and entrapping.

In this regard, it is well to realize that secured-frame therapy, however rare it is, is not only the ideal conditions for therapeutic cure; it also offers the only conditions of therapy that enables patients to express and experience their existential death anxieties in ways that can be interpreted and suitably processed. This type of therapeutic work is essential to coming to terms with these ever present, unconsciously disruptive anxieties and resolving them to the greatest extent feasible. Any therapy that has not helped a patient resolve or make peace with a portion of their existential death anxieties is an incomplete therapy. However, as we shall see, dealing with one form of these anxieties is feasible in time-limited treatments.

THE COMMUNICATIVE APPROACH AND FRAMES IN BRIEF THERAPIES

Applying unconsciously validated insights to short-term therapies is a valid effort because of incontrovertible evidence that whereas conscious views and experiences of ground rule interventions vary greatly, deep unconscious views and experiences do not (Langs, 1998). Clearly, all planned short-term psychotherapies inherently entail a basic departure from the ideal frame as defined—they are fundamentally deviant-frame therapies. Yet just as clearly, with few exceptions, every therapy being conducted in the world today is a deviant-frame therapy as well. One needs to look at the deeper, unconscious reasons for this state of affairs, after which one can explore the implications of the deviant-frame conditions for short-term therapy treatments. Before doing so, however, it is well to be clear that there is no intention here to discredit the time-limited treatment modality. There is an evident tension between the conscious need for this type of psychotherapy and deep unconscious experience—between social need and psychobiological effects. This conflict calls for very careful and unbiased explorations.

Ground Rules and Brief Therapies

Time-limited treatments in which there is a patient–therapist contract that includes an agreed on, limited number of sessions after which the therapy will be terminated, are classified as a distinctive form of therapy largely because they include a condition for treatment that is not part of the usual or more standard therapeutic contract. This indicates that even on the surface—manifestly—short-term therapies are conducted within a framework that is distinctive and likely to have notable effects. This suggests that the question of the influence of framework conditions on the treatment experience and its outcome should be of particular interest to therapists who work with this modified modality of treatment. It follows too that the more we understand about these effects the greater will be our understanding of the conscious and unconscious dynamics of the short-term treatments modality and how they are best practiced to offer an optimal therapeutic experience to the patient within the time constraints.

Applying the template of the ideal or secured frame to short-term psychotherapies then is certain to generate illuminating insights that could easily be verified by any mental health professional who brings the communicative-adaptive approach to his or her short-term therapy work with patients. For it so happens that without engaging in trigger decoding in response to one's own frame-related interventions—a method of linking images to their triggering events and the sole known means of accessing deep unconscious experience—none of the ideas that I present here can be directly experienced or truly appreciated for their soundness and import.

Frame Deviations and Brief Therapies

Time-limited psychotherapy is, as noted, inherently frame modified. In addition, it is almost always accompanied by additional departures from the ideal frame, for example, modifications in total privacy and confidentiality, departures from the relative anonymity of the therapist, and variations in the time and length of sessions. These conditions, as I indicated, foster predatory death anxieties in patients and equally intense predator death anxieties in therapists. Yet also, a forced termination can create a persecutory form of death anxiety that is experienced by both parties that is quite unlike the existential death anxiety seen in secured frame treatment settings.

The mobilization of these deep unconscious anxieties and experiences are observable in the unconsciously selected details of these frame-related impingements that appear in patients' dreams and other narratives. To enable the patient to experience a measure of deep healing in these areas, these narrative themes need to be decoded and interpreted in light of their frame-deviant triggers—the immediate and anticipated frame-deviant interventions of the therapist.

In this regard there is an unexplored and unsolved issue of considerable importance: Can the interpretation of patients' experiences of the impact and consequences of their short-term, deviant frames be sufficient to resolve and lead to deep healing in the absence of rectification of the frame modifications?

Ideally, healing occurs when frame alterations are both interpreted and corrected or rectified. The failure to rectify a frame modification is experienced deep unconsciously as a way of belying and undoing the offer by the therapist of a sound and unconsciously validated trigger decoded interpretation of patients' frame-responsive material. The stark contradiction between word and deed also is experienced as an attempt to confuse the patient and as a reflection of confusion if not madness in the therapist. Nevertheless, many short-term therapies arise because of clear social or financial need or in the absence of available alternative forms of treatment. There is therefore an unconscious appreciation for this aspect of the situation, even though we do not as yet know the extent to which it permits sound healing. Thus, one must appreciate the tension between the deviant frame and its necessity and between the deviant frame and the sound interpretation of its meanings. A great deal of clinical research is needed before therapists fully understand the ramifications of these problems and discover how to best resolve them.

Finally, there's the problem of paradoxical forms of relief from emotional symptoms. Humans are able to respond to therapist-evoked traumas and frame violations with a mobilization of adaptive resources that lead to some measure of self-healing. It is critical then to avoid the assumption that symptom relief has arisen from sound interventions and to determine the actual source of a patient's improved emotional state.

A CLINICAL ILLUSTRATION

A review of transcribed clinical material was made available to the contributors to this book. The transcriptions were from a brief therapy practiced in a hospital clinic where the therapist worked with a team of consultants who refer to each other as needed. This is a common workplace environment throughout the psychotherapy world. When the parameters of this work are compared with the ideal secure-frame therapy that is advocated here, this form of therapy in this location actually entails many frame modifications.

Therefore, the communicative approach impels therapists to analyze the patient's narratives for encoded perceptions about these modifications. However, in the available transcripts there was little in the way of encoded, narrative responses. This is not an uncommon finding in therapies in which a therapist works with manifest contents and surface meanings and tends to be rather active in making comments to his or her patient—comments that preclude the build up of narrative expressions. Indeed, the very characteristics of brief therapies include an active therapist working in a focused manner. Although it is acknowledged that this way of working may be effective within limits, there is also evidence that at times brief therapies are motivated by the therapist's own unconscious predilections. In these circumstances, the therapist's countertransference-based needs will preclude unconscious communications from patients that are strongly critical of the therapist's frame management activities and other interventions.

To demonstrate the communicative approach and its relevance to frame-related modifications, I turn now to a brief excerpt from this time-limited therapy. This excerpt reveals an encoded response by the patient, code named A, who is a young woman with uncontrolled diabetes. She was seen by a female therapist in a nine-session, time-limited therapy for noncompliance with her medical regime. The sessions were recorded and it is possible that prior to the session from which the excerpt came the therapist, without the patient's permission or knowledge, could have talked to the referring physician who works in the same clinic where the patient was being seen. The therapist may have used information received that way in her interventions to the patient. I state this because of what is known about staff protocols in similar settings and also by decoding the excerpt. However, this becomes evident as I explain the technique. Thus, any one or all of these frame modifications could become a trigger around which the patient will encode her unconscious responses.

We are looking at the last few minutes of the second session. The patient speaks of being an avid smoker and there ensues a discussion of her smoking habits, after which the patient mentions that her mother doesn't usually smoke, that her mother claims she never smoked, but actually did smoke before she met her husband (A's dad) and that she now has an occasional cigarette as a way of being rebellious. The therapist says that the patient is rebellious too, and the patient responds that she doesn't hide things much now because she's living on her own. She can smoke in her flat and do what she likes, to which the therapist comments that the patient is in control of things there. The patient agrees with that—she's more in control since she's been on her own. The therapist (T) then says that just before they end, she wonders who A feels most out of control with—is it her "mum" or her dad, or who?

The balance of the session continues:

A: [Responding to the therapist's question] Anyone, at different times. I don't think there's any ... it may be dad one day, my mum the next. There's two, well three including you. Two people I think I can say anything to, and that's my two friends, Sally and Kate.

T: All right, and they're the friends that talk ...

A: But even then, yes ... even, not Sally much, because, no, Sally has been quite open, she openly talks to me and she's been through quite a lot. She's anorectic and she's not happy with her parents, so she openly talks to me. She's an initiator I think, really, she'll openly talk to me, so I opened up more to her than to Kate, because.... Yeah, I will tell Kate things, but not necessarily everything, because, for one thing I know the person she is.

T: Do you feel that she disapproves of you?

A: Not that she disapproves, just that she does know, I think, she's come round when I've been at my mum's and my mum and her have sat chatting. And I'm sitting there thinking, please don't bring up a certain subject, because if she did, I know you're going to say something that I'm not going to want you to say. So, like I know that Sally would never do that. She'd never discuss anything that . . . you know, anything that we say is between the two of us.

T: Kate might not be confidential?

A: Yeah. Something, like you know, I'll still say more than I'd say to my family to her, but I don't trust her.

T: That's another example, just before we finish, of how in your family you're either blanked out or you have your space invaded. And lot's of what's been going on for you is a completely extreme version: Either I trust people, or I don't trust them at all.

A: Yes, that is true.

T: Either your family are completely and utterly quite overbearing and wondering what you're doing and making you do things for them, or they're blanking you out. And you feel. . . .

A: Yeah, I do wonder whether they do that because I get so annoyed at them when they. . . . They know it upsets me when they keep going on at me. If they do they just don't say anything and I feel like something. . . . It's like they think they're doing it for my benefit, but they think they can cross any lines then.

I suggest the following encoded scenario. The patient is responding deep unconsciously to the (possible or likely) therapist's discussions of her case with the referring physician and to the tape recording of her sessions through which the therapy is opened to others—third-party intruders. There's a hint of an unconscious perception that the therapist is not disclosing important information to or is keeping a secret from the patient in the story of the mother's hiding her behaviors in saying that she never smoked.

There follows from the patient an encoded perception about what would constitute a corrective or model of rectification regarding this frame violation that has mitigated against the ideal secure-frame requirement of much-needed privacy of the sessions. I'm referring to the patient's not having to hide things now because she has her own, private space (flat) and that she's freer to do things she likes to do under those conditions (in contrast to her needing to hide things and being less free when others are in her space). This is corrective in the sense that the patient is sending an encoded message to the therapist that she needs a private space where she can freely talk.

10. GROUND RULES

The patient then turns the discussion of being in control of things into a minimal story about whom she can and cannot communicate openly. Although A consciously places her therapist among those with whom she can do this, her encoded story about her friend Kate reveals a deep unconscious perception of the therapist as someone to whom she cannot reveal a great deal to because she has no boundaries about what can and cannot be said to third parties (represented as A's mother). In this context, the trusted friend Sally most likely is an encoded message offering another corrective message to the therapist—to make the therapy private so A can talk to her openly. The invasive actions of A's family, to which the therapist refers to manifestly, actually encodes (represents, symbolizes) disguised perceptions of how the therapist is behaving with the patient by recording what should, ideally, be private, unrecorded sessions and by (possibly) speaking to the referring physician about the patient.

The therapist's interventions are not informed by the communicative approach and therefore missed the accurate encoded perceptions of the frame modifications. Instead, the interventions are aimed solely in relating narratives to the patient's formulation (the Cognitive Analytic Therapy diagram) and of monitoring transference enactments. The effect is to work on the manifest level without attention to what is being encoded by A. The subsequent impact will be based on the therapist's overlooking the patient's needs for a secure-frame therapy.

In this light, one may say that these interventions fail to reflect an appreciation that patients accurately and unconsciously perceive the implications of the framework of therapy made available to them by their therapists. Because these perceptions are valid, it is important to realize that communications from patients should not to be thought of as solely, if at all, related to transferences. In this case, the added understanding of the patient's encoded meanings would alert the therapist to the unconscious implications of her own behaviors—here, her frame violations—and preclude the patient's tendency to deflect the harm that she, the therapist, is doing to the patient onto the patient's friends and family. Put another way, the trigger decoded unconscious meanings of this material would alert the therapist to her frame violations and to the patient's feelings of mistrust of the therapist. In contrast, the reading of A's manifest material holds others, including the patient herself, responsible for what's awry at the moment and the therapist's contributions to this disequilibrium. Manifest content therapists address one world—superficial, self-evident, defensive, denial based, and of little emotional power—whereas trigger decoding therapists address a very different one: deep, truly unconscious, far from obvious, nondefensive, and emotionally powerful.

Finally, it is clear that it is absolutely necessary to engage in a listening process that is organized around triggering events—therapists' interventions—to hear and appreciate encoded meanings. This world of deep unconscious experience and communication goes unheard when a therapist's attention is restricted to the manifest contents of patients' material and their extracted implications. The world of deep unconscious experience is a camouflaged world and a therapist needs to know how to look beyond the camouflage (the disguise) to see what's there but hidden. Put another way, what a therapist sees is based on the lenses the therapist uses—with a lens focused on manifest contents a therapist sees only the surface and the self-evident meanings of patients' material. By adding the decoding lens and using it, a therapist sees an otherwise unseen, nonmanifest world of great power and beauty—and of enormous importance to the basis for a patient's emotional problems and their insightful resolution. These insights also facilitate the therapist's learning from the patient about what constitutes sound therapy.

SUMMARY AND SOME POSSIBLE SOLUTIONS

As this discussion indicates, there's an important place for communicative-adaptive understanding and interpretive work in short-term therapies. Efforts to get in touch with patients' deep unconscious experiences of the therapist and therapy transactions in light of frame-related and other interventions are certain to enhance the therapeutic experience and outcome for the patient. Such efforts will also provide inevitable insights for the therapist that can lead to improvements in practice. This means that therapists should attend to identifying the most active triggers in a given session—whether they're frame modifying or moments of frame securing—and organize, decode, and interpret the patient's narrative material as deep unconscious perceptions of the actual meanings and impact that these triggers are having on the patient.

Subsequently, the therapist should rectify those departures from the ideal frame that can be corrected. This offers the patient (and the therapist) a secured-frame moment of healing and the activation of natural existential death anxieties under conditions that allow for the processing and resolution of those ever-present concerns.

One of the triggers might be the brief or short-term contract of therapy. For some patients, this may need to be changed to one that is open ended, at the patient's encoded request and directives in their narratives. A patient is greatly helped when a therapist is able to recognize and explore the unconscious basis for adverse behavioral effects of a time-limited therapy.

Practitioners of brief and short-term therapies are strongly advised to engage in self-processing activities to deeply understand and resolve the adverse effects of this pursuit where possible (Langs, 1993). Therapists have the advantage of being able to identify and process their own responses to critical triggers related to their work with time-limited patients. Unless a therapist trigger decodes their patient's imagery and brings it into awareness, these encoded perceptions register deep unconsciously in the therapist and their unconsciously perceived predatory quality registers and evokes self-punitive unconscious pressures. The result of this unconscious dialogue between patient and therapist may result in further acting out by the therapist in the form of further frame modifications—an effect that can be precluded only through sound self-processing. For example, a therapist may miss a session for whatever reason and the patient's subsequent narratives may reveal the accurate perception of the harm done by this absence. Unless decoded accurately, further frame modifications may occur such as the patient then being absent for a session to which the therapist then reacts by changing the appointment time.

Valid trigger decoding provides deep insight into the unconscious aspects of the therapy process. In this way, the healing that results from sound interventions serves as a countermeasure against the harm caused by the modified therapy frame. A therapist who conducts unconsciously validated short-term therapies is serving not only his or her patient but him or herself as well.

CONCLUDING COMMENTS

Short-term therapies appear to be a social necessity. This does not mean, however, that they are biologically or psychologically sound or inherently healing for all patients. As I've been indicating, the true nature of their effects needs to be understood in depth so ways of making the short-term treatment experience optimally rewarding and healing for both parties to therapy can be discovered. Their true nature can only be glimpsed by decoding narratives around real-life triggers.

Using insights derived from the communicative-adaptive approach, I have offered a series of ideas and suggestions that not only are likely to seem foreign to the reader but enlightening for how we might adjust technique in the interests of the patient. This approach may arise some anxiety, but a reasonable measure of anxiety is a great stimulus for growth and self-healing and for correcting flaws in how therapists carry out therapy. The reader must first engage in trigger decoding to verify, and even advance, the ideas presented in this chapter. Anyone with the courage and strength to take this step will then, I'm quite certain, be motivated to think carefully about the ground rules, boundaries, and frame of brief and short-term treatments in the light of decoding patients' narratives. These discoveries provide new ways to improve what those treatments can offer to both patients and therapists alike.

REFERENCES

Kuhn, T. (1962). *The structure of scientific revolution.* Chicago: University of Chicago Press.
Langs, R. (1993). *Empowered psychotherapy.* London: Karnac Books.
Langs, R. (1996). *The evolution of the emotion processing mind, with an introduction to mental Darwinism.* London: Karnac Books.
Langs, R. (1997). *Death anxiety and clinical practice.* London: Karnac Books.
Langs, R. (1998). *Ground rules in psychotherapy and counseling.* London: Karnac Books.
Langs, R. (1999). *Psychotherapy and science.* London: Sage.
Raney, J. (1984). Narcissistic defensiveness and the communicative approach. In J. Raney (Ed.), *Listening and interpreting* (pp. 465–490). New York: Jason Aronson.

CHAPTER

11

Countertransference and Its Management in Brief Dynamic Therapy

Charles J. Gelso
University of Maryland, College Park

> *We have begun to consider the "counter transference," which arises in the physician as a result of the patient's influence on his unconscious feelings, and have nearly come to the point of requiring the physician to recognize and overcome this countertransference in himself. . . . Anyone who fails to produce results in a self-analysis of this kind may at once give up any idea of being able to treat patients by analysis.*
> —Freud (1910/1957, pp. 144–145)

With this statement, Freud (1910/1957) placed the concept of countertransference (CT) into the theoretical mix of key constructs in psychoanalytic treatment. Yet Freud rarely addressed this construct over his long career, and in fact the concept was neglected for many years. CT was seen as something that was a hindrance to therapy, something to be done away with. Good analysts were considered to be sufficiently analyzed to the point that their work was not infected by this phenomenon. When seen in this light, it is not surprising that CT attained the status of a taboo topic.

This pejorative view of CT held sway for many years. However, as classical drive and ego analytic theories themselves broadened, and as other models became prominent within psychoanalysis, conceptions of CT also changed. The newer theories had a decidedly interpersonal or relational focus, even though intrapsychic events were still considered fundamental to analytic thinking and work. (See Pine's, 1990, discussion of the different schools of thought under the broad umbrella of psychoanalysis.) These models, which began emerging in the 1950s, more likely viewed CT as inevitable. Furthermore, within these conceptual systems CT was seen as having potential to aid as well as hinder therapy, depending on how the therapist dealt with his or her internal reactions. So broadened, CT has been theorized about with much greater frequency in recent decades, and a number of empirical studies have examined how CT relates to treatment process and outcome. This chapter briefly examines the varying conceptions of CT with an emphasis on the relational perspective. Some distinctions that facilitate an understanding of this complex construct, countertransference, are made, and the concept of CT management is introduced. Research on CT as it relates to treatment process and outcome is briefly summarized. The chapter concludes with clinical examples and suggestions to practitioners.

CONCEPTIONS OF COUNTERTRANSFERENCE

Over the years, it has been possible to delineate four interrelated conceptions of CT. In chronological order, these are the classical, totalistic, complementary, and relational perspectives. As we shall see, each perspective has a certain slant on CT and certain advantages. Each also has inevitable limitations.

The classical view springs from Freud's (1910/1957) beliefs about CT, as it is embodied in the quote given at the beginning of the chapter. CT is seen as, in effect, the therapist's transference to the patient's transference. In other words, it is the therapist's reaction (internal or behavioral) to the patient's transference, rooted in the therapist's own unresolved conflicts and issues. As an example, within the transference the therapist may be experienced by the patient as the uncaring and self-centered mother of the patient's inner world. The therapist consciously or unconsciously senses this reaction, and this stirs the therapist's own unresolved issues around not being a good enough mother, which in turn relate to deprivations the therapist experienced. The transference thus produces anxiety in the therapist. Lacking insight into this conflict, the therapist allays the anxiety by being overindulgent with the patient. In this way, the therapist's needs, rather than the patient's needs, have been taken care of. Such CT reactions obviously do not facilitate treatment and need to be worked through so that they do not become manifested in the treatment hour. Therapy proceeds most effectively in the absence of CT, that is, CT as seen in the preceding example.

What has become known as the totalist view of CT arose in reaction to the perceived narrowness of the classical position. Whereas the classical conception restricted CT to only those situations in which the therapist reacted transferentially to the patient's transference, the totalist conception was that CT included all the therapist's emotional reactions to the patient.

In this way, CT became seen as the totality of the therapist's emotional reactions and was thus equivalent to the therapist's experience of and reactions to the patient—the therapist's "subjectivity," to use Aron's (1991) term. This conception emerged in the 1950s (Heimann, 1950; Little, 1951) and was further developed subsequently (e.g., Kernberg, 1965).

In defining CT in such broad terms, the totalists went significantly beyond the conception of CT as conflict based. CT experiences were no longer something to be done away with, but rather such internal reactions were to be understood in the context of each ongoing therapeutic relationship. If so understood, CT would substantially benefit the patient and the work. Thus, the therapist's inner experience, the CT, often revealed subtle aspects of the patient's life and psyche. In other words, the feelings the therapist experienced with and toward the patient had much to say about how others reacted to the patient, what the patient stimulated in others, how the patient dealt with others, how the patient was treated by significant others earlier in his or her life, and of course how the patient reacted to significant others in childhood. As elsewhere discussed (Gelso & Hayes, 2002), the totalistic position gained support as analytic therapists increasingly worked with and theorized about severely disturbed patients, in particular those with borderline and narcissistic disturbances. When working with such patients, the experience of intense emotional reactions (e.g., hate and rage) is commonplace and perhaps inevitable, and it does not seem to be the therapist's unresolved conflicts that solely cause these intense reactions, according to totalists. Rather, such reactions are stirred to an important extent by the patient, often through primitive defenses, for example, projective identification (see clarification by Gabbard, 2001, and Gabbard & Wilkinson, 1994). It seemed wise to the totalists to consider intense therapist reactions under the broad umbrella of CT. In this sense, it is appropriate to view CT as a more general process and something that can facilitate the therapy process if the therapist is able to understand and use his or her feelings to guide responses to the patient.

Just as the classical view may be criticized for its narrowness, the all-encompassing nature of the totalist conception makes it scientifically suspect (Gelso & Hayes, 1998, 2002; Hayes & Gelso, 2001). It may be scientifically more meaningful to refer to the totality of the therapist's experience with the patient as simply the therapist's experience and reserve the term CT for such experience as it occurs under or is caused by certain conditions, for example, when patient material stirs the therapist's unresolved issues or conflicts with therapist personality factors. If the broad conception is maintained, then it would make sense to divide CT into different types. For example, the interpersonalist Kiesler (2001), dichotomized CT into subjective and objective types. The former refers to the irrational therapist reactions tied to his or her unresolved conflicts, whereas objective CT includes therapist emotional reactions that are expected and natural (not based on unresolved issues) with a particular patient.

A third conception of CT has been referred to as the complementary view (Epstein & Feiner, 1988). CT is seen as a complement or counterpart to the patient's transference or style of relating. Thus, patients "pull" for certain reactions in therapists, and therapists experience the impulse to respond to these pulls in certain ways. This conception was best articulated a number of years ago by Racker (1957, 1968) and is evident in modern interpersonal theory (Butler, Flasher, & Strupp, 1993; Kiesler, 2001; Levenson, 1995). Racker's (1957/1968) "law of tallion," for example, specifies that every positive transference is met with a positive CT, and every negative transference is met with a negative CT. Thus, the patient's transference and other material pull for accompanying therapist reactions. However, the effective therapist does not simply act out these reactions—does not act out *lex talionis* ("an eye for an eye, a tooth for a tooth"). Instead, he or she seeks to understand the dynamics within himself or herself and the patient and respond in ways that best facilitate the treatment process.

Although the complementary or counterpart view of CT captures the interpersonal aspect of CT better than the other conceptions, it too is limited. The focus on CT as pulls on the therapist originating in the patient's material or style does not take into account the therapist's defenses, unresolved conflicts, and more broadly, personality. In a word, it tends to ignore what the therapist brings to the table and how the therapist, along with the patient, cocreates relationship dynamics.

The *relational* conception of CT (e.g., Aron, 1996; Greenberg & Mitchell, 1983; Mitchell, 1988, 1997) is very similar to the complementary one but seeks more so to capture the deeply interactive nature of the CT. Originating more broadly from object relations theory, the relational perspective is often referred to as a two-person theory in contrast to more classical psychoanalytic theories that are viewed as one-person theories. Classical theories tend to view much of the therapeutic process as originating from the patient's defenses and psychopathology, with the effective therapist serving as a kind of empathic but neutral observer, one who stays outside of the patient's issues and offers well-timed, sensitive interpretations. The relational theorists, on the other hand, stress that whatever happens between therapist and patient is coconstructed. Both therapist and patient shape the nature of the transference, and the CT also is a joint creation. CT then is a product of the inevitable interaction of the patient's dynamics (including transference and other material) and the therapist's dynamics (including unresolved conflicts, personality patterns, needs, etc.).

One difficulty with this two-person perspective is the flip side of its very strength. That is, in its emphasis on cocreation, the fact that each person brings his or her own set of dynamics to the relationship may be neglected. Similarly, each person will behave in similar ways across relationships, and there is a core of each person (or a set of interconnected traits) that dictates this. Indeed, people who do not have this core, and who change extensively to fit the dictates of every situation and relationship, are seen as psychologically unhealthy in one way or another.

Although there is a difference in degree, it appears that psychoanalytic theorists from diverse persuasions now share some key relational propositions. For example, as Gabbard (2001) pointed out, most now agree that CT is always a joint creation involving contributions from both patient and therapist. Gabbard (2001) further stated that

> There is a remarkable degree of agreement that what the patient projects onto the clinician and what the clinician brings to the situation are both relevant to the end result of countertransference. There is also widespread agreement that the patient will inevitably attempt to transform the therapist into a transference object. The therapist then must work diligently to find a way out of the transference–countertransference enactment or projected role that the patient thrusts upon him or her. (p. 989)

There is also now general agreement that CT can be both a hindrance and an aid to treatment, depending on the extent to which the therapist gains insight into it and how the therapist deals with it in the work. Yet there remains one key source of contention among the different viewpoints: the extent to which the therapist's own unresolved conflicts are implicated. Although the therapist's subjective experience is always involved, and although all of this subjectivity is important, it may be best scientifically and clinically to restrict the definition of CT to those situations in which the therapist's personality and unresolved conflicts are implicated in one way or another (Gelso & Hayes, 1998, 2002). Otherwise one would need to divide CT into two types, as noted previously (Kiesler, 2001), or understand that CT is equivalent to the therapist's emotional experience or subjectivity (Aron, 1991). In the latter case, the term CT ceases to be especially meaningful. One could simply refer to the therapist's internal experience or subjectivity. However, clinical theorists would then likely have to come up with some new term (some variant of countertransference?) to capture situations in which the therapist's unresolved issues are implicated in his or her reactions! Be that as it may, what seems most important is that theorists, researchers, and clinicians be clear on the CT perspective they are employing. As I have elsewhere noted (Gelso & Hayes, 2002), it is too often unclear which of the conceptions, or which combination, is being used, and the conception often shifts, even within the same discussion!

SOME FURTHER DISTINCTIONS

An understanding of CT and its use in therapy is aided by some key distinctions that are a part of the literature on the complex construct.

Acute Versus Chronic Countertransference

This distinction was first made by Reich (1951). Acute CT refers to therapist responses made "under specific circumstances with specific patients" (Reich, 1951, p. 26). Reich asserted that this type of CT was based on the analyst's identification with the patient. For example, the patient's current relational struggles that stem from early trauma with a punitive father trigger the therapist's issues with her own father. As a consequence, the therapist identifies with the patient's struggles and becomes overly directive about the patient's need to be assertive in current relationships. Acute CT may reflect many therapist needs and may go well beyond identification. The basic point is that something in the patient's transference or nontransference communication hits on a soft spot in the therapist and stirs anxiety. What the therapist does with this anxiety will then affect the interaction for better or worse.

Chronic CT, on the other hand, reflects an ongoing need of the therapist that is part of his or her personality structure. It represents the unresolved issues that cut across patients and is manifested in essentially all of the therapist's work. A somewhat typical example of such chronic CT is the therapist who is excessively gratifying to all patients as a way of protecting from consciousness the therapist's experience of being chronically neglected in childhood. Other examples would be the highly active therapist whose excessive activity represents a defense against passive longings; the therapist who sees aggression everywhere as a defense against his or her own feared aggression; or the therapist who pushes patients too hard to improve out of the therapist's own achievement issues. It is true that patient transferences and other material may serve as a trigger to chronic CT, but such CTs are a "reaction waiting to happen" (Gelso & Hayes, 2002).

Countertransference as Internal State Versus Overt Expression

CT may be manifested in a wide range of ways, some representing the internal experience of the therapist and others representing overt behaviors. As an internal experience, CT may show itself as therapist anxiety, failure to recall clinical material, feelings states ranging from highly negative to highly positive, or the extremes of emotional intensity ranging from very high intensity to emotional flatness. Regarding overt behavior, therapist actions representing withdrawal, avoidance, or at times overinvolvement have often been studied empirically. Generally, overt CT behavior is seen is hindering treatment because it gratifies the therapist's needs, for example, through defending against anxiety, rather than providing what is needed to the patient. Internal CT, however, can aid the work if the therapist is able to understand his or her experience and grasp how this relates to the patient's inner life and behavior. From a relational perspective, the therapist continually seeks to understand how his or her inner experience comes from both what the patient stirs and what the therapist brings to the treatment hour.

Countertransference as Projection Versus Emotional Reaction

As is the case with both transference and CT, feelings, attitudes, and impulses connected to significant others early in one's life are often displaced and projected onto the other in the dyad. However, in many or perhaps most cases there is not a one-to-one connection between the current person and a single figure in the past. With respect to CT, it seems to be more often the case that material from the patient touches on areas of unresolved conflict, which arouses defensive reactions in the therapist. For example, the critical, hard-to-please patient may stir in the therapist unresolved conflicts around being not good enough. Although these feelings likely have their basis in early significant relationships, it does not seem to be the case that those early objects (e.g., the punitive and hard-to-please mother or father) are displaced or projected onto the patient. More likely, feelings about not being good enough get aroused in the therapist, and these are dealt with in either therapeutic or countertherapeutic ways in the treatment. The vastly different roles of therapist and patient are likely implicated centrally in the differing ways in which transference and CT operate. Because the patient is in the help-receiving role, he or she is more likely to make projections onto the therapist from significant others who were responsible for the patient's welfare. Because the therapist is in the help-offering role, projections and displacements of this sort are less likely. More likely is that patient material triggers responses tied to "soft spots" or sources of conflict in the therapist's psyche without the involvement of displacement or projection. It should be noted that these theoretical inferences are based on clinical experience and are in need of empirical scrutiny.

Management of Countertransference

The potential of CT to both hinder and aid treatment are two thematic constructs that, as Epstein and Feiner (1988) noted, have been intertwined like a double helix throughout the history of thought about CT. It is generally agreed that if CT, however defined, is to help rather than hinder, something must be done to, with, or about it. Internal CT reactions must be understood, controlled, or managed in one way or another, albeit imperfectly. In my theoretical work with my collaborators (Gelso & Hayes, 1998; Van-Wagoner, Gelso, Hayes, & Diemer, 1991), we have conceptualized the therapist factors that are implicated in effective management of CT such that it may benefit the work. These factors may be seen as constituents of CT management and they are transtheoretical. Elsewhere (Gelso & Hayes, 2002; Hayes & Gelso, 2001) the empirical studies have been reviewed that support the importance of these constituents and of CT management as a global construct. The five factors that have been proposed to be key parts of CT management are therapist self-insight, self-integration, anxiety management, empathy, and conceptualizing ability. These factors are briefly described in what follows.

Self-insight refers to the extent to which the therapist is aware of his or her own feelings in the work (including those that are countertransferential) and understands their basis in both the therapist's psyche and the relational matrix of the treatment dyad. The importance of self-insight is no more clearly seen than in Freud's (1910/1957) comment that "no psycho-analyst goes further than his own complexes and internal resistances permit; and we consequently require that he shall begin his activity with a self-analysis and continually carry it deeper while he is making observations of his patients" (p. 145). From a relational perspective, the task is even more daunting, for it involves insight into the self as part of the relational matrix and in this sense entails an understanding of joint influence.

Self-integration refers to two qualities. First, it includes the therapist's possession of an intact, basically healthy character structure, a sense of wholeness on the part of the therapist or at least a self that is more unified than disorganized. Second, in therapy self-integration manifests itself as a recognition of ego boundaries. In the process of merging with and separating from the patient (Gorkin, 1987), the therapist must be able to differentiate self from other, and this itself requires a stable identity. From a two-person, relational perspective, self-integration is especially important, for the therapist's experience is "necessarily shaped by the analysand's relational structure; he plays assigned roles even if he desperately tries to stand outside the patient's system and play no role at all" (Mitchell, 1988, p. 292).

Anxiety management is the third constituent of CT management. Anxiety itself is a signal that something is awry. At the same time, it is important that therapists allow themselves to experience anxiety and that they also possess the ego strength to control, understand, and manage this anxiety so that it does not bleed over, to too great an extent, into their responses to patients. Therapists who defend against the experience of anxiety are at once depriving themselves of a key source for understanding the patient and the interactional matrix, and they are increasing substantially the likelihood of CT acting out in the hour.

Fourth, *empathy,* or the ability to partially identify with and put one's self in the other's shoes, is seen as a central moderator of CT behavior. It facilitates the therapist's focus on the patient's needs despite difficulties the therapist may be experiencing with the work and the pulls to attend to the therapist's own needs. Also, empathy may be part of sensitivity to one's own feelings, including CT-based feelings, which in turn ought to prevent the acting out of CT (Peabody & Gelso, 1982; Robbins & Jolkovski, 1987). In other words, the emotional quality that fosters empathy toward others may be a basis for sensitivity toward one's self and one's feelings more generally. This quality or state of "in-tunedness" theoretically ought to prevent the acting out on the patient of conflict-based reactions.

Finally, *conceptualizing ability* reflects the therapist's ability to draw on theory in the work and grasp theoretically the patient's dynamics in terms of the therapeutic relationship. In Reich's (1951) terms, conceptualizing ability allows the therapist to take an "outside position in order to be capable of an objective evaluation of what he has just now felt within" (p. 25). In this sense, it is the observer side of Sullivan's (1954) famous statement about need for the therapist to be both a participant and an observer. Conceptualizing ability is especially helpful in conjunction with the therapist's self-awareness or insight into the CT dynamics. When standing alone, however, conceptualizing ability is not likely to foster CT management and in fact may impede it. In other words, in the absence of self-awareness, conceptualizing skill may simply reflect intellectualized understanding, which itself may create distance in the relational matrix. Interestingly, at least two experimental studies of CT (Latts & Gelso, 1995; Robbins & Jolkovski, 1987) support the idea that although conceptualizing ability is an aid to CT management when it combines with therapist CT awareness, it is a hindrance when it stands alone.

RESEARCH ON COUNTERTRANSFERENCE AND ITS MANAGEMENT

Over the decades, empirical research has trailed sadly behind clinical theory in this area. There are likely two basic reasons for this. First, psychoanalysis, the theoretical system in which the construct of CT has been embedded, has been largely indifferent to controlled empirical research during much of its life. Second, the construct itself is extremely complex, resorting as it does to unconscious processes residing in a complex relational matrix. Fortunately, in recent years things have been changing. To begin with, research on psychoanalytic constructs and treatments in general has increased dramatically.

In addition, laboratory research has allowed investigators to simplify the great complexity of the CT construct and to study questions that could not have been examined in the field. At the same time, in recent years investigators have conducted qualitative studies that, rather than simplifying as does laboratory research, have studied general questions and sought to tap participants' subjective experience around CT issues.

There have been three major reviews of the empirical literature during the past quarter century. The first was by Singer and Luborsky (1977) in which research on CT and on therapist emotional reactions in general was scrutinized and its relation to clinical theory analyzed. The other two reviews are recent, and have been conducted by myself in collaboration with Hayes. Hayes and Gelso (2001) examined research on the role of CT in therapy process and outcome with a focus on the clinical implications of the research. Gelso and Hayes (2002) reviewed the literature connecting CT to session and treatment outcomes. In the following, I summarize the key findings from these three reviews.

The Causes, Effects, and Prevalence of Countertransference

Although few studies had been conducted on CT per se by the time of Singer and Luborsky's (1977) review, a sizable number of investigations focused on therapist reactions to patients' or research participants' behavior. (I use the term *participants* because a number of these studies were laboratory simulations.) Based on a review of the existing research, Singer and Luborsky offered some major conclusions. They noted that much of the research supported the clinical literature. However, in keeping with the complementary and relational conceptions of CT, the actual stimulus value of the patient was found to matter substantially. Thus, patient behaviors elicited corresponding therapist behaviors, for example, patient hostility elicited therapist hostility. Singer and Luborsky (1977) suggested that "*more than the clinical literature would suggest, the patient influences the therapist to a marked degree and in predictable ways*" (p. 449). Naturally, the job of the effective therapist in treatment of any duration is to understand the feelings triggered by the patient and to then tailor responses to the patient that foster understanding and growth. The impulse may be to enact what the patient stimulus triggers, but, as noted earlier, *lex talionis* is not the effective way.

Over the past 25 years, the evidence has slowly accumulated to confirm solidly and extend another of Singer and Luborsky's (1977) conclusions that were based on few studies:

> Perhaps the most clear-cut and important area of congruence between the clinical and quantitative literatures is the widely agreed-upon position that

uncontrolled countertransference has an adverse effect on therapy outcome. Not only does it have a markedly detrimental influence on the therapist's technique and interventions, but it also interferes with the optimal understanding of the patient. (p. 449)

To this conclusion, I could add that uncontrolled CT also appears to impair the therapeutic relationship. In line with this, two studies (Ligiero & Gelso, 2002; Rosenberger & Hayes, 2002) have uncovered substantial relations between CT behavior in sessions and both therapist and clinical supervisors' (for doctoral trainees) ratings of the working alliances these therapists were able to form. For example, Ligiero and Gelso studied 50 clinical supervisors and their supervisees, who were graduate students in clinical and counseling psychology. These investigators found that supervisors' ratings of CT behavior during supervisees' therapy sessions predicted working alliances as rated by both therapist trainees and supervisors. The greater the amount of both positive and negative CT, the poorer were the working alliances these therapist trainees formed with their clients.

In the years since the Singer and Luborsky (1977) review, studies have also examined the patient and therapist factors that create CT feelings and behavior. In these studies, CT is usually conceptualized as implicating unresolved conflicts or issues in the therapist, in one way or another. Although there is usually a patient trigger to CT, research has not identified any particular class of patient reactions that serve as triggers. That is, no class of behaviors (e.g., aggression) stands out above other classes (e.g., dependency) in triggering CT in therapists, nor, with one exception, have therapist factors been found. The exception is that therapist level of trait anxiety seems to underlie CT reactions. Therapists with greater anxiety are more likely than those with less anxiety to avoid patient affect, inaccurately recall material from the session, and avoid patient feelings toward the therapist (Gelso & Hayes, 2002). Whereas neither patient or therapist factors, in themselves, appear to heavily influence CT, the interaction of patient qualities or reactions with therapist factors does play a significant role. Consistent with a relational perspective, whether or not any given patient factor serves as a trigger depends on the therapist and his or her conflicts and issues. For example, in two laboratory studies (Gelso, Fassinger, Gomez, & Latts, 1995; Hayes & Gelso, 1993), the sexual orientation of a role-played client (lesbian, gay, or heterosexual) had no effect of behavioral, affective, or cognitive indexes of CT. However, in both studies, when therapist trainees completed a paper-and-pencil measure of homophobia prior to the experiment, it was found the their measured level of homophobia correlated with their avoidance of the client's material (the measure of CT behavior) when interacting with the gay or lesbian client actor or actress.

One may raise the question of how common CT is. Naturally the answer depends on the particular conception of CT being studied. If we take a totalist perspective, the answer is clear. CT constantly occurs in every session. It cannot not occur! However, if one uses a more restrictive definition, one in which the therapist's unresolved issues are a necessary aspect of CT, then the frequency of occurrence of CT becomes a meaningful question. Although only one study has addressed this question, it is worth noting. Hayes et al. (1998) studied eight experienced therapists who were identified as experts by their peers, and who treated one patient for between 12 and 20 sessions. Despite a more restrictive definition of CT, these theoretically heterogeneous therapists identified CT as occurring in 80% of their 127 sessions, and it appeared that CT was prominent in each case. Findings such as these provide strong disconfirmation for the Freudian myth that effective therapists do not experience CT (Spence, 1987). Notably, Hayes et al. (1998) also found strong evidence in these cases for the proposition that CT can both hinder or aid treatment and that therapist self-understanding around internal CT reactions was a key factor in determining if CT benefited or impeded the work.

Research on Countertransference Management

The hindering and helping effect of CT brings us to the topic of CT management, for this topic is the only one on which research to date has examined the conditions under which CT may be beneficial to the work. Several studies (see review by Gelso & Hayes, 2002) have been conducted over the past decade on CT management, and the general conclusion has been that therapists' ability to manage CT has a desirable effect on treatment process and outcome. Specifically, the extent to which therapists exhibit in their sessions the five factors noted earlier (self-insight, self-integration, anxiety management, empathy, conceptualizing skill), individually or especially when combined, is meaningfully related to the reduction of CT behavior, the therapeutic working alliance, session quality, and treatment outcome. It should be noted that this line of work is still in its early stages and is not extensive. Although no more than a dozen studies have been conducted on the topic, the results are generally promising. Work on the topic of how CT can aid therapy may well represent the growing edge in this area of inquiry.

COUNTERTRANSFERENCE IN BRIEF RELATIONAL PSYCHOTHERAPY

It has become part of clinical lore that the tactics and techniques of long-term therapy need to be modified if brief work is to be effective. For example, for many years researchers have suspected that the therapist needs to be more active in brief therapy and formulate a central issue that is to be the focus of the work (Gelso & Johnson, 1983). There is much clinical wisdom driving such modifications, if not clear scientific support. However, in the area of CT, I suggest that there is essentially no difference between brief and long-term therapy. In each of these formats, it is imperative that the therapist attend closely to his or her own feelings and behavior, even as the therapist is following the dictates of his or her theory during the hour.

As noted earlier, however, from a relational perspective it is not enough for the therapist to pay attention to only his or her own feelings and behavior. The therapist must also consider what impact his or her behavior (including the more subtle, nonverbal behaviors) has on the patient and must also allow himself or herself to be affected by the patient so as to best understand the patient's impact and the dynamics of that impact. In this sense, Freud's (1912/1958) suggestion is still very apt when he says that the analyst "must turn his own unconscious like a receptive organ towards the transmitting unconscious of the patient" (p. 115) as the best way to deeply understand the patient. In sum, the therapist needs to be attending to how the participants cocreate a dynamic interchange of affects, thoughts, and enactments.

The Case of June

When reading and reflecting on the transcript of three sessions of therapy with June, I was sharply aware of the difficulties in making inferences about CT from such material. One cannot look into another's psyche from such material, especially given the fact that cultural differences between the participants and myself can affect the accuracy of any observer inferences. Having noted this caveat, I comment briefly on the therapist and then focus mostly on how I might think about CT if I were the therapist behaving as the therapist behaved with this particular patient.

Briefly, the therapist achieved the psychotherapeutic tasks of developing a focus for the work by articulating the key dynamic issues in this patient: her tendency to passively withdraw from conflict situations such that she ended up feeling blank, as well as the ways in which June contributed to situations in which she ended up feeling insignificant. Taken together, one might consider this the core conflictual relationship theme in June's life (Luborsky, Popp, Luborsky, & Mark, 1994). The following excerpt from Session 6 illustrates the core theme and an interaction between patient and therapist about their relationship (6-79 is, e.g., Session 6, Segment 9).

Q: 6-79: She blanks you out, true. What do you do? You accept it. That's your part in it. That's what we are changing.
A: 6-80: Yeah. That's perfectly right, I accept it.
Q: 6-81: I'm not putting words in your mouth [laugh].

A: 6-82: No, no, that is right. But if there is a conversation and if I actually say something, involve myself in it, she'll knock me back. There'll be some criticism and I'll just get tearful. I think sod it you've done it again, and think why do I bother. The whole time I just think it's not worth the fight, and it feels like a fight. To actually have a part in a conversation feels like a fight. My friend is very talkative as well but she doesn't seem to have that power over me. I interrupt her at times but I can never do that to Vicky cause it just doesn't work. She just doesn't hear you, she just carries on. Where as my friend will stop, will involve me. She does, like Vicky, have a lot to say. So I'm often the quiet party but at least I can get a word in now and then. I don't feel anything like the blanked out I feel as I do with Vicky.

Q: 6-83: And how does that relate to being here? How does it all relate to our relationship?

A: 6-84: I don't know. I was really sorry that . . . I know it's not your fault . . . I couldn't come last week because of this happening the Wednesday before. It was one week that I feel that I really could have done with it. I was coming this week blizzards or what. I was . . . I don't know. This morning I decided to come on my own because

Q: 6-85: So it was a practical thing.

The therapist maintained the core theme as the focal point around which the sessions pivoted. The therapist also seemed sensitive to some transference possibilities and other relational dynamics between her and June, although she withdrew immediately when June did not pick up on the therapist's relational comments. At other times, however, the therapist seems to dissuade potential transference and other relational material from the patient. For example, in Session 6 when June expresses worries that she has too readily taken in the therapist's views (Segments 68–71), the therapist seems to dismiss this possibility, thus dissuading the unfolding of potentially important relational material that would connect the treatment dynamics to June's dynamics and behavior outside of treatment.

Q: 6-67: You took your sister's mood on board like it was your mood. The way in which if you feel blanked out you sort of say, all right then I'll blank out, I'll disappear.

A: 6-68: Another thing she said was that basically anything I say when I come back from here, is what you put into my mouth . . . And she says that any one who goes to a psychiatrist, there's this thing again. She has a real phobia about me seeing psychiatrists and psychotherapists and what have you.

Q: 6-69: mm.

A: 6-70: She said it's you know, I'm only saying what you've basically told me to say, or you've told me I'm feeling, what you've told me to feel. But, that made me think to be honest that, that did make me think.

Q: 6-71: mm, mm, is it true?

A: 6-72: Yeah. And I don't know. I know exactly what I feel. What I've said today and ... you know, you've just said it. We've agreed on it rather than you saying what's happened. I've told you what's happened. You know, you've put no ideas into my mind that weren't there already.

Q: 6-73: In past weeks you thought I could have put ideas in your mind?

A: 6-74: Or that I've just gone along with what you've ... cause I can't honestly, I can't remember that.

Q: 6-75: What you blank it out.

A: 6-76: Yeah. And I don't know whether I've just gone along with what you've said, agreed ... I don't know. I hope not. I hope I haven't done that cause otherwise if I'm just listening and agreeing then what's the point me coming up here.

Q: 6-77: mm, that's right.

A: 6-78: I'm sure I haven't. But once it's said it stuck, and you do keep going over it.

Q: 6-69: mm. I wonder what that's about though. I mean these words for example, on here, are all your words aren't they.

A: 6-70: There's no doubt about that. I've done that.

Q: 6-71: Your words, "don't matter, blanked out, rejected, passive, bottle things up, feeling to extreme, feeling exploited, feeling easily replaceable, angry, numb, jealousy, hate, rebellious, stubborn." They're all your words aren't they. They're not my words.

A: 6-72: No, no. I do know I've said them. I knew that. I read that back to myself. I said it a couple of times and I keep reading it back and I know they're all my words. It's just like, it's almost like she was saying you ... I said them, but you put them there.

Q: 6-73: But she could also be saying that it's not valid because I put the ideas and words into your mind. You're so blanked out that I can come along ... you turn up every week, and I can suggest these things to you that you agree with.

As I read the transcript and placed myself into the role of the therapist, my experience with June most often involved a sense of admiration coupled with some wishes to come to the patient's rescue and solve her problems for her. These feeling were stirred by June and seem to relate to the silent transference that is unfolding in this case, perhaps revolving around her hidden wish to be taken care of in ways it seems she did not experience in her early years or even now. The rescue fantasies, however, are also partly my own issue, stemming from wishes to be the good parent and tied to conflicts about being taken care of. This is an example of the relational dynamics of CT—how they are stirred by the transference and nontransference material, but also how the therapist's issues serve as a hook to which the patient's projections can stick. My task as June's therapist would be to control the CT based urge to rescue (which would inhibit her constructive change) and instead help her understand how her withdrawal stimulates others to take over. The transference around these issues may or may not be dealt with directly, depending on June's capacity for insight. Also, when time is short, as in this nine-session case study, the therapist needs to decide what issues can be most effectively dealt with in light of the time constraints.

As noted, one cannot really know the CT that is occurring from transcripts of only three sessions. However, if I were behaving as was June's therapist in certain portions of the work, I would be defending against my anxiety, for example, about not being helpful enough. For example, in Session 8, in the segment where June expresses worries about her problems returning after the therapy ends, the therapist seems to not want to hear this but instead seems to want to talk June out of her fears of relapse.

> Q: 8-47: I would see everybody, absolutely every patient I ever see, they all have a follow-up session with me. And that's how we practice it here. So, and it's more than three months at the end of the therapy, but we could see one another as soon as I got back from maternity leave to review you and see what's going on.
>
> A: 8-48: But, God forbid, what if I got right back to square one. What would then happen?
>
> Q: 8-49: I'd give you a right good telling off. I don't think that I agree with the view that people need therapy for 16 years or something every week. I don't agree with it. I think it makes people inappropriately dependent. They think I can only change if I'm seeing this person and actually that's not true, and it is certainly not true for you.

This one is also an example:

> A: 8-85: I should be. I am. I am, but in order to stay in control, do I just have to steer clear?

Q: 8-86: But you're having some 'time out' aren't you, to get your health in order really, your psychological health in order. So things changed in order for you to extract yourself from the family a bit more, stand back a bit more. And yes, you will eventually go back to them, hopefully not so much as before, but in a slightly more constructive way, reflected in your phone calls with Dad for example. The old self-destructive feelings aren't going to go overnight after 7 hours of psychotherapy.

A: 8-87: No.

Q: 8-88: But the difference is you know what to do about it. Because you've already done it. You've separated from your family. Does that make sense?

A: 8-89: Yes. It doesn't make perfect sense.

Q: 8-92: Am I better because I'm not seeing them? No you're not seeing them, because you're better.

A: 8-93: Yes.

Q: 8-94: And then of course you will go back and you'll think, Oh God, Vicky's so popular. But you decide if you are going to be more in control and positively assertive. Or whether you're going to passively go home and bottle things up and have a bottle of wine, and go to sleep in the armchair, it's up to you, isn't it?

A: 8-95: Yeah.

Q: 8-96: On one level, you are going to be on your own, because I'm not going to be here. But what we've done together, is going to be there.

When a therapist engages in such behavior, he or she could be defending against anxiety about patient's relapse, especially considering that the work was limited to seven sessions due to the therapist's pregnancy. For many therapists (and I would be among them), a CT response of this sort is unlikely to be a response to the patient's transference or other material but instead would reflect a more chronic CT around letting others down and abandoning others, perhaps related to personal feelings about abandonment. Again, I have no way of knowing if such CT defenses were operating in this particular therapist. At the same time, the therapist is just so active and persuasive around this concern about relapse that it creates doubts in me that she is closely monitoring her CT at that point. It is possible, however, that the therapist's persuasiveness and the support it entails actually is helpful to the patient, and perhaps this is what the therapist is consciously hoping and believing. Sometimes anxiety-based CT can actually benefit the patient, as long as it also conforms to what the patient needs at a given time.

CONCLUSION

The therapist's subjectivity, including CT reactions, is a universal and vital aspect of the psychotherapy relationship. Transcending its early status as a taboo topic, CT has been vigorously theorized about in recent decades, and despite theoretically based differences in how CT has been defined and conceptualized, there are currently many points of consensus. Empirical efforts have also increased in recent times. Regardless of one's theoretical inclinations, the evidence suggests that it is important for therapists to monitor their subjective reactions and to manage them so that they can devise the most effective responses to their patients. This conclusion is at least as apt for brief therapy as for longer term treatment, for in brief work the therapist does not have the luxury of time that would permit recovery from therapeutic mistakes tied to the CT. In addition, in brief treatments the sense of time urgency created by the need for brevity and patient change in a short period of time may create unique CT issues that require therapist attention and management, as well as empirical study and understanding.

From a relational perspective, the therapist's task around the CT is more daunting than in the classical approaches, for it entails understanding of the complex relational matrix cocreated by both participants—the ways in which each participant in the drama of dynamic therapy affects and is affected by the other's transference and nontransference material. This relational perspective is fertile ground for both theoretical and empirical advances in the years ahead.

REFERENCES

Aron, L. (1991). The patient's experience of the analyst's subjectivity. *Psychoanalytic Dialogues, 1,* 29–51.

Aron, L. (1996). *A meeting of minds.* Hillsdale, NJ: Analytic.

Butler, S. F., Flasher, L. V., & Strupp, H. H. (1993). Countertransference and the qualities of the psychotherapist. In N. E. Miller, L. Luborsky, J. P. Barber, & J. P. Docherty (Eds.), *Psychodynamic treatment research: A handbook for clinical practice* (pp. 342–360). New York: Basic Books.

Epstein, L., & Feiner, A. H. (1988). Countertransference: The therapist's contribution to treatment. In B. Wolstein (Ed.), *Essential papers in countertransference* (pp. 282–303). New York: New York University Press.

Freud, S. (1957). Future prospects of psychoanalytic therapy. In J. Strachey (Ed. and Trans.), *The standard edition of the complete works of Sigmund Freud* (Vol. 11, pp. 139–151). London: Hogarth Press. (Original work published 1910)

Freud, S. (1958). Recommendations to physicians practicing psychoanalysis. In J. Strachey (Ed. and Trans.), *Standard edition of the complete works of Sigmund Freud* (Vol. 12, pp. 11–120). London: Hogarth. (Original work published 1912)

Gabbard, G. O. (2001). A contemporary psychoanalytic model of countertransference. *Journal of Clinical Psychology, 57,* 983–992.

Gabbard, G. O., & Wilkinson, S. M. (1994). *Management of countertransference with borderline patients*. Washington, DC: American Psychiatric Association.

Gelso, C. J., Fassinger, R. E., Gomez, M. J., & Latts, M. G. (1995). Countertransference reactions to lesbian clients: The role of homophobia, counselor gender, and countertransference management. *Journal of Counseling Psychology, 42*, 356–364.

Gelso, C. J., & Hayes, J. A. (1998). *The psychotherapy relationship: Theory, research, and practice*. New York: Wiley.

Gelso, C. J., & Hayes, J. A. (2002). Countertransference and its management. In J. C. Norcross (Ed.), *Psychotherapy relationships that work: Therapist contributions and responsiveness to patient* (pp. 267–284). New York: Oxford University Press.

Gelso, C. J., & Johnson, D. H. (1983). *Explorations in time-limited counseling and psychotherapy*. New York: Columbia University Press, Teachers College Press.

Gorkin, M. (1987). *The uses of countertransference*. New York: Aronson.

Greenberg, J., & Mitchell, S. A. (1983). *Object relations in psychoanalytic theory*. Cambridge, MA: Harvard University Press.

Hayes, J. A., & Gelso, C. J. (1993). Counselors' discomfort with gay and HIV-infected clients. *Journal of Counseling Psychology, 40*, 86–93.

Hayes, J. A., & Gelso, C. J. (2001). Clinical implications of research on countertransference: Science informing practice. *Journal of Clinical Psychology, 57*, 1041–1052.

Hayes, J. A., McCracken, J. E., McClanahan, M. K., Hill, C. E., Harp, J. S., & Carozzoni, P. (1998). Therapist perspectives on countertransference: Qualitative data in search of a theory. *Journal of Counseling Psychology, 45*, 468–482.

Heimann, P. (1950). Countertransference. *British Journal of Medical Psychology, 33*, 9–15.

Kernberg, O. (1965). Notes on countertransference. *Journal of the American Psychoanalytic Association, 13*, 38–56.

Kiesler, D. J. (2001). Therapist countertransference: In search of common themes and empirical referents. *Journal of Clinical Psychology, 57*, 1053–1063.

Latts, M. G., & Gelso, C. J. (1995). Countertransference behavior and management with survivors of sexual assault. *Psychotherapy, 32*, 405–415.

Levenson, H. (1995). *Time-limited dynamic psychotherapy*. New York: Basic Books.

Ligiero, D. P., & Gelso, C. J. (2002). Countertransference, attachment, and the working alliance: The therapist's contributions. *Psychotherapy: Theory/Research/Practice/Training, 39*, 3–11.

Little, M. (1951). Countertransference and the patient's response to it. *International Journal of Psychoanalysis, 32*, 32–40.

Luborsky, L. L., Popp, C., Luborsky, E., & Mark, D. (1994). The core conflictual relationship theme. *Psychotherapy Research, 4*, 172–183.

Mitchell, S. A. (1988). *Relational concepts in psychoanalysis*. Cambridge, MA: Harvard University Press.

Mitchell, S. A. (1997). *Influence and autonomy in psychoanalysis*. Hillsdale, NJ: Analytic.

Peabody, S. A., & Gelso, C. J. (1982). Countertransference and empathy: The complex relationship between two divergent concepts in counseling. *Journal of Counseling Psychology, 29*, 240–245.

Pine, F. (1990). *Drive, ego, object, and self: A synthesis for clinical work*. New York: Basic Books.

Racker, H. (1957). The meanings and uses of countertransference. *Psychoanalytic Quarterly, 26*, 303–357.

Racker, H. (1968). *Transference and countertransference*. New York: International Universities Press.

Reich, A. (1951). On countertransference. *International Journal of Psychoanalysis, 32*, 25–31.

Robbins, S. B., & Jolkovski, M. P. (1987). Managing countertransference feelings: An interactional model using awareness of feeling and theoretical framework. *Journal of Counseling Psychology, 34*, 276–282.

Rosenberger, E. W., & Hayes, J. A. (2002). Origins, consequences, and management of countertransference: A case study. *Journal of Counseling Psychology, 49,* 221–232.
Singer, B. A., & Luborsky, L. (1977). Countertransference: The status of clinical versus quantitative research. In A. S. Gurman & A. M. Razin (Eds.), *Effective psychotherapy: A handbook of research* (pp. 433–451). New York: Pergamon.
Spence, D. (1987). *The Freudian metaphor.* New York: Norton.
Sullivan, H. S. (1954). *The psychiatric interview.* New York: Norton.
VanWagoner, S. L., Gelso, C. J., Hayes, J. A., & Diemer, R. (1991). Countertransference and the excellent therapist. *Psychotherapy, 28,* 411–421.

CHAPTER

12

Maintaining the Therapeutic Alliance: Resolving Alliance-Threatening Interactions Related to the Transference

Dawn Bennett
Clinical Psychology Service, Blackburn, England

Glenys Parry
Professor of Applied Clinical Therapies, University of Sheffield, England

The therapeutic alliance is of vital importance for successful psychotherapy. A good alliance means that the therapist and patient agree on the goals and tasks of therapy and develop an affective bond in which the patient works purposefully and the therapist shows empathic understanding and involvement (Bordin, 1979). A strong alliance does not mean, as Garfield (1995) pointed out, "comfort, sociability and enjoyment of the relationship" (p. 49). On the contrary, patients in a good alliance may be able to express more negative emotion.

The importance of resolving threats to the therapeutic alliance in psychotherapy is widely acknowledged. For example, Safran and Muran (1996), who listed general principles of the therapeutic alliance in brief therapy, advised that vicious cycles of transference and countertransference enactments should be minimized and that alliance ruptures must be detected early on and addressed. Of course, these two principles are closely related, as threats and ruptures to the alliance commonly arise from a reenactment with the therapist of the patient's own repetitive dysfunctional pattern of interpersonal relating. Resolving such enactments to repair alliance ruptures is a key therapeutic task. It allows other work to proceed that would otherwise reach an impasse. Most crucially, the resolution of an alliance rupture linked to a transference–countertransference enactment is in itself therapeutic, a corrective emotional experience (Alexander & French, 1946).

In this chapter, we describe the development and refinement of a model of how therapists practicing cognitive analytic therapy (CAT) competently resolve transference-related ruptures or challenges to the therapeutic alliance, and we illustrate the model by clinical example.

PROCESS FACTORS AND PSYCHOTHERAPY OUTCOME

The quality of the therapeutic alliance is the process factor with the strongest and most consistent relation to outcome (Orlinsky, Grawe, & Parks, 1994). The alliance represents a common therapeutic factor or "pantheoretical process variable" operating in all forms of psychotherapy (Horvath & Greenberg, 1994). It has been defined in terms of three elements; the bond between patient and therapist and the extent to which they agree on the goals of therapy and on the tasks proposed to reach these goals (Bordin, 1979). One of the key skills in a psychotherapist (of any school or discipline) is to develop a satisfactory therapeutic relationship, as patients vary in this capacity (Bearden, Lavelle, Buysse, Karp, & Frank, 1996).

Therapists differ in their skill in this regard, which may be one reason why the impact on outcome of individual therapists is greater than that of therapy type (Luborsky et al., 1986). Strupp (1980) observed that a major factor distinguishing poor outcome cases was therapists' difficulty establishing good therapeutic alliances with their patients because of a tendency to become caught in negative interactional cycles in which, for example, they responded to patient hostility with their own counterhostility. This was supported in a more systematic study (Henry, Schacht, & Strupp, 1986) in which negative complementary cycles distinguished treatment failures from treatment successes. The therapists in these studies were well trained and experienced but not immune to engaging in potentially destructive interpersonal process.

ALLIANCE THREATENING TRANSFERENCE REENACTMENTS

The term *enactment* refers to events occurring within the dyad that each party experiences as the consequence of behavior in the other (McLaughlin, 1991). The idea that patients and therapists often enact the type of interpersonal patterns characteristic of the patient's other relationships has been a central theme in psychoanalytically oriented approaches to therapy. The phenomenon, typically discussed in terms of transference and countertransference, is understood in different terms by different theoretical traditions. The psychoanalytic concept has evolved toward an interpersonal perspective with the therapist, an involved, not invulnerable participant (Kiesler, 1986).

Regardless of the different conceptualizations of the transference, many share the view that the transference is an interactional process, which provides information about problematic relationship patterns in the patient's life (Foreman & Marmar, 1985; Safran, Crocker, McMain, & Murray, 1990; Safran & Muran, 1996). Exploration of the way in which both therapist and patient are contributing can provide an understanding that would otherwise be unavailable. Some theorists have warned against the countertherapeutic effects of failing to recognize or colluding with patients' maladaptive relationship patterns (Henry, 1998; Strupp, 1998).

There has been an increasing research focus on ruptures to the alliance, both as markers for mutative events (important change-inducing events) in psychotherapy and as an indicator of therapist skill. Safran and Muran (1996) and Kivlighan and Shaughnessy (1995) have modeled how these events can be resolved, focusing on therapist skill in managing the alliance.

RESEARCH STRATEGY

As researchers, we are conducting a program of research on therapist competence in CAT which includes this key competence of how therapists identify and resolve ruptures to the alliance due to the emergence of maladaptive interpersonal patterns in the therapeutic relationship, that is, in the transference and countertransference.

Our research strategy has two aspects: first to focus on a patient group in which therapist competence and incompetence are most likely to be related to outcome (borderline personality disorder [BPD]). Patients with BPD frequently fail to engage with offered treatment (Waldinger & Gunderson, 1984), they do not improve spontaneously in the short term (Stone, 1993), and their clinical state is highly responsive to therapeutic errors (Shearin & Linehan, 1993). These findings point to the problem of forming and maintaining a treatment alliance with patients with BPD.

Secondly, naturalistic performances of real clinicians working in routine United Kingdom National Health Service settings were studied so that the findings would be more applicable to clinicians and provide information on clinical effectiveness (Aveline, 1997; Goldfried & Wolfe, 1998). Bearing in mind Waltz, Addis, Koerner, and Jacobson's (1993) exhortation that competencies must be examined in relation to a prespecified performance standard, we studied competencies in the context of a specific technique required in CAT. However, the key competence has applicability beyond any specific technique to many relational therapies.

CAT

CAT (Ryle, 1995a, 1977; Ryle & Kerr, 2002) is widely practiced in the United Kingdom and is developing in other parts of Europe. It is a brief, focused psychotherapy, typically between 8 and 25 sessions, which integrates cognitive behavioral and psychoanalytic (object relations) principles. CAT formulates maladaptive, repetitive sequences of cognition, emotion, behavior, and their consequences (called *procedures*), which are problematic to the extent that the patient's aims are not achieved and not revised. CAT theory also asserts that mental representations of self–other relationship patterns become the basis of the procedures governing intrapersonal (how the patient relates to himself or herself) as well as interpersonal relationships. In practice, CAT therapists are trained to share written and diagrammatic formulations of these maladaptive or problematic procedures with patients to aid their recognition and revision.

IDENTIFYING AND RESOLVING ALLIANCE THREATS IN CAT

In CAT, early formulation (in the form of a letter and a diagram) is a central technique and a shared tool. As it describes the nature and origin of the problematic patterns of relating, the therapist can use it to predict problematic patterns that may occur in the therapy relationship. A major element of the formulation is a diagram mapping the procedural sequences. The diagram is constructed around a core self-state within which the underlying procedural patterns of either self-to-self or self-to-other are depicted as reciprocal role procedures (RRPs). The reciprocal nature of these patterns is depicted as opposite poles in which one pole is enacted and the other elicited. They also govern self-management and the I–me relationship. For example, "preoccupied and unavailable in relation to anxiously striving"; "mocking and sneering in relation to humiliated and shamed."

Precise identification of maladaptive reciprocal procedures is the basis for the flexible application of interventions explicitly targeted on the procedures requiring revision. Formulation is a tool used by the patient for self-monitoring and used by the therapist to aid the recognition of transference and countertransference and thereby understand and guide the process of therapy. CAT defines *transference* as the enactment of the patient's RRPs in the therapeutic relationship. The patient is seen as exerting pressure on the therapist to enact one pole of a particular RRP, whereas *countertransference* is understood as the therapist's awareness of this or his or her tendency to respond to this pressure. Every reciprocal procedure described in the diagram may be enacted by the patient in relation to the therapist or may be induced in, or perceived to be played by, the therapist (Ryle, 1995b). The form of a patient's participation in therapy therefore reflects and is determined by their available RRPs. A transference enactment is therefore an example in a specific context of a more general RRP. Accurate formulation of a patient's interpersonal patterns can be achieved within the time limitations imposed by clinical practice (Bennett, 1998; Bennett & Parry, 1998), which is important because CAT depends on the accuracy and completeness of the formulation to identify and resolve enactments of procedures.

An example of a reciprocal role enactment threatening the therapeutic alliance:

> A patient arrived late. He said he hadn't given "much thought" to issues suggested by the therapist and he had considered not continuing in therapy. "I don't feel involved somehow ... to be honest, earlier this week I didn't want to carry on." The therapist began to explore what had triggered this feeling, but the patient could not think of anything. All the therapist's efforts to discuss and explore the feeling in more depth met with vague, unfocused responses, such as "yeah it could be" or "I don't know, I guess so" or shrugs. The therapist began to feel irritated and started to challenge the patient. He interpreted the patient's unwillingness to work in therapy as a form of hostility toward the therapist and linked this to unresolved aggression and hostility toward his father. The patient rejected this interpretation and then became very silent.
>
> This patient described an early experience of a strict father and school experience against which he rebelled, allowing the therapist to identify an RRP of "controlling and demanding in relation to trapped and rebellious." Reenactments of this reciprocal role in the therapeutic relationship may take the form of the patient responding to perceived demands or therapist interpretations by feeling trapped and rebelling. The therapist may feel irritated, redouble interpretive effort, and come to occupy the controlling role. If unrecognized, this reenactment would undermine the working alliance and limit any therapeutic progress.

For patients with BPD in which dissociation and multiple core or self-states are major features, the formulation process is more complex. The explicit aim in CAT is to create in the patient the capacity for continuous self-observation. The use of the formulatory tools by patient and therapist is central to achieving this aim, with the formulation taking the form of a diagram showing the various self-states and the procedures by which the patient switches between them. Although specific techniques may be used to modify or control particular procedures, the combination of self-observation in relation to the diagram with the collaborative, noncollusive relationship provided by the therapist are thought to be the crucial mechanisms of change.

The depiction of the patient's maladaptive procedural sequences in a formulation using a diagram and other tools enables CAT therapists to anticipate and recognize procedures that might occur within the therapeutic relationship. Once recognized, the therapist can engage the patient in resolving these alliance-threatening RRPs, and in doing so, foster new interpersonal learning.

RESEARCH STUDY: THE EMPIRICALLY DERIVED MODEL OF ENACTMENT RESOLUTION

Sample, Measures, and Session Selection

We wished to identify sessions likely to contain RRPs occurring in the therapeutic relationship (referred to as *RR enactments*) that threatened the therapeutic alliance and were competently resolved by the therapists. We therefore sampled "good outcome" cases and studied the course of therapy to locate sessions containing these alliance-threatening events.

The sample population consisted of patients whose scores on measures of clinical outcome met criteria for statistically reliable and clinically significant psychotherapeutic change (Jacobson & Revenstorf, 1988; Jacobson & Truax, 1991). Patients in a quasi-naturalistic research project of CAT for BPD at Guy's Hospital, London completed the Therapy Experience Questionnaire (TEQ) after each session (Ryle, 1997). The TEQ is a measure of their experience of the therapeutic relationship, which has been shown to be sensitive to fluctuations in the therapeutic alliance (Ryle, 1995b). TEQ scores were plotted and median smoothing (Jackson, 1989) was adopted to identify sessions for which TEQ scores were unusual in relation to the underlying trend in scores.

Figure 12.1 illustrates the variation in TEQ scores in an 18-session therapy, ranging from −13 in Session 1 when the patient expressed ambivalence about therapy due to mistrust of others to +32 in Session 9 when the patient reported procedural understanding and change. Smoothing displays a gradually more positive therapy experience from Sessions 1 to 9 then deterioration and final recovery to the level of the early therapy phase. There was an enactment spanning Sessions 10 to 13 when the patient felt abandoned following negotiation of the final number of sessions. Session sampling began at Session 5 as therapeutic work with the diagram is only fully established then, included one session prior to an alliance fluctuation, and continued until the smoothed curve returned to stable values. The selected sessions from this therapy were therefore 5 to 15.

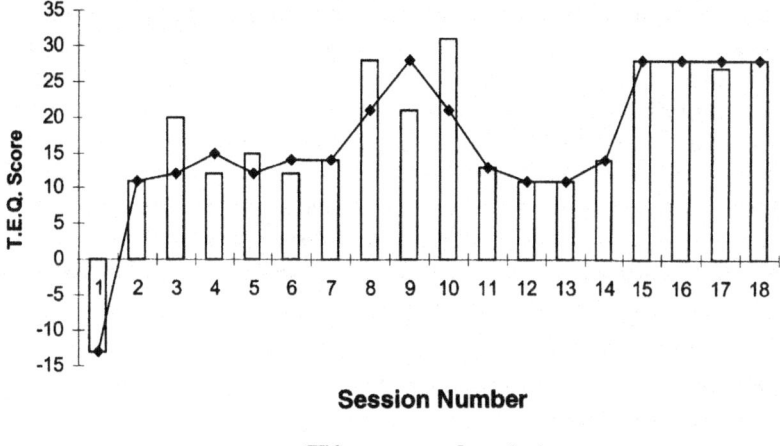

FIG. 12.1. Therapy Experience Questionnaire (TEQ) scores and smoothing in an 18-session therapy.

Identification of Markers of Alliance-Threatening Enactments

Three raters independently listened to the audiotaped sessions to locate markers—evidence of an RR, as identified in the formulatory diagram, being enacted within the patient–therapist interaction. Raters had referral and assessment details, the diagram and the selected session audiotapes, and were required to locate the observed procedure on the diagram. In-session enactments of RRPs for each patient–therapist pair produce individualized markers. Such markers, specific to the individual case, differ from approaches that list specific patient behaviors such as negative feelings, avoidance, or high levels of compliance as signs of impairment in the alliance (Agnew, Harper, Shapiro, & Barkham, 1994; Safran et al., 1990; Safran & Murran, 1996). RR enactments for which there was independent agreement between at least two of three raters (presence of an enactment and its location on the diagram) were selected for task analysis.

Task Analysis (Greenberg, 1984a, 1984b)

Task analysis is a process research strategy involving the detailed study of key in-session events to specify the processes patients use to resolve particular problems in psychotherapy. It is guided by theoretical and clinical understanding and in this current context, the aim was to understand task resolution and to build explanatory models of the processes involved. The initial step (the rational analysis) was to construct a hypothetical idealized performance representing the clinician or researcher's best understanding of how resolution was achieved. This then guides the rigorous observation and description of actual task performances (the empirical analysis), identifying the strategies used and the characteristics of successful performances. The ideal performance model was then compared to the actual performances in an iterative manner (the rational–empirical comparison), moving back and forth between the data and the hypothetical model until a refined performance model was built.

The Rational Analysis: The Ideal Model for Enactment Resolution

The key therapeutic task in postreformulation sessions for CAT therapists is collaborative work with the patient on recognition and revision of their problematic procedures, including in-session procedural enactments. Therapist interventions are considered helpful only to the extent that the therapist does not collude or reciprocate the patient's RRPs and engages with the patient to understand enactments. The therapist is aided by the CAT diagram. On the basis of CAT theory and clinical experience, it was decided that the most effective intervention would involve the therapist focusing on the enactment while resisting reciprocation. The central task would then be to facilitate linking and explanation of the enactment by referring to the shared reformulatory tools.

A theoretically based model of the ideal stages of successful RR enactment resolution was constructed by Dawn Bennett, Anthony Ryle, and David Shapiro, a clinician and researcher familiar with the events paradigm but with limited experience of CAT. The model drew on relevant psychotherapy research and theory, the view of expert CAT therapists, clinical experience, observations of relevant task performances, and empathizing with the therapist and patient through self-directed questions such as "What would I do now?". The resulting rational ideal model provides preliminary understanding of the possible performance components, strategies, and sequences. On identifying evidence of an RR enactment occurring in the patient–therapist interaction, the model (Fig. 12.2) hypothesizes five stages for performance. In the first, there is an acknowledgment of the in-session event by the therapist, making the enactment event explicit by directing the patient's attention to the therapeutic relationship or acknowledging the patient's expressed feelings; the second stage is an exploration and collaborative clarification of their respective understandings. In the third, linking and explanation stage, the therapist invites or proposes how the enactment may be linked to the reformulation, other shared tools or

Marker
Evidence of enactment of patterns identified in reformulation in the patient-therapist interaction

↓

1. Acknowledgement

↓

2. Exploration

↓

3. Linking & Explanation

↓

4. Negotiation

↓

5. Consensus

There are an additional three stages constituting:

↓

6. Further explanation

↓

7. New ways of relating/exits

↓

8. Closure

FIG. 12.2. The rational ideal model.

metaphors, relationships with others, childhood memories or earlier examples in therapy. Negotiation of the patient's acceptance and understanding is elaborated, and doubts and disagreements are explored in the fourth stage. A consensus agreement is reached about the in-session event, its association to other relationships, or its origin in the past. Following this resolution, there may be three additional stages: The procedure is related to the whole reformulation (extension or further explanation); alternatives and exits are explored (new ways of relating); and the therapist affirms the focus of therapy on the therapeutic relationship and the possibility of change (closure). While working toward resolution the therapist does not collude, that is reciprocate, the expected role in the enacted RR. This model is not fixed or linear and it is assumed that cycling within and between stages will occur. It is a "best guess" at what may be required for resolution and thus is a framework to guide empirical analysis. A fuller description of the premises that led to the model can be found in Bennett (1998).

The Empirical Analysis: Observation of Resolution Performances

Following each identified marker, the task performances were broken down into elements and systematically developed into descriptive accounts of the components and stages of each resolution performance. This contrasts with studies using a finite number of resolution performances classified as the most successful resolutions (Rice & Sapiera, 1984; Greenberg, 1984b). We included all reliable markers of RR enactments to examine successive attempts at resolution within each case, as this may convey how therapists and patients achieve resolution rather than just what they do.

The Rational–Empirical Comparison: Model Building

Cumulative revisions were made to the ideal model by three judges (Dawn Bennett, Glenys Parry, and Anthony Ryle), experienced CAT therapists, trainers, and supervisors, culminating in the refined performance model. Each cycling, from the conceptual stages of the ideal model through a detailed inspection of a resolution performance, as located in the transcripts, produced a more informative and refined map of the stages that patient and therapist moved through to achieve successful resolution. This phase reflects two model-building principles (Morris, 1967). First, model development is considered a process of progressive enrichment or elaboration of the ideal model to reflect the complexity of the actual situation. Second, in this iterative process, as each new version of the model is tested, a new version is produced that leads to a subsequent test. Progressive cycling between the ideal model and empirical observations continued provided that cycles produced new findings. When the addition of further cases did not add any substantially new discoveries or refinements, the process was judged to have reached a saturation point (Greenberg & Newman, 1996).

RESULTS: THE REFINED MODEL OF RRP ENACTMENT RESOLUTION

Working through the pool of good outcome cases on a case-by-case basis, the sampling strategy led to the inclusion of 107 markers and their associated enactment resolution performances from 66 sessions of four good outcome cases. Resolved enactments were characterized by the presence of both an explicit statement of understanding, for example, "I can see what you are saying there and I agree. So I am still running away," and an affective shift suggesting full emergence from the state of the enactment, for example, "[laughing] That's why I slagged you off last week ... not caring for me enough."

Partial resolution was characterized by some cognitive awareness, but emotional and behavioral aspects of the enactment were still present (e.g., "I don't know but I've been thinking about it"). Unresolved enactments were characterized by the absence of either resolution marker. On this basis, raters classed 57 (52%) enactments as resolved, 37 (34%) as partially resolved, and 15 (14%) unresolved.

There was confirmation in each of the four cases for the eight stages of the ideal model. Case 1 added 16 refinements, Case 2 confirmed 13 of these and added a further 3, Case 3 confirmed all 19 refinements added by the previous cases and contributed 1 further refinement, and Case 4 provided confirmation for 19 of the 20 refinements but did not add anything further. Sampling stopped at this point.

The final empirical model for resolution of the RR enactments is depicted in Fig. 12.3. It is referred to as the performance model, as it indicates the therapists behaviors and so forth that constitute a competent performance in recognizing and resolving the RR enactment.

Refinements to the Rational Model

The systematic comparison between the rational model and the empirical analysis led to a number of amendments to the rational model, although the stages and their sequence remain the same. Figure 12.3 shows the refinements made to the model in Fig. 12.2.

Tangential Steps. Sometimes therapists moved the focus away from the enactment before returning to it. For example, a therapist could acknowledge a therapy event that may reflect an enactment (e.g., patient being consistently late) but then allow space for discussion of outside events or establish a reality base to the enactment (the patient's explanation) at the acknowledgment stage then explore whether lateness reflected an enactment of an RRP. These and other interventions attend to the alliance by addressing the patient's reports and concerns. It seemed that only by allowing space for patients' accounts of enactments are successive attempts at resolution possible. Therapists repeatedly cycled between stages, for example, resolution did not proceed beyond the linking stage without securing consensual acknowledgment of the in-session experience. Therapists and patients were observed to cycle through deepening levels of understanding, emotional awareness, and assimilation, demonstrating the inadequacy of a

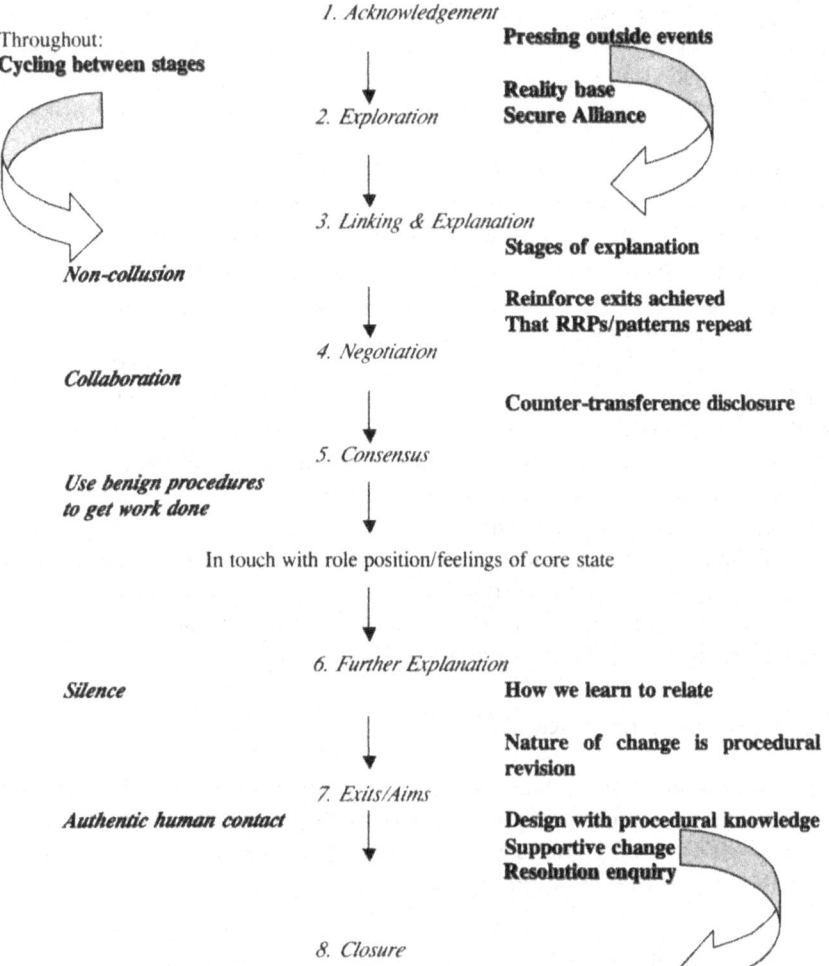

FIG. 12.3. Refined performance model. RRP = reciprocal role procedures.

linear stage model. An enquiry to assess resolution occurred after consensus, facilitating, if necessary, a second cycle through the model.

A New Stage Following Consensus Recognition. Therapists and patients focused on understanding and assimilating previously warded off feelings associated with the RR that had emerged between them. Therapists validated the patient's experience and used the diagram to explain why the problematic experiences had not been assimilated.

Within the Explanatory and Negotiation Stages. Therapists offered CAT understandings of the patient's situation; the recurrent nature of procedures as patterns of relating that fail to be revised and that the patterns can occur in any relationship, including that with the therapist. Therapists used countertransference disclosure to illustrate and explain the emergence of RRPs within the therapy relationship. They also explained how patients developed and perhaps needed the procedures as survival strategies, understandable given the patient's history.

Within the Exit Stage, Therapists Facilitated the Patient's Engagement in Change. Therapists explained and reinforced alternatives to the problematic procedures that the patient could engage in with others and with the therapist. They used procedural knowledge to design and anticipate difficulty with or rejection of these alternatives, anticipating how the patient's procedures would facilitate or inhibit engagement with homework. Therapists also used supportive interventions as the patient engaged in the difficult process of procedural revision. They explained that change involves revising procedures and predicted the consequences of continued use of damaging procedures.

A Series of Refinements Classed as Heuristic Guiding Principles. The collaborative and noncollusive therapeutic stance that was held to characterize the ideal model was observed and elaborated. Therapists used phrases that specifically enlisted patients' participation, verified their understandings, and invited patients' views throughout. Therapists used patients' unproblematic procedures (e.g., a responsible, working-hard procedure) to achieve the work of therapy while being alert to the possibility of problematic or maladaptive procedures being enacted (e.g., "responsible patient" becoming "anxiously striving to please the therapist"). Noncollusion involved refraining from enacting a damaging procedure or pointing it out and providing a rationale about why this occurred (metacommunication).

Two further principles were identified: First, silence facilitated a self-observing capacity with subsequent contributions by the patient advancing the work of therapy. Second, the therapist offered reflective and linking statements within an empathic and respectful relationship when the therapist was in tune with the patient's experience and affect. Therapists used self-disclosure and showed vulnerability and aspects of their real self in the service of modeling a new way of being to the patient. This authentic stance provided a new role procedure available for internalization. Therapists consistently disconfirmed patient's negative self-expectations. One therapist engaged at this authentic level particularly at points of therapy- and life-threatening transference enactments.

The Pattern of Resolution of Transference-Related Alliance Ruptures

The complete refined performance model was not observed in every selected RR enactment. Successful resolution did require the patient's engagement in acknowledging the enactment and establishing and exploring meanings. Resolution work was never able to proceed to the stage of linking without first achieving this. For some enactments, this was successfully achieved, whereas for others, if the patient was unsure or disengaged, the therapist cycled through the early stages of the model and if the patient disagreed, the therapist invited and then elaborated the patient's view. For most enactments, these interventions were sufficient to preserve an alliance, engage the patient, and proceed to linking.

Links to the diagram were offered or invited in all resolution performances and therapists ensured that the patient understood the pattern that was the enactment and its origins. The consensus stage was not always clearly distinguished, but all successful resolution performances contained a patient statement of recognition of the enactment. At the point of resolution, patients spontaneously disclosed feelings associated with the role they had experienced with the therapist and the historical basis to these feelings (often previously warded off). Premature attempts by therapists to explore such feelings were unsuccessful. This did not occur in every performance but occurred for all patients at some point in therapy. Therapists offered their perception of the patient's affect following resolution as an opportunity for assimilation ("I guess you may have felt ..."). Only if enactments were acknowledged and consensus achieved did work proceed to the exit stage in which new procedures and patterns of relating to self and others were considered. Each resolution performance contained at least one supportive explanatory intervention in which the therapist offered hope for the possibility of change.

For enactments that had been difficult to resolve and characterized by successive resolution attempts such as repeated cycling and negotiation, therapists gave more attention to the exit stage. They ensured that the patient understood the rationale and need for alternatives to damaging interpersonal procedures and planned these carefully to prevent failure.

Collaboration, noncollusion, and silence were observed in all four cases. Therapists paid attention to the extent to which their own styles and therapeutic techniques could reenact a maladaptive procedure with the patient. If the therapist reciprocated a procedure, they explained this using the diagram and countertransference disclosure. When an enactment is not resolved through the model stages, the therapist used the real relationship explicitly to challenge and replace the destructive procedures, make contact with the patient, and secure an alliance.

TESTING THE MODEL

We predicted that therapists in poor outcome cases would fail to resolve enactments and that their resolution performances would be characterized by an absence of model-consistent interventions. Thirty-five enactments from a total of 16 sessions from two poor outcome cases (deterioration on two or more self-report measures) were sampled. In contrast to the good outcome cases in which over half the enactments were resolved, only 1 of the 35 enactments from poor outcome cases was classed as resolved, with a further 7 partially resolved. Therapists in poor outcome cases did not detect the majority of enactments and there was evidence for unrecognized collusion. In summary, the two therapists involved did not adhere to the model (Fig. 12.3). The way in which they did not is summarized in Table 12.1.

TABLE 12.1
Characteristics of Resolution Performances
of Therapists of Poor Outcome Cases

The majority of enactments were not detected or recognized:
- If detected, resolution performance did not proceed beyond the linking stage of the performance model.
- Although present, acknowledgment and exploration was incomplete in that they lacked the reflective focus on feelings, tentative style, and cycling of the refined model.
- Little use of the reformulation, specifically the diagram, in the linking stage.
- Evidence for only 4 of the 20 refinements (made to the model by therapists of good outcome cases), and their form was partial.
- No evidence of negotiation. Therapists ended resolution attempts with supportive gestures when they met patient disagreement.
- Little evidence of the consensus stage of the refined model. Therapists may have successfully linked some enactments to patterns in other relationships, but there was little evidence for exploring the patients understanding of links or reaching a shared understanding considered characteristic of the consensus stage.
- No evidence for the consistent work in the later stages of the model: further explanation, exits, or closure. Proposed exits were not designed with knowledge of the patients' procedures and lacked explanations that could facilitate the patient's engagement.
- Little evidence of the heuristic guiding principles. Therapists were not tentative, negotiating, or collaborative, nor did they use silence or the authentic relationship in which the therapist was in tune with painful feelings.
- Evidence for unrecognized collusion, whereby the therapist reciprocated the patient's reciprocal role procedures and failed to acknowledge this. Some instances of reciprocation served to preserve the alliance (but there was no evidence that these were intentional), whereas others led to ruptures in the alliance (therapists failed to identify their own contribution).
- Evidence for patients having more awareness of some enactments than the therapist, as if the therapist lacked an implicit cognitive map to guide their performance.

Resolution of RR Enactments and the Therapeutic Relationship

Therapists of good outcome cases were able to recognize 84% of the RR enactments when they occurred. There was an average of 1.62 enactments in each session and a range of 1 to 4 enactments per session. When these therapists recognized an enactment, they acknowledged that this had occurred and attempted to resolve the majority of enactments through a focus on the therapeutic relationship. They moved to outside events when these were pressing but always returned to the focus on the therapeutic interaction. In contrast, therapists in the poor outcome cases only recognized 34% of enactments, and when they did recognize an enactment, there was an emphasis on outside events. Poor outcome therapists maintained this outside focus even on those occasions when the patient was explicit in their expression of negative feelings toward the therapist. This finding is consistent with Sachs (1983) who observed that failing to address patient's negative attitudes toward either the therapist or therapy and passive acceptance of problematic aspects of the patient's behavior, such as evasiveness, was highly associated with negative therapeutic outcome.

In one of the poor outcome cases, in response to an enactment and explicit disengagement of the patient, the therapist focused repeatedly on prescriptive interventions, which the patient rejected. For example, the therapist offered solutions for an interpersonal dispute with a neighbor while the patient felt unsupported and overlooked and became dismissive. This reenacted an RR in which the patient experienced any failure to offer total understanding and support as rejection. This became a major threat to the alliance.

This seems to be a similar phenomenon to that described by other researchers in which dogged adherence to technique in the face of a deteriorating alliance is associated with poor outcomes or the patient leaving therapy prematurely. Piper et al. (1999) describe a nonproductive pattern characterized by a high level of transference interpretation despite patient resistance in the final session of those prematurely dropping out of time-limited, interpretive, individual psychotherapy in a randomized clinical trial. Castonguay, Goldfried, Wiser, Raue, and Hayes (1996) also found that some cognitive therapists attempted to resolve alliance problems by increasing their adherence to cognitive therapy rationale and technique.

Resolution of alliance-threatening transference enactments is dependent on therapists' ability to identify their presence. There was a significant difference in therapist's ability to do this in the good and poor outcome cases. Therapists of poor outcome cases infrequently used the diagrammatic formulation for linking in-session enactments. Failing to use the diagram as an aid to recognize and resolve enactments may partly reflect inaccuracy of the diagram. Although we have shown that it is possible to develop a succinct but comprehensive and accurate formulation based on information from the first three sessions (Bennett, 1998; Bennett & Parry, 1998), not all diagrams are of this quality. In other cases, therapists and supervisors need to revise the diagram. All the enactments identified by raters in the good outcome cases were located on the patient's respective diagrams. In contrast, only half of the enactments in the poor outcome cases were represented on the respective diagrams. This difference was significant and has important implications for training and supervision. An important implication for CAT and indeed any other brief psychodynamic psychotherapy is that practice should allow for revision of the formulation during therapy as needed. It is therefore considered good CAT practice that when an affect or event cannot be located on the diagram, revise the diagram. This guards against the possibility of the therapist and patient engaging in an RR enactment that cannot be related to the formulation. It is important here to distinguish between all the procedures represented on the diagram and the focus of therapy. A therapy may focus on one or two of the most damaging procedures within the context of a more complex diagram.

APPLICATIONS AND IMPLICATIONS OF THE MODEL

The emphasis in brief dynamic psychotherapies on developing a formulation for the focus of the work with the patient is supported by the work summarized in this chapter. A good formulation helps the therapist predict and recognize possible damaging procedures and transference enactments as they appear in therapy. In CAT, this formulation can be in written and diagrammatic forms. Another key feature of brief therapy is that of collaboration to engage the patient's reflective capacities, which is a central mechanism of change. This collaborative stance models a respectful and new relationship for patient internalization. We suggest that these general points are applicable to any brief psychodynamic psychotherapy.

The resolution performance model is not a rigid prescription or intervention manual but a system to sensitize therapists to these enactment events and the skillful technical interventions associated with successful resolution. This is a way to encourage "responsive matching" (Frank & Spanier, 1995) in which therapists skillfully match their response to the changing needs of the patient, which reflects intuition and the ability to modify technique when required, a key feature of effective therapists. However, it is important to determine when responsive matching is inherently dangerous and driven by countertransference rather than reflecting flexibility and therapeutic responsiveness. The empirically derived refined performance model offers a way to guide selection of interventions at particular points in the progress of enactment resolution. In this way, psychodynamic therapists can become familiar with the flexible, responsive use of techniques guided by formulation.

Applications of the empirically derived model has been the focus of our subsequent research and we have developed guidelines for therapist performance and a training pack for trainers and therapists; developed and piloted a measure of therapy competence in managing alliance threatening RR enactments for use in training, supervision, and research (The Therapist Intervention Checklist; Bennett, Parry, & Ryle, 1999); and evaluated a training method of intensive supervision in model-specific interventions ("microsupervision").

SUMMARY AND CONCLUSIONS

The kind of research summarized here demonstrates how qualitative accounts of psychotherapy process can lead beyond the particulars of individual cases to descriptions of patterns. Qualitative accounts contribute to a systematic, replicable, and theoretically appropriate method of selecting material likely to increase understanding of how therapist performance has an impact on outcome. The particular value and contribution of task analysis, as was evident here, was the intensive fine-grained tracking of therapeutic process guided by a rational framework. The process of empirically refining a model guided by theory and experience has formalized some of the nuances of the clinical process, often referred to as *intuitive clinical wisdom* (Rice & Greenberg, 1984). Knowledge about what works in psychotherapy must be rooted in clinical observation and draw on the experience and wisdom of the practicing clinician, but it must also have empirical verification (Goldfried & Wolfe, 1998). The methodological sophistication of the change-process paradigm offers the opportunity for continuing to forge such collaboration.

Such research has a number of limitations. The findings may relate only to the cases under study. In part, the issue of generalizability across other patient–therapist dyads is a challenge to task analysis as a methodology. Although we focused on CAT, we envisage that the findings and the model will be applicable across theoretical orientations.

In distinguishing between good and poor outcome cases and presuming that competent performance was more likely to be observed in good outcome cases, we were influenced by the assumption that there is an association between competence and outcome. However, although there is a relation between therapist skill and better outcomes, it is not a strong one—some patients improve regardless of the therapist's expertise, and some may progress slowly no matter how skillful the therapist may be (Beutler, Machado, & Neufeldt, 1994). It can be argued that one would not logically expect to see a linear relation between the amount of a given active ingredient in therapy and the therapeutic outcome because therapists adapt and respond to the needs of the patient (Stiles & Shapiro, 1994). In view of this, the results (showing such clear differences between the therapists of good and poor cases) are surprising. One reason may be that the relation between competence and outcome is easier to observe in the patient group under study, as people meeting diagnostic criteria for BPD are unlikely to improve spontaneously and tend to respond negatively to therapist errors. We also suggest that by going beyond proxy measures of competence (e.g., years of experience or training), the resolution model provides a means of observing a much clearer association between competence and outcome. Of course, it remains possible that the model encompasses client difficulty as well as therapist competence, as they are difficult to disentangle, and both are associated with outcome (Waltz et al., 1993).

The model describes what therapists in good outcome cases were doing, and we showed that therapists in poor outcome cases did not follow it. However, this research design does not allow generalizations about the relation between model-consistent process components and outcomes. To test the validity of the refined performance model would require a demonstration that the hypothesized mechanisms of change do predict treatment outcomes. This would involve blind rating of whether or not the process components of the model were present, then examining the relationship to outcome in a large enough sample for adequate statistical power.

Replication is the key to these shortcomings and we would recommend that others replicate the procedure, with a new set of cases, to test the refined performance model. Unfortunately, task analysis is labor intensive. An alternative way would be to use the checklist of therapist competencies derived from the model and apply it to actual therapist performance to test whether performance relates to outcome. This makes the research replicable and of potential clinical value. It is currently being undertaken in a randomized controlled trial of CAT.

In the light of these caveats, the model should not be seen as the definitive account of competent enactment resolution performance. On the other hand, it contributes to our knowledge of therapist competence in a way that is falsifiable, generalizable, and replicable.

REFERENCES

Agnew, R. M., Harper, H., Shapiro, D. A., & Barkham, M. (1994). Resolving a challenge to the therapeutic relationship: A single case study. *British Journal of Medical Psychology, 67,* 155–170.

Alexander, F., & French, T. M. (1946). *Psychoanalytic therapy: Principles and application*. New York: Ronald Press.

Aveline, M. O. (1997). The limitations of randomized controlled trials as guides to clinical effectiveness with reference to the psychotherapeutic management of neuroses and personality disorders. *Current Opinion in Psychiatry, 10,* 113–125.

Bearden, C., Lavelle, N., Buysse, D., Karp, J. F., & Frank, E. (1996). Personality pathology and time to remission in depressed outpatients treated with interpersonal psychotherapy. *Journal of Personality Disorders, 10,* 164–173.

Bennett, D. (1998). *Deriving a model of therapist competence from good and poor outcome cases in the psychotherapy for borderline personality disorder*. Unpublished doctoral dissertation, University of Sheffield, Sheffield, England.

Bennett, D., & Parry, G. (1998). The accuracy of reformulation in cognitive analytic therapy: A validation study. *Psychotherapy Research, 8,* 405–422.

Bennett, D., Parry, G., & Ryle, A. (1999). *Development of a measure of therapist competence in resolving transference enactments which threaten the therapeutic alliance*. Unpublished report. Mental Health Foundation.

Beutler, L. E., Machado, P. P., & Neufeldt, S. A. (1994). Therapist variables. In A. E Bergin & S. L. Garfield (Eds.), *Handbook of psychotherapy and behavior change* (pp. 229–269). New York: Wiley.

Bordin, E. S. (1979). The generalizability of the concept of the working alliance. *Psychotherapy: Theory, Research and Practice, 16,* 252–260.

Castonguay, L. G., Goldfried, M. R., Wiser, S., Raue, P. J., & Hayes, A. M. (1996). Predicting the effect of cognitive therapy for depression: A study of unique and common factors. *Journal of Consulting and Clinical Psychology, 64,* 497–504.

Foreman, S. A., & Marmar, C. R. (1985). Therapist actions that address initially poor therapeutic alliances in psychotherapy. *American Journal of Psychiatry, 142,* 922–926.

Frank, E., & Spanier, C. (1995). Interpersonal psychotherapy for depression: Overview, clinical efficacy and future directions. *Clinical Psychology: Science and Practice, 2,* 349–369.

Garfield, S. L. (1995). *Psychotherapy: An eclectic-integrative approach* (2nd ed.). New York: Wiley.

Goldfried, M. R., & Wolfe, B. (1996). Psychotherapy practice and research: Repairing a strained alliance. *American Psychologist, 51,* 1007–1016.

Goldfried, M. R., & Wolfe, B. E. (1998). Toward a more clinically valid approach to therapy research. *Journal of Consulting and Clinical Psychology, 66,* 143–150.

Greenberg, L. S. (1984a). Task analysis: The general approach. In L. Rice & L. S. Greenberg (Eds.), *Patterns of change: The intensive analysis of psychotherapy process* (pp. 124–148). New York: Guilford.

Greenberg, L. S. (1984b). A task analysis of interpersonal conflict resolution. In L. Rice & L. S. Greenberg (Eds.), *Patterns of change: The intensive analysis of psychotherapy process* (pp. 67–123). New York: Guilford.

Greenberg, L. S., & Newman, F. L. (1996). An approach to psychotherapy change process research: Introduction to the special section. *Journal of Consulting and Clinical Psychology, 64,* 435–438.

Henry, W. P. (1998). Science, politics, and the politics of science: The use and misuse of empirically validated treatment research. *Psychotherapy Research, 8,* 126–140.

Henry, W. P., Schacht, T. E., & Strupp, H. H. (1986). Structural analysis of social behaviour: Application to a study of interpersonal process in differential psychotherapeutic outcome. *Journal of Consulting and Clinical Psychology, 54,* 27–31.

Horvath, A. O., & Greenberg, L. S. (1994). Introduction. In A. O. Horvath & L. S. Greenberg (Eds.), *The working alliance: Theory, research and practice* (pp. 259–286). New York: Wiley.

Jackson, P. R. (1989). Analysing data. In G. Parry & F. N. Watts (Eds.), *Behavioural and mental health research: A handbook of skills and methods* (pp. 55–80). London: Lawrence Erlbaum Associates.

Jacobson, N. S., & Revenstorf, D. (1988). Statistics for assessing clinical significance of psychotherapy: Issues, problems and new developments. *Behavioural Assessment, 10*, 133–145.
Jacobson, N. S., & Truax, P. (1991). Clinical significance: A statistical approach to defining meaningful change in psychotherapy research. *Journal of Consulting and Clinical Psychology, 59*, 12–19.
Kiesler, D. J. (1986). Interpersonal methods of diagnosis and treatment. In J. D. Cavenar (Ed.), *Psychiatry. Vol. I* (pp. 1–23). Philadelphia: Lippincott.
Kivlighan, D. M., & Shaughnessy, P. (1995). Analysis of the development of the working alliance using hierarchical linear modeling. *Journal of Counseling Psychology, 42*, 338–349.
Luborsky, L., Crits-Christoph, P., McLellan, T., Woody, G., Piper, W., Imber, S., & Liberman, B. (1986). Do therapists vary much in their success? Findings from four outcome studies. *American Journal of Orthopsychiatry, 56*, 501–512.
McLaughlin, J. T. (1991). Clinical and theoretical aspects of enactment. *Journal of the American Psychoanalytic Association, 39*, 595–614.
Morris, W. (1967). On the art of modelling. *Management Science, 13*, 77–114.
Orlinsky, D. E., Grawe, K., & Parks, B. K. (1994). Process and outcome in psychotherapy: Noch einmal. In A. E. Bergin & S. L. Garfield (Eds.), *Handbook of psychotherapy and behaviour change* (4th ed., pp. 270–376). New York: Wiley.
Piper, W. E., Ogrodniczuk, J. S., Joyce, A. S., McCallum, M., Rosie, J. S., O'Kelly, J. G., & Steinberg, P. I. (1999). Prediction of dropping out in time-limited, interpretive individual psychotherapy. *Psychotherapy, 36*, 114–122.
Rice, L. N., & Greenberg, L. S. (Eds.). (1984). *Patterns of change: Intensive analysis of psychotherapy process.* New York: Guilford.
Rice, L. N., & Sapiera, E. P. (1984). Task analysis of the resolution of problematic reactions. In L. N. Rice & L. S. Greenberg (Eds.), *Patterns of change: Intensive analysis of psychotherapy process* (pp. 29–66). New York: Guilford.
Ryle, A. (Ed.). (1995a). *Cognitive analytic therapy: Developments in theory and practice.* Chichester, England: Wiley.
Ryle, A. (1995b). Transference and countertransference variations in the course of the cognitive analytic therapy of two borderline patients: The relation to the diagrammatic reformulation of self states. *British Journal of Medical Psychology, 68*, 109–124.
Ryle, A. (1997). *Cognitive analytic therapy and borderline personality disorder: The model and the method.* Chichester, England: Wiley.
Ryle, A., & Kerr, I. B. (2002). *Introducing cognitive analytic therapy: Principles and practice.* Chichester, England: Wiley.
Sachs, J. S. (1983). Negative factors in brief psychotherapy: An empirical assessment. *Journal of Consulting and Clinical Psychology, 51*, 557–564.
Safran, J. D., Crocker, P., McMain, S., & Murray, P. (1990). Therapeutic alliance rupture as a therapy event for empirical investigation. *Psychotherapy, 27*, 154–165.
Safran, J. D., & Muran, J. C. (1996). The resolution of ruptures in the therapeutic alliance. *Journal of Consulting and Clinical Psychology, 55*, 379–384.
Shearin, E. N., & Linehan, M. M. (1993). Dialectical behaviour therapy for borderline personality disorder: Treatment goals, strategies and empirical support. In J. Paris (Ed.), *Borderline personality disorder: Etiology and treatment* (pp. 285–318). Washington, DC: American Psychiatric Association.
Stiles, W. B., & Shapiro, D. A. (1994). Disabuse of the drug metaphor: Psychotherapy process outcome correlations. *Journal of Consulting and Clinical Psychology, 62*, 942–948.
Stone, M. H. (1993). Psychotherapy with schizotypal borderline patients. *Journal of the American Academy of Psychoanalysis, 11*, 87–111.
Strupp, H. H. (1980). Success and failure in time-limited psychotherapy: Further evidence. Comparison IV. *Archives of General Psychiatry, 37*, 947–954.
Strupp, H. H. (1998). The Vanderbilt I study revisited. *Psychotherapy Research, 8*, 17–29.

Waldinger, R. J., & Gunderson, J. G. (1984). Completed psychotherapies with borderline patients. *American Journal of Psychotherapy, 38,* 190–202.

Waltz, J., Addis, M. E., Koerner, K., & Jacobson, N. S. (1993). Testing the integrity of a psychotherapy protocol: Assessment of adherence and competence. *Journal of Consulting and Clinical Psychology, 61,* 620–630.

PART

IV

ENDING AND EVALUATING

CHAPTER

13

Ending Therapy: Processes and Outcomes

Denise P. Charman
Anne C. Graham
Victoria University

In the psychotherapy literature, ending therapy is referred to as *termination* and the final phase of therapy is the *termination phase*. The length of this phase is determined in large part by the length of the therapy, with the last 10% to 25% of therapy considered as the termination phase (Gelso & Woodhouse, 2002). The negotiation of termination can be problematic for patient and therapist alike. It can be tempting for therapists to avoid the ending by either continuing indefinitely or by delaying discussion of a forthcoming ending. Indeed, many trainees avoid negotiating the termination phase by not discussing it at all with the patient until the last session (Bostic, Shadid, & Blotcky, 1996). Patients too may avoid termination, for example, by dropping out prematurely or fleeing into health (Malan, 1979).

The end of therapy, and the last session in particular, can come about in a variety of ways. Ideally, the last session, especially in long-term therapies, comes about as part of a "natural ending" (Wittenberg, 1999, p. 342), a planned response to the patient's decreased need for therapy. Patient and therapist work toward a set date and the final session becomes the last in a carefully considered process. Unfortunately, a natural ending is relatively rare. Many psychoanalysts acknowledge that the majority of analyses end because the patient moves to another city, runs out of money, impulsively quits, or agrees with the analyst that a stalemate has been reached (Malcolm, 1982). The trend toward brief, time-limited therapies has meant that more therapies commence with a termination date already set. Nevertheless, many therapies end "by default" (Budman & Gurman, 1988, p. 6). A meta-analysis of

125 psychotherapy studies showed that the mean dropout rate varied from 36% to 51% (Wierzbicki & Pekarik, 1993) and, for trainees at least, 35% ended as forced terminations (de Bosset & Styrsky, 1986). In short, a planned negotiated end of therapy is the exception rather than the rule.

Regardless of the way the ending comes about, it is important to consider how to successfully negotiate termination, the associated dynamics, and the therapeutic tasks to be accomplished. Marx and Gelso (1987) found that patient satisfaction with termination of therapy was most strongly related to how termination proceeded. However, termination procedures may depend on the success of the therapy. Quintana and Holahan (1992) asked counselors to compare termination in a successful and an unsuccessful counseling case (with similar duration of brief therapy). Success was indicated by therapists' rating improvement in feeling, behavior, self-understanding, and overall change. The unsuccessful cases were not to be premature terminations or dropouts. Quintana and Holahan (1992) found that therapists undertook more termination behaviors with the successful cases. With unsuccessful cases, there was less frequent discussion of the end of counseling, less review of the course of counseling, less activity bringing closure to the relationship, and less discussion of the counselee's affective reactions to termination.

This chapter considers termination issues by considering the experience of the patient and therapist, the empirical research, and what the therapist can do to facilitate a therapeutic ending. These themes are illustrated by reference to the last two sessions of the case study referred to throughout this book.

CONCEPTUALIZING THE EXPERIENCE OF TERMINATION

The experience of patients (and indeed therapists) during the termination phase is frequently shaped by a past history of painful endings in which the course of events could neither be influenced nor understood. The experience of endings in psychotherapy taps into these past experiences and connects with a range of existential human anxieties about ending and separation. Wittenberg (1999) characterized these anxieties as pertaining to infantile, child, adolescent, and adult levels of psychic life:

> On an infantile level, [these anxieties] are about being abandoned, starving, left to die, disintegrating; on a child level, they are, in addition, about feeling lost, unable to cope on one's own and being thrown back into a state of terrifying helplessness; on a adolescent level they include having to take on adult responsibilities; and on an adult level, any ending also makes us acutely

aware of the passing of time, the end of a period of our life bringing us a step nearer to death, the end of our lifetime. (p. 340)

Within the psychoanalytically oriented therapy literature, termination has usually been conceptualized as an experience of loss. The goal of therapy and the implications for termination have been described as being "individualization which implies making a clean cut, permanent break with the therapist which enacts a death-like experience" (Lee, 2000, p. 50). The concept of termination as loss has received some support in the (rather scant) research literature. Marx and Gelso (1987) found, in a university counseling center, that the amount of termination work undertaken (as reported by the counselee) was related to closeness to the counselor, loss as a theme of counseling, and number of sessions. The counselee's rating of the importance of discussing reactions to termination was predicted by loss as theme of counseling, closeness to counselor, and loss history. Boyer and Hoffman (1993) also found in a study of 117 psychologists that their affective reaction to termination was predicted by their own history of loss, as well as their perceptions of their clients' sensitivity to loss.

An alternative conceptualization views termination as a weaning process, implying that the end of therapy, although a loss, is also an opportunity for development and transformation (Quintana, 1993). This view is consistent with theories emphasizing the process of internalization in which the patient "transforms real or imagined regulatory interactions with [the therapy] environment, and real or imagined characteristics of [the therapy] environment into inner regulations and characteristics" (Schafer, 1968, p. 9). In this view, aspects of the therapist and the therapy process are internalized by the patient who then continues to have access to these representations beyond the end of therapy. This internalization process is seen as necessary for successful termination. Whether termination is conceptualized as loss or as weaning, the way in which therapy ends will have implications for internalization and adjustment after therapy, either for the mourning process or else (or as well as) for the incorporation and utilization of the gains that have been made and a new image of self as a result of growth in therapy.

NEGOTIATED ENDINGS

Natural Endings and Long-Term Therapy

Natural endings occur when the patient experiences an ongoing decline in his or her need for therapy, and both patient and therapist begin to sense that the therapeutic endeavor is coming to an end. Behavioral referents that indicate that therapy is sufficient have been identified by Kramer (1986) who surveyed 20 psychotherapists about the types of termination cues they used. The signs indicative of ending included (a) patients no longer idealize or depreciate their therapists but rather begin to relate to them more as equals; (b) patients seem to need less input, evaluation, and interpretation from the therapist and seem to have internalized the therapist; (c) patients start to space out sessions further apart in time; and (d) patients consistently have less to talk about in sessions.

In long-term therapies that progress to a natural termination, anxieties about ending may be moderated because much therapeutic work about endings has already taken place. Temporary endings, such as holiday breaks, provide opportunities to experience, observe, and work to understand the ways in which the patient responds to endings and separations (Malan, 1979). A natural end to therapy is likely to be approached with some sense of readiness, but this is fluctuating and ambivalent. There is pleasure and pride in the work done and the developments achieved, alternating with doubt and anxiety about future challenges. There may be profound sadness and regret at leaving a valued relationship, as well as gratitude and some envy of the future patient who will take one's place. (In group therapy, a patient's leave-taking can be further complicated by the remaining patients' envy of his or her readiness to leave.)

Nevertheless, despite the mutual agreement inherent in a natural termination, once a final date has been set, the patient often appears to regress. The therapist then needs to consider whether this is a real setback or a final reworking and consolidation (Wittenberg, 1999). The therapist needs to be alert to destructive efforts to demonstrate that the patient needs to stay in therapy. The depth of reaction often makes termination difficult for therapist and patient alike. Difficulties include ambivalence, regression, and other negative affects, reexperiencing of previous losses, expression of a need for more treatment, and therapist and patient experiences of sadness (Fortune, Pearlingi, & Rochelle, 1992).

Planned Endings and Brief Therapies

Audits of therapy have consistently shown that most patients receive less than 10 sessions (Budman & Gurman, 1988; Seligman, 1995). Even with these few sessions, many patients report improvements. Therefore, one might expect that if brief therapies were planned at the outset to be only about 10 sessions, they would terminate in a planned way. Whenever this occurs and the patient completes a therapy as planned, Budman and Gurman (1988) referred to this as brief therapy "by design" (p. 6).

There is a range of views about the extent to which the intense emotional reactions elicited by endings in longer term therapies are replicated in brief and time-limited psychotherapies. Gustafson (1995) argued that endings in brief therapies were largely uneventful provided the beginning and middle of the therapy had proceeded properly. However, he stressed the importance of careful assessment of suitability for brief therapy. In contrast, Malan (1979) argued that termination issues might be seen in their most concentrated form in brief therapies. In Mann's (1973) time-limited therapy, resolution of the separation at the end of the therapy is seen to be the key to the therapeutic effect. Mann and Goldman (1982, p. 71) referred to the patient's awareness of "the shadow of termination" from just after the midpoint of the therapy. Wittenberg (1999) thought that entering therapy with a time limit made a big difference because the reality of the time limit is consciously and unconsciously worked at throughout the therapy. She also argued that knowing the time limit influenced how patients proceeded in the therapy. Less disturbed patients may respond to the time limit by working intensively and making the most of the time. They reach termination with a sense of having achieved a lot (though the ending may still be regretted). More disturbed patients may feel the need to protect themselves from becoming too deeply engaged and may be unable to use the therapeutic time fully. The restricted engagement protects the patient from feared intense or overwhelming responses to termination.

Research investigating termination experiences in brief therapy has shown that positive feelings may outweigh painful or negative feelings (Gelso & Woodhouse, 2002). Typical positive feelings include feeling healthy, proud, and calm. In Quintana and Holahan's (1992) study, these adjectives were used by 59% to 79% of responding counselors when describing the termination reactions of patients who had experienced a successful therapy. When asked for their feelings about ending counseling, at least half of the counselees in Marx and Gelso's (1987) study checked positive adjectives such as calm, alive, good, and satisfied. Whereas approximately one third indicated some anxiety by selecting feelings such as afraid, alone, or nervous, far fewer checked negative adjectives indicating depression and hostility. Only 10% were dissatisfied with how counseling came to an end, with a further 25% being neutral. These figures are consistent with those from Mohr (1995) who reported that 10% to 30% might experience negative outcomes.

These relatively positive experiences of termination are consistent with theories that view termination as development or transformation. This does not mean however that therapeutic work on reactions to termination can be neglected. When Marx and Gelso (1987) inquired about termination experiences after brief counseling (an average of 10 sessions), counselees indicated it was important or very important even in this brief work to be able to discuss their reactions to ending.

ENDINGS BY DEFAULT

Patient Dropout

Many therapies are not brief "by design" but are instead brief "by default" (Budman & Gurman, 1988, p. 6). It appears that only a proportion of patients remain after 6 to 10 sessions even if more sessions were planned at the outset. A patient-initiated premature end of therapy is referred to as *patient dropout*. However if an early end is mutually agreed, then this is considered early termination rather than dropping out.

To identify the variables associated with psychotherapy dropout, Wierzbicki and Pekarik (1993) conducted a meta-analysis of 125 studies. They found that increased risk of dropout was significantly associated with minority race, low level of education, and low socioeconomic status. History of deliberate self-harm has also been associated with dropping out (Hillis, Alexander, & Eagles, 1993). It is possible that, in these groups, extratherapeutic factors might mitigate against therapy attendance, such as the cost of travel, competing family crises or responsibilities, or poor physical health. It is more likely that the therapist has not tailored the therapy to suit the needs of these groups (Joyce & McCallum, chap. 4, this volume). Dropping out was not related to diagnosis, duration of illness, history of alcohol abuse, or family history of psychiatric illness (Hillis et al., 1993).

Piper (1998) argued that dropout could be a manifestation of failure of therapy or deterioration of the therapeutic relationship. He reported that the last sessions of dropouts in the study were characterized by too many transference interpretations or too great an adherence to a manual at the expense of the relationship or the patient's opportunity to explore. In this study, the patients expressed thoughts about dropping out early in (what was to become) the last session and therapist and patient appeared to get into conflict. It remains unclear what led patients to thoughts of dropping out, nor is it known how therapist beliefs, behaviors, countertransference, and so forth contributed toward the (apparent) change in technique that took place when the patient made such an announcement. It is possible that the patient dropping out may be a healthy response to an unhealthy therapeutic environment. Indeed the patient may be acting on an accurate perception about the therapy and the therapist (Langs, 1998); for example, the therapist may be conveying an unconscious communication to have therapy end.

A more positive view of dropout is apparent if we accept the figures provided by Howard, Moras, Brill, Martinovich, and Lutz (1996) on dose-response effect. This effect demonstrates that by the eighth session 50% of patients have shown measurable improvement. Similarly, in a meta-analysis of the value of psychotherapy, Smith, Glass, and Miller (1980) showed that positive impacts occurred in the first 6 to 8 sessions. Consequently, it is plausible that patients have dropped out for positive reasons. They may have had their initial expectations fulfilled and their symptoms improved.

Forced Endings

When the therapist seeks to end the therapy prematurely, this becomes, for the patient, a forced ending. The reasons for early termination may be related to the therapy or to personal reasons such as therapist pregnancy (as in the case discussed throughout this book). Often, forced endings are initiated because of extratherapeutic factors such as limitations imposed by funding agencies, short internships, placements or training rotations, and relocation (Bostic et al., 1996). These endings are considered forced endings for the patient who has no choice but to end before achieving their treatment goals. This type of ending is common especially among trainees and was the most common reason for termination in a study of psychiatric residents in which 35% of cases were forced terminations (de Bosset & Styrsky, 1986).

Forced endings are problematic for therapists, with only 16% of psychiatric residents reporting satisfaction with their therapy terminations (Bostic et al., 1996), although this figure includes all terminations not just forced ones. Teyber (2000) suggested that unresolved separation anxieties or guilt about letting someone down in the context of forced termination are the most common forms of countertransference difficulty. Reproachful, angry, rejecting, and helpless responses in the patient (or the therapist's anticipation of such responses) often elicit guilt and defensiveness in the therapist. Therapist conflicts about stopping the therapy can lead to a delay in giving the patient clear information about the termination date or can result in the therapist colluding with the patient in avoiding discussion of termination issues. If the therapist just disappears, this "sends an unhealthy message about relationship, therapeutic or otherwise, since avoiding or neglecting the real relationship prompts hostile patient responses not based on transference" (Bostic et al., 1996, p. 350).

For patients, forced endings more closely mimic the characteristics of past painful endings and usually evoke distressing emotions associated with these past separations, as well as representing a real disappointment in the present (Teyber, 2000; Wittenberg, 1999). Patient responses to forced termination are likely to include shock, anger and blaming, intense grief and sadness, and feelings of being helpless, abandoned, and needy. In any case, the manifest reactions to terminations are likely to be only part of the overall reaction (Baird, 1999).

> Whatever the initial reaction of a patient to the forced termination, it is likely that his or her reaction is more complex and layered than first seems to be the case. A patient who is in touch with only sadness over the loss of the therapist may find it more difficult to acknowledge anger toward the therapist for causing that loss; one who is in touch with only the rage may be reluctant to feel the tender feelings and the sadness behind the anger. Indifference can alternate with strong feelings of separation anxiety. (Penn, as cited in Baird, 1999, p. 153)

Clinical opinion holds that forced terminations are harder for patients than natural endings and the few studies available offer some support for this. Patients in forced terminations were less able to move toward more positive activities outside of therapy (Fortune et al., 1992), and they experienced more negative affect. Some patients abruptly leave therapy in retaliation or to avoid the painful experience of being left (Malan, 1979).

If a termination is forced, when should the patient be advised? In an interesting study by Gould (1978, as cited in Gelso & Woodhouse, 2002), patients whose therapist informed them that they would be leaving at the end of the year appeared relieved to find out that they would not be in therapy indefinitely. Moreover, knowing the end date did not seem to pose a difficulty for patients in investing in the therapeutic work. All patients who were informed of the end date stayed in treatment for the duration. On the other hand, some patients who were informed near the end of therapy did not return to sessions once they were told.

To manage the impact of forced termination on the therapist and the patient, Gelso and Woodhouse (2002) argued that a forced ending be transformed into time-limited therapy in which the patient is told from the earliest opportunity when therapy will end. (This occurred in the case study referred to throughout this book.) Patients need to know much about the departure to maintain some control over their reactions, transference based or otherwise. In addition, providing a patient with the opportunity to make decisions about the continuation of therapy, such as the therapist did with the case study referred to throughout this book, can facilitate a sense of control over the "trauma of rejection" (Gelso & Woodhouse, 2002, p. 350).

Supervision during a phase of forced termination is particularly important because of the potential countertransference difficulties, which may cloud the therapist's understanding of the client's needs. Relevant here is the evaluation of the patient's need for referral. Historically, 33% to 66% of

13. ENDING THERAPY **283**

patients have been referred on (Bostic et al., 1996) even though patients may benefit from a period between therapists to consolidate the work done and to reevaluate the issues for a new therapy. Unfortunately there is some evidence that trainee therapists receive less extensive supervision in cases of forced termination than in cases of natural termination (de Bosset & Styrsky, 1986).

TERMINATION PROCESSES IN THE CASE STUDY

To examine the process of termination in the case under discussion in this book, a review of the themes in the final two sessions (Sessions 8 and 9) was undertaken.

The Second-to-Last Session

Much of the work of the termination phase occurs before the last session. Interestingly, in the Piper (1998) study of the last sessions of a sample of dropouts, the patients announced quite early in the session that this was to be their last. This phenomenon implies that the penultimate session may shed light on the dynamics that were salient when the patient formed the intention to finish. From clinical experience also, patients often seem to work through termination issues prior to the last session, which then becomes a process of goodbye.

Early in Session 8 the patient stated that she had been able to express her feelings safely in the therapy and that she had not "blanked them out." She expressed positive themes in relation to her family and friends but expressed an anxiety about fear of going backwards, that is, a return of the symptoms. She needed her therapist to support her. The therapist reflected on the relationship and indicated that changes had happened and that these were evident in the way in which the patient had taken control in the session and how she now recognized her rebelliousness can, if exerted negatively, prevent her from consolidating the changes. These themes of blanking out, control, and rebelliousness were integral to the patient formulation and they were also addressed as and when evident in the patient's reaction to termination.

The therapist acknowledged that the shortened nature of the planned therapy was due to her going on maternity leave. She addressed possible fantasies that the patient might have had about the termination and arranged for a review with extra sessions if the patient wished to have them. The therapist assured the patient that she did not need to get sick again to have the sessions but that they would be available regardless. The patient was reminded that she knew what to do and that it was she who was in control. There was a strong statement to the effect that the patient was going to be on her own because the therapist was not going to be there, but what they had done (together) was going to be there. The business matters to be concluded in the last session were anticipated.

The Last Session

The last session began with concerns about being out of control versus in control and taking responsibility. The patient then expressed her fear of slipping back once therapy had ended. In response, the therapist acknowledged the brevity of the therapy and that changes were not yet fully consolidated, while encouraging the patient's efforts and reminding her of progress made. With a focus on looking ahead, the patient was concerned that taking responsibility and staying well would bring increased expectations (losing the sick role and being pressured to get a job). The idea was "terrifying." The therapist suggested that "we'll cross that bridge" later. With a sense of pressure eased, the patient fantasized that she may do it! She may succeed so well and be so busy that she can "only spare five minutes" to see the therapist. In a safe, humorous way, this comment conveyed the patient's consciousness of the limited time the therapist had for her. Progress was reviewed, with the therapist's theme being, "you're doing well," and the patient's theme being, "yes that's true but . . . but I may slip back, I may still need you." Indicating she would be writing to the referring doctor, the therapist asked the patient if there was something she wanted conveyed. The patient's message was "don't bully me." Therapist and patient reviewed the patient's increased understanding of her past angry and resentful stance in relation to medical contact. (Although not stated overtly, one wonders if this mirrored changes in the patient's stance in therapy.) This discussion culminated in mutual warmth and laughter, followed by a quick retreat from closeness.

The next part of the session focused around a discussion of whether or not the patient was going to have a blood test to monitor her diabetes. This seems at one level to be a retreat from the emotional experience of the here and now while still concerned with the issue of how the patient will do in the future. The interchange is reminiscent of a parent farewelling an adolescent leaving home. The therapist-mother says let me do something, arrange something for you before you go. There will be a memento (test result) that the patient-adolescent can take away. The patient is reluctant and concerned about getting a poor result. Testing is confronting and she doesn't want to be remembered as doing poorly. After some to-and-fro, the therapist and patient return to a more here-and-now expression of feeling. There followed some lighthearted banter that conveyed an enjoyment of each other's company while providing a light camouflage of the warmth and sadness between them. The therapist reminded the patient they had "half a minute left to say goodbye." The patient acknowledged the therapist's help and thanked her. The therapist acknowledged the patient's effort and persistence, which enabled the patient to acknowledge this too. The therapist mentioned the follow-up appointment and thanked the patient for letting her tape the sessions (for leaving her with a memento too).

Case Review

Although this was in fact a forced ending (in the context of brief therapy), the themes of the last two sessions were similar to those of a natural ending. The interrelated issues of "Am I ready?, Will I slip back?, Will future challenges be too hard?" were the main focus of the work in Session 8 and these continued into Session 9. This occurred in a context of acknowledging the work done together and the changes achieved. The other main issue in the final session was the question of how to say goodbye. If there was any reexperiencing of previous separations this was not overtly evident, except insofar as the patient thought back over the nature of her previous relationships with doctors. Doubt and anxiety alternating with confidence, together with feelings of warmth and gratitude, were the predominant emotions. In Wittenberg's (1999) terms, the main anxieties were at the child and adolescent levels (managing on her own and being expected to take on adult responsibilities). Intense anger and grief were not apparent, although the patient signaled her awareness of the limited time offered to her (and threatened that next time she may be too busy for the therapist). There is a sense from the therapist as well as the patient of wanting to remember and be remembered. The overall picture is consistent with research findings, including Fortune et al. (1992), who found that negative reactions among patients were weak or absent, the strongest reaction being positive affect (pride, independence, accomplishment), evaluation of success, evaluation of therapy experience, and positive flight. Least strong were regression, denial and recapitulation, and expression of a need for further treatment. Therapists expressed strongest reactions as pride in the client's success and pride in their own skill; least strong were relief, doubt about their effectiveness, doubt about the client's progress, and reexperiencing of previous losses. Positive valuations outweighed negative.

THERAPIST TASK IN THE LAST SESSIONS: TO OPTIMIZE THE WORK DONE

The process of working through the ending needs time and cannot be left to the final session. Nevertheless, the work of the therapist continues to the last moment of the last session. Sullivan (1970) wrote that the job of the interviewer was "to see that the person gets something out of the interview" (p. 209). This is also the aim of the termination phase of therapy, that is, the patient should get something out of termination. A therapeutic ending requires that the therapist clearly and unambiguously acknowledge the reality of the ending and also talk with the patient about it, including the ways in which it may evoke thoughts and feelings from other painful endings in the past (Teyber, 2000). If the patient makes no reference to the end or its significance, the therapist needs to remind the patient that there are "3 weeks or three sessions to go," and so forth, with a specific date on the calendar nominated as the last session. If nothing is said, then the therapist may need to ask what the patient feels about the ending (Jacobs, 1989).

Ending therapy is an opportunity to reexamine the legacy of past endings and also a real here-and-now separation. Both aspects need to be acknowledged. The therapist should not feel afraid about encouraging the patient to bring both positive and negative feelings into the open. Teyber (2000) recommended that the therapist invite the patient to share angry, disappointed, or sad feelings. In relation to positive feelings, Fortune et al. (1992) argued that therapists should savor rather than question and interpret their own and their patients' sense of pride and accomplishment and that such an approach may help to reinforce patients' sense of mastery. This is in contrast to the practice of interpreting motives (e.g., Bostic et al., 1996). Whether to question gently or simply acknowledge may depend on the therapists' understanding of the realistic versus distorted basis for the feelings expressed. During this work of consolidation, the therapist needs to be especially alert to the possible reappearance of maladaptive interpersonal patterns encapsulated in the initial formulation.

The work of the termination phase essentially involves "looking back," "looking forward," and "saying goodbye" (Marx & Gelso, 1987, p. 7). Looking back encompasses a review and evaluation of the therapy. Questions that might be asked include, In what ways has the patient changed? What new understanding has been acquired? What changes are still hoped for? (Jacobs, 1989). Similarly, Bostic et al. (1996) suggested canvassing developments in personal capacity to love and work, acceptance of self and capacity to observe the self and analyze situations, as well as changes in presenting problems and their precipitants. In this final phase, the therapist should avoid disturbing the patient deeply and aim to preserve self-esteem. The person should leave with hope and an improved grasp on what has been the trouble (Sullivan, 1970).

Looking forward involves aiming to consolidate the work done, to facilitate internalization, and to anticipate challenges ahead. Feelings of sadness at the end need to be distinguished from return of depression, and relief (because the therapeutic work has in part been painful and disruptive) needs to be distinguished from wish to avoid intimacy in the relationship.

Further ups and downs in the course of life should be anticipated and special requests dealt with, for example, to plan a review session or to finalize a letter to the referrer. Teyber (2000) recommended that therapists acknowledge ways in which the therapy remains unfinished. The therapist may offer a plan for subsequent therapy contact if needed. In particular, if consolidation of some gains for the patient has not been achieved then further plans need to be put into place. In the process of saying goodbye, patients share with the therapist their feelings about ending and about the therapy. Patients may also ask about how therapy works. The real relationship becomes apparent when the patient feels that he or she and the therapist are relating more like equals than at earlier times. The therapist and patient then undertake a formal leave-taking.

Using their Termination Behavior Checklist, Marx and Gelso (1987) showed that a range of termination behaviors (e.g., setting a date for the final session and tapering off the frequency of the sessions) predictably occur during the termination phase. However, none of the items were checked by more than 50% of the counselees in their study and some were checked by as few as 13%. This study was of personal-social counseling in a university setting and many counselees may simply have dropped out naturally and termination not come about in a planned manner. Even so, the proportion not checking the termination behaviors is a sobering reminder that these therapist behaviors need to be explicitly taught in psychotherapy training.

SUMMARY AND CONCLUSIONS

Ending therapy is generally considered a difficult time for therapist and patient alike. Anxieties about ending can lead both therapist and patient to avoid the topic, thus resulting in a discrepancy between psychotherapy theory and actual practice. This is a precautionary alert for termination issues to be addressed openly and in a timely manner. Significant therapeutic gains can come from attention to both the real therapist–patient separation and the reevocation of past endings. Termination has traditionally been conceptualized as an experience of loss. However, this stance can overlook the processes of consolidation and internalization, which keep the therapy alive in the patient.

REFERENCES

Baird, B. N. (1999). *The internship, practicum, and field placement handbook: A guide for helping professions* (2nd ed.). Upper Saddle River, NJ: Prentice Hall.

Bostic, J. Q., Shadid, L. G., & Blotcky, M. J. (1996). Our time is up: Forced terminations during psychotherapy training. *American Journal of Psychotherapy, 50,* 347–359.

Boyer, S. P., & Hoffman, M. A. (1993). Counselor affective reactions to termination: Impact of counselor loss history and perceived client sensitivity to loss. *Journal of Counseling Psychology, 40,* 271–278.

Budman, S. H., & Gurman, A. S. (1988). *Theory and practice of brief therapy.* New York: Guilford.

de Bosset, F., & Styrsky, E. (1986). Termination in individual psychotherapy: A survey of residents' experience. *Canadian Journal of Psychiatry, 31,* 636–642.

Fortune, A. E., Pearlingi, B., & Rochelle, C. D. (1992). Reactions to termination of individual treatment. *Social Work, 37,* 171–178.

Gelso, C. J., & Woodhouse, S. S. (2002). The termination of psychotherapy: What research tells us about the process of ending treatment. In G. S. Tryon (Ed.), *Counseling based on process research: Applying what we know* (pp. 344–369). Boston: Allyn & Bacon.

Gustafson, J. P. (1995). *The dilemmas of brief psychotherapy.* New York: Plenum.

Hillis, G., Alexander, D. A., & Eagles, J. M. (1993). Premature termination of psychiatric contact. *International Journal of Social Psychiatry, 39,* 100–107.

Howard, K. I., Moras, K., Brill, P. L., Martinovich, Z., & Lutz, W. (1996). Evaluation of psychotherapy: Efficacy, effectiveness, and patient progress. *American Psychologist, 51,* 1059–1064.

Jacobs, M. (1989). *Psychodynamic counselling in action.* London: Sage.

Kramer, S. A. (1986). The termination process in open-ended psychotherapy: Guidelines for clinical practice. *Psychotherapy, 339,* 526–531.

Langs, R. (1998). *Ground rules in psychotherapy and counselling.* London: Karnac Books.

Lee, R. R. (2000). Self psychology: Termination. *Australian Journal of Psychotherapy, 19*(2), 40–55.

Malan, D. H. (1979). *Individual psychotherapy and the science of psychodynamics.* London: Butterworths.

Malcolm, J. (1982). *Psychoanalysis: The impossible profession.* New York: Penguin.

Mann, J. (1973). *Time-limited psychotherapy.* Cambridge, MA: Harvard University Press.

Mann, J., & Goldman, R. (1982). *A casebook in time-limited psychotherapy.* New York: McGraw-Hill.

Marx, J. A., & Gelso, C. J. (1987). Termination of individual counseling in a university center. *Journal of Counseling Psychology, 34,* 30–39.

Mohr, D. C. (1995). Negative outcome in psychotherapy: A critical review. *Clinical Science: Science and Practice, 2,* 1–27.

Piper, W. E. (1998, June). *The therapist's contribution to the dropout phenomena: Therapist technique, style, and perceived alliance.* Paper presented at Society for Psychotherapy Research, 29th Annual Meeting, Snowbird, Utah.

Quintana, S. M. (1993). Toward an expanded and updated conceptualization of termination: Implications for short-term, individual psychotherapy. *Professional Psychology: Research and Practice, 24,* 426–432.

Quintana, S. M., & Holahan, W. (1992). Termination in short-term counseling: Comparison of successful and unsuccessful cases. *Journal of Counseling Psychology, 39,* 299–305.

Seligman, M. E. P. (1995). The effectiveness of psychotherapy: The *Consumer Reports* study. *American Psychologist, 50,* 965–974.

Smith, M. L., Glass, G. V., & Miller, T. I. (1980). *The benefits of psychotherapy.* Baltimore: Johns Hopkins University Press.

Sullivan, H. H. (1970). *The psychiatric interview.* New York: Norton.

Teyber, E. (2000). *Interpersonal process in psychotherapy: A relational approach* (4th ed.). Belmont, CA: Brooks/Cole.

Wierzbicki, M., & Pekarik, G. (1993). A meta-analysis of psychotherapy dropout. *Professional Psychology: Research and Practice, 24,* 190–195.

Wittenberg, I. (1999). Ending therapy. *Journal of Child Psychotherapy, 25,* 339–356.

CHAPTER

14

Termination, Posttermination, and Internalization of Therapy and the Therapist: Internal Representation and Psychotherapy Outcome

Elizabeth G. Arnold
Private Practice

Barry A. Farber
Teachers College, Columbia University

Jesse D. Geller
Private Practice

In 1963, Edelson described the question of termination as "... not how to get therapy stopped, or when to stop it, but how to terminate so that what has been happening keeps on 'going' inside of the patient" (p. 23). The problem of termination, Edelson (1963) wrote, is not only one of helping the patient to achieve independence; rather, it is a problem of "facilitating achievement, by the patient, of the ability to 'hang on' to the therapist" in the therapist's physical absence, "in the form of a realistic intrapsychic representation ... which is conserved rather than destructively or vengefully abandoned following separation" (p. 23).

This transformation of a relationship between patient and therapist, or self and object, in the external world of the treatment room into a relationship within the patient's internal representational world occurs through a process of internalization (Atwood & Stolorow, 1980; Behrends & Blatt, 1985; Loewald, 1960). Through internalization, "the subject transforms real or imagined regulatory interactions with [the] environment, and real or imagined characteristics of [the] environment into inner regulations and characteristics" (Schafer, 1968, p. 9). An internalized representation of the therapist, therefore, reflects the processes by which the interactions and relationship with the therapist in the external environment eventually become elements of the patient's character or self.

The processes of internalization and representation are regarded as fundamental to psychological development at all points throughout the life span (e.g., Freud, 1917/1963; Loewald, 1962; Meissner, 1981; Schafer, 1968). They are also theorized to play a pivotal role with regard to therapeutic change, as patients use the person of the therapist as a new object (Behrends & Blatt, 1985; Loewald, 1960), thereby effecting changes in the self in relation to this new object. This creative use of the object, crucial to the earliest processes of self-formation (Summers, 1997), is equally necessary in the ongoing development, differentiation, and structuralization of the self (Loewald, 1960).

Empirical investigation into the processes of internalization and representation of the therapist offers a potential deepening of the interrelation between current theories of therapeutic change and researchers' ability to test and further develop this theoretical understanding, thereby integrating it with clinical practice. Although the hypothesis that psychotherapeutic change is mediated by the processes of internalization is widely accepted (Atwood & Stolorow, 1980; Horvath & Symonds, 1991; Loewald, 1960; Luborsky, 1984; Orlinsky, Geller, Tarragona, & Farber, 1993; Orlinsky & Howard, 1986), there has been surprisingly little research, until recently, on the ways in which it occurs. In part, this is due to the fact that because patients' representations of the therapist and of therapy "occur most noticeably outside therapy sessions, they have not been viewed as part of the therapeutic process; and since they are not overtly related to symptoms or explicitly involved in adaptive functioning, they have found no place in outcome research" (Orlinsky & Geller, 1994, p. 424). In other words, the clinical phenomena attributed great theoretical importance have yet to be widely embraced as potential areas of valid scientific inquiry.

Additionally, the evaluation of therapeutic effects need not be restricted to the time of termination but should include follow-up after a significant time interval. Psychoanalytic writings indicate that the fate of the therapist representation and the psychological work patients engage in following termination are critical in determining the extent to which the beneficial effects of therapy endure following the cessation of formal meetings (Bergmann, 1988; Bernard & Drob, 1989; Geller, 1987; Geller & Farber, 1993; Loewald, 1988). Although such follow-up is not routinely done, it is necessary if we define outcome in term of therapy's lasting impact.

Under ideal conditions, psychotherapy can be brought to a natural completion. The issues of separation and mourning often present with the termination of therapeutic relationships are experienced and shared and there is mutual agreement that a patient is ready to leave both the therapist and the treatment. In actuality, many factors conspire to prevent a timely and mutual ending, including the often temporary nature of treatment at training clinics and the advent of managed care networks with their limited access to mental health services. Given the real constraints within which many treatments are conducted, this chapter aims to present an overview of recent research on factors (i.e., treatment length and manner of termination) that may impact patients' future consolidation of treatment gains.

INTERNALIZATION AND REPRESENTATION: GENERAL CONCEPTS

Two independent theoretical traditions, namely psychoanalysis and cognitive-developmental psychology (e.g., Bruner, 1964; Piaget, 1954; Vygotsky, 1962), focus on the interrelated processes of representation and internalization. The "evolving approach to studying the construction, forms, and functions of patients' representations of their therapy and therapists, is based on a selective integration of these two theoretical traditions" (Orlinsky & Geller, 1994, p. 425). A focus on the concepts of self-representation and object representation has become central to an increasing number of psychotherapeutic schools and approaches. Whether referred to as "representations" in psychodynamic theory, or as "schemas," "scripts," or "mental models" in more cognitive conceptualizations, these contents of experience are seen as templates that guide feelings and behavior and direct expectations and interpretations of events.

These self-representations and object representations are believed to develop simultaneously in an interactive dialectic as a result of differentiating from and internalizing aspects of relationships with significant others (Atwood & Stolorow, 1980; Behrends & Blatt, 1985; Mahler, Pine, & Bergman, 1975; Schafer, 1968). Inherent in every representation, therefore, is a sense of the self, the other, and the interrelationship (Blatt & Shichman, 1983; Stern, 1985).

Beginning with Freud (1917/1963), this process of internalization has been theoretically linked with mourning, specifically with managing experiences of separation and loss through reconstructing lost objects internally. Mourning, wrote Loewald (1988), involves the "gradual relinquishment of a cherished relationship with another person and its internalization" (p. 156), meaning an "increasing dissolution of the relationship as one with an external object . . . leading to an absorption into the very fabric of the subject" (pp. 156–157). In this way, termination and internalization are intimately related.

The first step in the process of internalization has been viewed as the establishment of a gratifying involvement with another person. The next step is the development within the patient of the need-gratifying functions of the relationship when they are disrupted through the inevitable "cleavages, rifts, and discontinuities in interpersonal relationships that can instigate the process of internalization" (Behrends & Blatt, 1985, p. 21). This perspective places less emphasis on internalization as a means of mourning the loss of the object and redefines it as a means of maintaining the self's coherence in light of the inevitable and required disruptions in human relationships.

In the context of the therapeutic relationship, the significant interactions between patient and therapist—encompassing moments of closeness as well as experiences of empathic failure or discontinuity—can lead to changes in a patient's internal representational world. These modifications in the very templates that guide feelings, expectations, interpretations of events, and behavior, illustrate the meaning of structural change in psychotherapy and are discernible and measurable in an individual's changing representations of others (or objects) and of self.

INTERNAL REPRESENTATIONS AS INDICATORS OF THERAPEUTIC CHANGE

Change in an individual's internal representations has been seen as "one of several intrapsychic concomitants of successful treatment" (Kavanagh, 1985, p. 547). Just as realistic and well-integrated internal representations play a crucial role in psychological health and adaptation, chaotic, static, underdeveloped, or distorted representations are significantly implicated in psychopathology. Although representations of self and other may become somewhat fixed as psychic structures, they are often amenable to modification through psychotherapy. Psychoanalytic theory credits such structural change to the patient's internalization of the therapeutic relationship, which in turn effects change in the patient's experience of self and resultant self-representation. This effect allows one to link "the study of patients' representations to the traditional domain of outcome research" (Orlinksy & Geller, 1994, p. 438).

A number of approaches to empirically assessing internalized representations have emerged in recent years as they are revealed in the content of responses to various kinds of projective instruments; through the use of attachment theory to delineate different types of adult relational patterns; through a focus on the structural or formal qualities of the representation, as exemplified by the work of Blatt and colleagues (Bers, Blatt, Sayward, & Johnston, 1993; Blatt & Blass, 1990; Blatt, Wein, Chevron, & Quinlan, 1979; Blatt, Wiseman, Prince-Gibson, & Gatt, 1991; Diamond, Kaslow, Coonerty, & Blatt, 1990; Gruen & Blatt, 1990), evoked through written descriptions of self and significant others and with various dimensions of the narrative descriptions then scored using scales grounded in developmental theory (e.g., Blatt, Bers, & Schaffer, 1992; Blatt, Chevron, Quinlan, Schaffer, & Wein, 1992; Geller et al., 1992); and through use of the Therapist Representation Inventory (TRI; Geller, Cooley, & Hartley, 1981–1982), a series of paper-and-pencil self-report measures that examines the forms and functions of patients' internalized representations of their therapist and the therapeutic relationship.

These approaches have been shown to provide important information about the "kinds of interpersonal relationship patterns to which individuals are predisposed and about the nature and severity of psychological disturbance" (Geller et al., 1981–1982, p. 131).

It is theorized that change in representations over the course of treatment is predicated on normative models of development. With progression of treatment, just as in earlier normative cognitive-developmental sequences, representations of self and other begin to have a clearer sense of boundaries and separateness (Blatt, Wild, & Ritzler, 1975), more complete self–other differentiation (Blatt & Blass, 1990), and indications of a greater degree of empathic relatedness than at the beginning of treatment (Blatt et al., 1991; Diamond et al., 1990). Indeed it has been empirically demonstrated that patients' self-descriptions become less constricted and contain an increasing number of modes and dimensions (Bers et al., 1993), indicating the inclusion and integration of various components of the self-representation. Additionally, research has shown that patients' self-descriptions, evaluated at intake and at termination from treatment, have demonstrated decreased self-criticism and harsh judgment directed at the self; at the same time, self-descriptions have become more benevolent, accepting, and caring, expressing significantly more positive self-regard and self-esteem at time of termination than at intake, prior to treatment (Arnold, Farber, & Geller, 2000).

It is expected that such empirical changes will parallel independent measures of therapeutic change such as changes in symptoms and behavior. The question remains as to what degree these changes are maintained and even improved on in the absence of the therapeutic relationship, posttermination.

"AFTERWORK" AND THE THERAPIST REPRESENTATION

Termination is, ideally, an "organic outcome of the treatment process itself" (Loewald, 1988, p. 155). From the perspective of the processes of internalization, treatment can be considered optimal if the patient is capable of sustaining aspects of the therapeutic dialogue posttermination.

Internalization of the therapeutic dialogue, reflected in an increased capacity for self-analysis and in an emerging ability to meet experiences with increased flexibility, engenders "mutual confidence" (Oremland, Blacker, & Norman, 1975, p. 820) in both therapist and patient that the process of psychotherapy will continue after they stop physically meeting and working together. This perspective was first expressed by Freud (1937/1963) in his belief that following termination of a successful analysis, the "processes of ego-transformation will go on of their own accord" and the patient will bring "new insight to bear" on all "subsequent experience" (p. 267). The formal termination of psychotherapy, therefore, does not and should not imply the cessation of the therapeutic process.

The term *afterwork* (Bernard & Drob, 1989) refers to the psychological work that patients engage in posttermination. In what they describe as a hypothesis-generating investigation, Bernard and Drob interviewed patients ($n = 10$) 5 months to 7 years following termination from therapy. They found that what remained with former patients ($n = 10$) were enduring changes in perspective and an internalization of the processes patients associated with the overall therapy experience, such as imagining the types of questions the therapist might ask and asking these questions of themselves. Patients described an active quality to their memories of the therapist and the therapeutic relationship, which they continued to use in their day-to-day lives posttermination. These patients appeared to have integrated the therapeutic process into their own ways of being, experiencing it as a part of themselves rather than as still associated with the person with whom they first developed it.

Internalization of the therapist and the therapeutic relationship seems to involve both cognitive, functional aspects (e.g., increased problem solving or analytic skills or both as a result of treatment), as well as affective components of the relationship, as patients internalize "in the sense of identifying with, the therapist's benevolent feelings and attitudes" toward his or her self (Geller & Farber, 1993, p. 167). In expressing what seemed most critical about their treatment experiences, former patients cited "incidents or exchanges which gave evidence of their therapists' concern, commitment and acceptance . . . the implication is that the sine qua non for effective therapy (at least as perceived by patients) is a high-quality relationship between patient and therapist" (Bernard & Drob, 1989, p. 368). Research focusing on patients' representations of their therapists and therapy is thus given a place of paramount importance in investigating the process of therapeutic change and in understanding treatment's lasting impact.

RESEARCH ON THERAPIST REPRESENTATION

An ongoing research project (Arnold, 1998; Arnold et al., 2000; Barchat, 1989; Bender, 1996; Bender, Farber, & Geller, 1997; Farber & Geller, 1994; Geller et al., 1981–1982; Geller & Farber, 1993; Honig, 1989; Honig, Farber, & Geller, 1997; Rosenzweig, Farber, & Geller, 1996; Wzontek, Geller, & Farber, 1995) is investigating ways in which current and former patients "construct, retain, use, and relinquish different types of internalized representations of their therapists and the therapeutic relationship" (Geller & Farber, 1993, p. 166) in extratherapeutic situations, such as between psychotherapy sessions and posttermination. This investigation emphasizes therapy's aftereffects engendered by patients' ability to both consolidate and learn to use therapeutic gains independent of the therapist's physical presence.

Two instruments have been developed to study patients' internalized representations of the therapist. The Therapist Representation Inventory or TRI (Geller et al., 1981–1982) emphasizes the developmental complexity of patients' representations, the sensory modalities evoked in forming them, and the functional value they serve for the patient, both during the treatment course and following termination. The Intersession Experience Questionnaire (Orlinsky & Tarragona, 1986) focuses on patients' representations between therapy sessions and was designed for repeated use over the course of ongoing treatment. The remainder of this chapter focuses on the TRI, as it can be used to investigate representations over the course of ongoing psychotherapy as well as long after treatment has formally ended.

Orlinsky and Geller (1994) described how research into patients' representations can be seen to constitute an important bridge between the traditional domains of therapeutic process and outcome. These representations, for example, connect the direct experience of in-session therapeutic process to the patient's subsequent personality and behavior in situations outside of therapy. With regard to outcome variables, patients' representations in later stages of treatment may reflect a growing identification with the therapist's knowledge, attitudes, and behavior, from which autonomous self-analytic functions may develop.

Research with the TRI has yielded interesting distinctions between current and former patients (Geller et al., 1981–1982; Geller & Farber, 1993) and between genders (Farber & Geller, 1994; Honig, 1989) in terms of the therapist representation. It has also highlighted differences in the forms and functions of therapist representations associated with length of time in treatment (Bender et al., 1997; Geller & Farber, 1993; Rosenzweig et al., 1996) and self-perceived outcome (Geller et al., 1981–1982; Wzontek et al., 1995).

The TRI is a set of three self-administered measures designed to investigate the content, forms, and functions of patients' representations of their therapists and of the therapeutic relationship. First, the content of patients' written descriptions of their therapists can be scored with Geller et al.'s (1992) or Blatt, Chevron, et al.'s (1992) scales (or both) for assessing narrative descriptions.

Second, three forms of the therapist representation are assessed using a subscale of the TRI called the Therapist Embodiment scale (TES; Geller et al., 1981–1982): a Haptic form emphasizing kinesthetic and tactile-perceptual qualities of the representation (i.e., what it feels like to be in the room with the therapist); an Imagistic form composed essentially of visual images of the therapist; and a Conceptual form reflecting real or imagined conversations with the therapist (Geller et al., 1981–1982). These three factors, corresponding to Bruner's (1964) delineation of representational form into "action," "imagery," and "language," are thought to be "separable systems through which information about the world is processed and inner schemas of the world are constructed" (Geller et al., 1981–1982, p. 130). A more recent factor analysis validated three dimensions of patients' formal representations that correspond closely to the initial factors. They have been termed Somatic, Imagistic, and Conversational-Conceptual (Schaffer & Geller, 1995).

Third, the Therapist Involvement scale (TIS; Schaffer & Geller, 1995), the third subscale of the TRI, assesses five functions of patients' representations of their therapists (Schaffer & Geller, 1995). Each function denotes a specific affective-interpersonal theme characterizing different aspects of the patient–therapist relationship. Factor 1, the Wish for Reciprocity, expresses preoccupation with the person of the therapist and the wish for a relationship that transcends the roles of therapist and patient. It is comprised of 10 items such as "I wish I could be friends with my therapist," and "I imagine our talking to each other outside of the therapy office." Factor 2, Failure of Benign Internalization, is characterized by disappointment in the therapist and expectation that the therapist will be disapproving and the inability to use representations of the therapy relationship in situations outside therapy. It comprises six items such as "I try not to think about my therapist," and "In stressful situations, I don't seem to be able to use what I previously used in therapy." Factor 3, Longing for Gratifying Aspects of the Therapy Relationship, captures the essence of a positive transference. It reflects the wish to use the therapeutic relationship as a model for other relationships (e.g., "I wish more of my relationships were like the one with my therapist"), the wish to make the therapist proud, and the experiences of mourning the loss of the therapist in his or her absence. It contains six items. Factor 4, Continuing the Therapeutic Dialogue, reflects patients' ability to use the therapist representation in personal situations. It is made up of four items such as "When I am having a problem, I try to work it out with my therapist in mind." Factor 5, Negative Involvement, is made up of only two items. These items reflect malevolent or persecutory images and the defense associated with them (e.g., "I imagine my therapist hurting me in some way").The five functions were based on a factor analysis and correspond closely to the six factors of the original standardization study: Wish for Reciprocity, Failure of Benign Internalization, the Effort to Create a Therapist Introject, Mourning, Continuing the Therapeutic Dialogue, and Sexual and Aggressive Involvement (Geller et al., 1981–1982).

Geller et al.'s (1981–1982) initial standardization study was conducted with 206 participants, psychotherapists themselves, in either current or previous treatment. All participants were found to evoke the forms and functions of therapist representation most often and experience it most vividly under conditions of needfulness, using the representation for help in mitigating painful feelings such as sadness, anxiety, depression, and guilt (forms and functions noted previously). Use of these representations was more frequent for patients in ongoing treatment as compared to those who had terminated. A smaller percentage of all patients, both current and former, brought their therapists to awareness when experiencing a need for relatedness, as in times of loneliness, alienation, or dealing with a sense of loss.

Patients who described the most vivid representations also tended to be more involved with these representations, as demonstrated by a significant positive correlation between the TES and TIS portions of the TRI. They felt more satisfaction with their therapists and were more likely to feel they were being helped. The most characteristic function served by the therapist representation was in patients' desire to identify with the therapist and gain the therapist's approval. This was evident in frequently endorsed statements such as "I would like my therapist to be proud of me," and "I try to solve my problems in the way my therapist and I worked on them in psychotherapy."

Using this same participant group, Geller and Farber (1993) explored factors affecting the nature and use of therapist representations both between sessions and after termination. They found that the greater the number of sessions attended, the greater the likelihood that patients will use representations of the therapist to continue the work of therapy following termination. (Participants' numbers of sessions ranged from 4 to 2,000. The median number of sessions attended was 238; the mean was 370.) They also found positive therapeutic outcome to be significantly associated with representations that were primarily visual in nature and that reflected a wish to Continue the Therapeutic Dialogue. Patients who did not experience therapeutic improvement were most often those who failed to form a benign representation of the therapist.

With the subsample of 66 patients currently in treatment in the aforementioned sample, Farber and Geller (1994) studied gender differences in the representation of the therapist. Their findings suggest that women were more likely than men to keep their therapist in mind (and for longer periods of time) when working on problems outside of therapy. Additionally, they were more likely both to use these representations to plan for their next session and to miss their therapists between sessions. This finding was specific to female patients with male therapists. Men's representations have been found to characteristically reflect the wish for a more egalitarian relationship with the therapist (Honig, 1989) regardless of therapist gender.

In the subsample of patients who were no longer in treatment, a feeling of satisfaction with their therapist and the belief that they had benefited from treatment was strongly associated with access to kinesthetic modes of representation. Additionally, there was a significant positive correlation between self-perceived outcome and the TIS factor Mourning (which, in the new factor analysis, is subsumed within the factor Longing for Gratifying Aspects), reflecting experiences of the loss of the therapist. In contrast, current patients were higher on all functions of the TIS except this one.

This finding was replicated in a study of 60 former psychotherapy patients, 6 months to 5 years after termination (Wzontek et al., 1995). Participants had been in individual treatments ranging from 6 months to 5 years, with a mean of slightly over 19 months. Wzontek et al. (1995) found that the highest TIS factor posttermination was Mourning. The next most highly endorsed factor was Continuing the Therapeutic Dialogue, reflecting patients' use of the therapist representation following termination to continue the process of psychotherapy. Former patients' use of the therapist representation to continue the therapeutic dialogue was significantly correlated with their feelings of satisfaction with their therapists and their belief that treatment was helpful to them. Although Wzontek et al. found no significant differences in the forms or themes of therapist representation associated with either length of treatment or length of time since termination, they concluded that these nonsignificant findings may have resulted from the cross-sectional design employed: Data was collected at only one point in time, thereby obscuring longitudinal trends or change over time.

MANNER OF TERMINATION AND ITS RELATIONSHIP TO OUTCOME

The manner in which the therapeutic relationship is brought to a close would be expected to have a major influence on the degree to which gains are maintained and further growth promoted posttermination (Levinson, 1977) and on the potential fate of the intrapsychic image of the therapist after termination (Bergmann, 1988).

Wzontek et al. (1995) explored the relationship between forms and functions of therapist representations using the TRI and former patients' self-reported reasons for termination (i.e., "therapist left," "problem had been solved," "ambivalence or unhappiness regarding the treatment," and "external reasons such as relocation or financial difficulty"). Participants were recruited from a mental health clinic affiliated with a graduate program in clinical psychology. Patients currently in treatment who had been in psychoanalysis or who had been hospitalized for psychiatric reasons were excluded from the study. Those who met the criteria were mailed questionnaires and a cover letter.

Wzontek et al. (1995) found differences in the functional themes characterizing the representations of the four groups differing in self-reported reasons for termination. Although no two groups differed statistically on any one function, these findings suggest that patients who left therapy for different reasons did in fact use their image of the therapist in different ways. The "therapist left" group tended to score higher on each of the six functions, suggesting that patients whose therapy was ended prematurely and who felt positively about their experiences in therapy were more involved with their images of the therapist following termination. Endings due to the patient's "ambivalence/unhappiness" or "relocation/financial" were correlated with lower function scores, suggesting that patients who ended their own treatments prematurely were characterized by lesser degrees of affective involvement.

Arnold (1998) investigated manner of termination and its potential impact on long-term outcome. She investigated longitudinal changes in representations of both self and therapist by examining data at two points in time: at termination from weekly treatment (Time 1) and again at a follow-up point, an average of 9 years posttermination (Time 2). The manner of termination was defined in three possible ways: "mutual agreement between you and your therapist," "your discontinuation of therapy," or "therapist's discontinuation of therapy," with the last being the forced termination. Only half of the patients who described their terminations as forced at Time 1 agreed to be included in the follow-up phase of the study. In contrast, 70% of those patients who left treatment on their own initiative and 79% of those who described their termination as mutual at Time 1 agreed to participate at Time 2.

Of the patients who described their termination as forced, use of the Haptic form of the therapist representation was a distinctive characteristic at Time 1. This TRI form emphasizes the kinesthetic qualities of the representation (i.e., what it feels like to be in the room with the therapist). This particular subgroup made significantly greater use of this form than other patients, as if trying to hold onto the therapist in a uniquely bodily or kinesthetic way. This correlation was no longer evident at follow-up, most likely due to the fading strength of the Haptic or kinesthetic form over time.

In terms of symptomatology at Time 2, patients who described their termination as forced were significantly higher than other patients on Interpersonal Sensitivity, a dimension measured by the Symptom Checklist–90–Revised (Derogatis, 1983), which is a widely used symptom checklist. This symptom dimension is characterized by agreement with such statements as "feeling others do not understand you or are unsympathetic," "feeling inferior to others," "feeling that people are unfriendly or dislike you," and "feeling critical of others."

It is entirely possible that patients with a ready propensity for interpersonal sensitivity might define their termination as forced when other patients would not. If, based on therapist training requirements, a time-limited treatment is understood from the start, some patients might later define this as a mutual ending, whereas others might conceptualize the experience as one of being left. It is equally likely, however, that a unilateral, potentially unresolved termination may really leave some patients with some sense of inferiority and damage. The association found here, between forced termination and heightened interpersonal sensitivity, clearly suggests the need for further study. It highlights potentially iatrogenic effects inherent in certain models of termination, suggesting that the manner in which treatment is brought to a close may indeed be crucial to long-term outcome.

ENDURING QUALITIES OF THE THERAPIST REPRESENTATION

What is the fate of the therapist representation? What qualities endure over time? The following findings (Arnold, 1998) focus on the period of time between patients' formal termination from psychotherapy and a research follow-up an average of 9 years later. The mean treatment length was 45.7 sessions, with a range from 7 to 193 sessions, though length of treatment did not prove to be a variable with significant effect.

The thematic structural dimensions of the therapist representation, expressed through the content of written descriptions of the therapist, stayed fairly constant in the years between termination and follow-up. Descriptions at both points in time suggest that patients kept their awareness of the therapist at the level of observable behaviors, primarily describing actions the therapist engaged in and statements made. It was uncharacteristic, on average, for patients to tie these observations to potential motivations or other aspects of the therapist's internal world, such as imagining what the therapist might think or feel about them. Additionally, it was rare for patients to describe the therapist as a person existing and changing over time, although this dimension increased slightly between termination and follow-up. Rather, the contents of the therapist description at termination and follow-up seemed to illustrate that the structural qualities of the object were preserved as constant and predominantly unchanged for the patient group as a whole.

Differences were found between the enduring, relatively unchanging nature of the structural qualities of the therapist representation as described previously and the fate of its more sensory forms. These differences lend support to the delineation of the therapist representation into three separable systems (Bruner, 1964; Geller et al., 1981–1982) through which individuals encode and retain information about the external world. Although all three forms of the representation, Imagistic, Haptic, and Conceptual, were characteristic to some degree at termination, these qualities of the therapist representation were found to fade significantly over time. Imagistic, Haptic, and Conceptual forms of representation, primarily dependent on sensory modalities in their creation, seem dependent on this source of information for their continued maintenance over time. The most profound dissipation over time was seen in the Haptic form, the bodily, kinesthetic, and emotional experience of what it had felt like to be with the therapist.

DESCRIPTIONS OF SELF AND THERAPIST IN RELATION TO OUTCOME (SUCCESSFUL INTERNALIZATION VS. "FAILURE OF BENIGN INTERNALIZATION")

For the majority of participants, self-representation continued to undergo progressive, statistically significant growth in the time period between termination and follow-up (Arnold, 1998). Patients ($n = 28$) presented an increasingly multidimensional view of themselves, describing multiple personal and professional roles and the challenges inherent in attempting to move flexibly between them. Expressions of internal, emotional experiences increased, with former patients reacting to the ongoing events and situations of their lives with pride, frustration, sadness, and hope, as well as with an increased awareness of time as a context in which their growth and change occur. At follow-up, a majority of participants evidenced an attitude of increased tolerance and benevolence toward themselves and expressed greater satisfaction with their interpersonal relationships.

At follow-up, a number of the dimensions of self-description were found to be significantly correlated with a dimension used in the assessment of therapist descriptions. This dimension, termed *De-Illusionment* (Geller et al., 1992), assesses one's capacity to constructively cope with the inevitable flaws, contradictions, and disappointments inherent in another—in this case in the therapist or the therapeutic relationship. In contrast to disillusionment, which is often characterized by rage or despair, De-Illusionment conveys "an attitude of understanding and forgiveness, at times even approaching a contemplative appreciation of the universality of imperfection and conflict" (Geller et al., 1992). Elevated scores on this dimension indicate an ongoing, active struggle to balance the positive aspects of the former therapist with negative ones (e.g., a therapist's often frustrating silence or lack of reciprocal sharing). For this sample of former patients, the continuing attempt to integrate and balance aspects of the therapist representation was significantly and positively correlated with their own experience of satisfaction in relationships with others and with their increasing experience of self as existing in and changing over time (Arnold, 1998).

Enduring positive feelings for the therapist, seen in the majority of former patients' written descriptions characterizing the therapist as a positive ideal or role model at follow-up, was associated with a distinct function of the enduring therapist representation (Arnold, 1998). The relationship between continued positive regard for the therapist and the use of the therapist representation for purposes of continuing the therapeutic dialogue, approached significance and is worthy of mention. Continuation of the therapeutic dialogue suggests that patients are using the representation "as a means of sustaining the work of therapy in the physical absence of the therapist" (Geller et al., 1981–1982, p. 142). This function has been repeatedly linked with patients' feelings of satisfaction with their therapists and their belief that therapy has been helpful to them (Geller et al., 1981–1982; Geller & Farber, 1993; Wzontek et al., 1995). The posttermination research findings support these studies in again highlighting an enduring function of successful internalization while additionally linking it to a specific structural or content dimension of the therapist description, namely a positive affective bond with the therapist.

Positive regard for the therapist's human, fallible qualities appears to be linked to a lasting, useful, beneficial, and accessible internalization of the therapeutic relationship. Conversely, unresolved negative feelings about the therapist as assessed through written descriptions of the therapist appear to be significantly correlated with the failure to achieve a cohesive, beneficial, and enduring internal representation. TIS statements such as "I feel as though I were never in therapy," "I don't remember very much of what my therapist said in our talks together," or "I think my therapist would be disapproving of me," indicate the characteristic difficulty some patients have in forming and using constructive representations of the therapeutic relationship. The distinct factors of the TIS appear to be useful in separating distinct subgroups of patients, as an elevated score on the factor Failure of Benign Internalization is in fact characteristic of patients with negative outcomes.

This failure of benign internalization, already associated with a negative view of the therapist, was also significantly linked with expressions of disappointment in one's self and a more general sense of failure in one's relationships with others (Arnold, 1998). Certain self-descriptions collected at follow-up illustrate this link between a negative therapist introject, a negative appraisal of self, and generally poor quality interpersonal relationships. As one patient wrote, "I am uncomfortable in many situations. Feelings of inferiority dominate my life. I have never been able to acquire a useful therapist–client relationship. I often wish I could live my life over again."

Failure of benign internalization can be regarded as a negative outcome measure and in fact has been found to have significant negative correlation with self-perceived outcome in therapy (Geller & Farber, 1993; Wzontek et al., 1995). Links between Failure of Benign Internalization and certain longstanding personality attributes were reported by Bender (1996). She found that the more patients manifested aspects of avoidant, dependent, passive–aggressive, self-defeating, and schizotypal character styles, the greater the likelihood that these patients would be unable to internalize helpful aspects of the therapy relationship.

The specific symptom dimensions of many of these character pathologies, often manifested by patients in terms of characteristic thoughts and feelings, have also been examined (Arnold, 1998). Failure of Benign Internalization was found to be significantly and positively correlated with numerous Symptom Checklist–90–Revised symptom dimensions such as Obsessive–Compulsive (e.g., "repeated unpleasant thoughts that won't leave your mind"), Interpersonal Sensitivity (e.g., "feeling that others do not understand you or are unsympathetic"), and Depression (e.g., "feelings of worthlessness"). The inability to internalize a positive, soothing representation of another was found to be significantly associated with heightened physical and psychological distress.

Psychotherapy effectively alters "inner psychic structure ... to the extent that [it] maximize[s] the conditions allowing for the creation of 'benignly influential' and enduring subjective representations of the therapy relationship" (Geller et al., 1981–1982, p. 127). The failure to create a benign internalization may emanate from a patient's fixed and negatively tinged internal representational world, from the vantage point of which it is difficult to experience, extract, and internalize positive aspects of relationships with new others in the external world. Meeting new experiences with rigid perceptual structures is characteristic of numerous clinical disorders and is problematic particularly for their self-perpetuating nature. Alternatively, however, the failure to create a benign internalization may be the result of the therapist's failure to maximize the conditions allowing for such an internalization to occur.

Rather than concluding that psychotherapy does not work for seemingly intractable character difficulties, it is expected, perhaps optimistically, that persistent, long-term focus on the specific representational world of the patient—in terms of transference, in psychodynamic terms, or schema modification, in more cognitive terms—could have some result. This emphasizes the importance of the therapist's role in focusing treatment. It addresses the clinical importance of using assessment measures focused on aspects of outcome more precise than general symptom reduction as well.

CLINICAL SIGNIFICANCE OF RESEARCH ON REPRESENTATIONAL CHANGE

This chapter focuses on termination and on the process of internalization in psychotherapy as a potential vehicle for long-term change. In this regard, its purpose has been to explore the aspects of the therapeutic relationship that can be emotionally and functionally portable for patients as they move onward into their lives, independent of their therapists, following termination. The idea of portability suggests movement from one place to another. The process of internalization embodies this type of psychological movement, whereas the process of termination from the treatment relationship necessitates it.

Termination, like other endings or losses of relationship, forces an individual to "repair, modify, expand, or intensify preexisting internalizations" of the lost or absent object to hold onto a "sense of inner connection and meaningful relation to that object, and to maintain this connection over time" (Gaines, 1997, p. 550). Distinct from mapping the process of representational change over the course of an ongoing therapeutic relationship, studying former patients who are independent of the physical presence of their former therapists places us firmly within their internal representational worlds. This vantage point allows unique access to those facets of the original relationship that have endured the transformation, from a relationship in the external world into a meaningful inner relationship.

The research presented here indicates that a majority of patients engage in some form of psychological afterwork following their termination from treatment. They continue to use representations of their therapist and the therapeutic relationship, although the nature of their engagement with these representations changes. Different structural and formal dimensions (forms of the therapist representation) appear to be created and maintained in differing ways, with the structural aspects of the therapist representation remaining constant through time as the more sensory dimensions fade.

It is notable that patients' characterization of the therapist as a positive presence is positively correlated with their use of the therapist representation for purposes of continuing the therapeutic dialogue. Positive regard for the therapist is significantly, negatively correlated with the failure of benign internalization as well.

When the condition of positive involvement is not met and the patient does not form a satisfying affective bond with the therapist, there appears to be no impetus to internalize the therapist's functions. In this sense, the perception of the therapist as a negative or ineffectual other is directly related to the failure to internalize as well as to negative therapeutic outcome. One's negative perception of the therapist is often a function of a fixed internal representational world (although it may also indicate a realistic perception of an ineffectual clinician). The ability to hold on to an experience of the therapist as a trustworthy other, even in times of substantial therapeutic conflict and negative emotion, is a necessary precondition for effective treatment.

These findings highlight the dual nature of the conditions necessary for therapeutic change. Effective treatment seems to be a function of internalization of the therapist's sensitivity to and acceptance of the patient, as well as internalization of the functions provided by the therapist within the context of the relationship itself. Internalization of the therapist's functions is discerned through patients' ability to continue the kind of dialogue characteristic of therapy in the therapist's absence. This function, initially provided to the patient by the therapist, is done within the context of a specific type of relationship. It appears that the internalization of aspects of the relationship itself, specifically of the therapist's benevolent attitude toward the patient, provides the context for internalization of function.

The human qualities of the therapist, seen in the degree to which the therapist is regarded as a positive ideal, are associated with the degree to which the therapeutic dialogue is continued internally following termination. This directs our focus to the quality and nature of the patient–therapist relationship itself as the locus of change. It emphasizes the value of measures such as the TRI, which direct a spotlight onto the internal arena. This is necessary in the ability to link theories of therapeutic change with empirical testing of these theories. One only internalizes in the absence of that which will be internalized. Thus, the notion of psychotherapy process of necessity includes extrasession exploration and, specifically, the assessment of long-term effects posttermination.

The reader might like to consider writing a description of your own therapist. Consider how you might characterize the affective tone of your description. What functions might your therapist representation serve? Under what conditions might you find yourself thinking about your therapist? What important differences might you expect from brief versus long-term psychotherapy? What might account for the lack of distinction between brief and long-term treatments in terms of the therapist representation?

REFERENCES

Arnold, E. G. (1998). *A follow-up study of post-termination effects of psychotherapy on self-representation, representation of the therapist, and symptomatology.* Unpublished doctoral dissertation, Teachers College, Columbia University, New York.

Arnold, E. G., Farber, B. A., & Geller, J. D. (2000). Changes in patients' self-representation over the course of psychotherapy. *The Journal of the American Academy of Psychoanalysis, 28,* 449–466.

Atwood, G., & Stolorow, R. (1980). Psychoanalytic concepts and the representational world. *Psychoanalysis and Contemporary Thought, 3,* 267–290.

Barchat, D. (1989, June). *Representations and separations in therapy: The August phenomenon.* Paper presented at the annual meeting of the Society for Psychotherapy Research, Toronto, Ontario, Canada.

Behrends, R., & Blatt, S. J. (1985). Internalization and psychological development throughout the life cycle. In A. J. Solnit, R. S. Eissler, & P. B. Neubauer (Eds.), *The psychoanalytic study of the child* (Vol. 40, pp. 11–39). New Haven, CT: Yale University Press.

Bender, D. (1996). *The relationship of psychopathology and attachment to patients' representations of self, parents, and therapist in the early phase of psychodynamic psychotherapy.* Unpublished doctoral dissertation, Teachers College, Columbia University, New York.

Bender, D., Farber, B. A., & Geller, J. D. (1997). Patients' representations of therapist, parents, and self in the early phase of psychotherapy. *The Journal of the American Academy of Psychoanalysis, 25,* 571–586.

Bergmann, M. (1988). On the fate of the intrapsychic image of the analyst after termination of the analysis. In A. J. Solnit, P. B. Neubauer, S. Abrams, & A. S. Dowling (Eds.), *The psychoanalytic study of the child* (Vol. 43, pp. 137–152). New Haven, CT: Yale University Press.

Bernard, H., & Drob, S. (1989). "Afterwork": A clinical phenomenological report. *Psychiatric Quarterly, 60,* 359–369.

Bers, S., Blatt, S., Sayward, H., & Johnston, R. (1993). Normal and pathological aspects of self-descriptions and their change over long-term treatment. *Psychoanalytic Psychology, 10,* 17–37.

Blatt, S., Bers, S., & Schaffer, C. (1992). *The assessment of self-description.* (Available from S. J. Blatt, 25 Park Street, New Haven, CT 06519)

Blatt, S. J., & Blass, R. B. (1990). Attachment and separateness: A dialectical model of the products and processes of development throughout the life cycle. In A. J. Solnit, P. B. Neubauer, S. Abrams, & A. S. Dowling (Eds.), *The psychoanalytic study of the child* (Vol. 45, pp. 107–127). New Haven, CT: Yale University Press.

Blatt, S. J., Chevron, E. S., Quinlan, D. M., Schaffer, C. E., & Wein, S. (1992). *The assessment of qualitative dimensions of object representations.* (Available from S. J. Blatt, 25 Park Street, New Haven, CT 06519)

Blatt, S. J., & Shichman, S. (1983). Two primary configurations of psychopathology. *Psychoanalysis and Contemporary Thought, 6,* 187–254.

Blatt, S. J., Wein, S., Chevron, E., & Quinlan, D. (1979). Parental representations and depression in normal young adults. *Journal of Abnormal Psychology, 88,* 388–397.

Blatt, S., Wild, C., & Ritzler, B. (1975). Disturbances of object representations in schizophrenia. *Psychoanalysis and Contemporary Science, 4,* 235–288.

Blatt, S., Wiseman, H., Prince-Gibson, E., & Gatt, C. (1991). Object representations and change in clinical functioning. *Psychotherapy, 28,* 273–283.

Bruner, J. S. (1964). The course of cognitive growth. *American Psychologist, 19,* 1–15.

Derogatis, L. (1983). *SCL–90–R: Administration, Scoring, and Procedures Manual.* Towson, MD: Clinical Psychometric Research.

Diamond, D., Kaslow, N., Coonerty, S., & Blatt, S. J. (1990). Changes in separation-individuation and intersubjectivity in long-term treatment. *Psychoanalytic Psychology, 7,* 363–397.

Edelson, M. (1963). *The termination of intensive psychotherapy.* Springfield, IL: Thomas.

Farber, B. A., & Geller, J. D. (1994). Gender and representation in psychotherapy. *Psychotherapy, 31,* 318–326.

Freud, S. (1963). Mourning and melancholia. In P. Rieff (Ed.) & J. Riviere (Trans.), *General psychological theory* (pp. 164–179). New York: Collier Books, Macmillan Publishing Company. (Original work published 1917)

Freud, S. (1963). Analysis terminable and interminable. In P. Rieff (Ed.) & J. Riviere (Trans.), *Therapy and technique* (pp. 233–271). New York: Collier Books, Macmillan Publishing Company. (Original work published 1937)

Gaines, R. (1997). Detachment and continuity: The two tasks of mourning. *Contemporary Psychoanalysis, 33,* 549–571.

Geller, J. D. (1987). The process of psychotherapy: Separation and the complex interplay among empathy, insight, and internalization. In J. Bloom-Feshbach & S. Bloom-Feshbach (Eds.), *The psychology of separation through the life-span* (pp. 151–219). San Francisco: Jossey-Bass.

Geller, J. D., Cooley, R. S., & Hartley, D. (1981–1982). Images of the psychotherapist: A theoretical and methodological perspective. *Imagination, Cognition and Personality, 1,* 123–146.

Geller, J. D., & Farber, B. A. (1993). Factors influencing the process of internalization in psychotherapy. *Psychotherapy Research, 3,* 166–180.

Geller, J. D., Hartley, D., Behrends, R., Farber, B. A., Andrews, C., Marciano, P., Bender, D., & Brownlow, A. (1992). *Thematic patterning scale of object representations II.* (Available from J. D. Geller, Yale University Department of Psychology, New Haven, CT)

Gruen, R., & Blatt, S. (1990). Change in self- and object representation during long-term dynamically oriented treatment. *Psychoanalytic Psychology, 7,* 399–422.

Honig, M. (1989). *The effect of level of object representation on patients' internalized representations of their therapists during the beginning phase of treatment.* Unpublished doctoral dissertation, Teachers College, Columbia University, New York.

Honig, M., Farber, B. A., & Geller, J. D. (1997). The relationship of patients' pre-treatment representations of mother to early treatment representations of their therapist. *Journal of the American Academy of Psychoanalysis, 25,* 357–372.

Horvath, A. O., & Symonds, B. D. (1991). Relation between working alliance and outcome in psychotherapy: A meta-analysis. *Journal of Counseling Psychology, 38,* 139–149.

Kavanagh, G. (1985). Changes in patients' object representations during psychoanalysis and psychoanalytic psychotherapy. *Bulletin of the Menninger Clinic, 49,* 546–564.

Levinson, H. (1977). Termination of psychotherapy: Some salient issues. *Social Casework, 58,* 481–489.

Loewald, H. W. (1960). On the therapeutic action of psychoanalysis. In *Papers on psychoanalysis* (pp. 221–256). New Haven, CT: Yale University Press.

Loewald, H. W. (1962). Internalization, separation, mourning, and the superego. *Psychoanalytic Quarterly, 31,* 483–504.

Loewald, H. W. (1988). Termination analyzable and unanalyzable. In A. J. Solnit, P. B. Neubauer, S. Abrams, & A. S. Dowling (Eds.), *Psychoanalytic study of the child* (Vol. 43, pp. 155–166). New Haven, CT: Yale University Press.

Luborsky, L. (1984). *Principles of psychoanalytic psychotherapy.* New York: Basic Books.

Mahler, M., Pine, F., & Bergman, A. (1975). *The psychological birth of the human infant.* New York: Basic Books.

Meissner, W. W. (1981). *Internalization in psychoanalysis.* Madison, CT: International Universities Press.

Oremland, J., Blacker, K., & Norman, H., (1975). Incompleteness in "successful" psychoanalyses: A follow-up study. *Journal of the American Psychoanalytic Association, 23,* 819–844.

Orlinsky, D., & Geller, J. D. (1994). Patients' representations of their therapists and therapy: New measures. In N. Miller, J. Docherty, & L. Luborsky (Eds.), *Psychodynamic treatment research* (pp. 423–466). New York: Basic Books.

Orlinsky, D. E., Geller, J. D., Tarragona, M., & Farber, B. (1993). Patients' representations of psychotherapy: A new focus for psychodynamic research. *Journal of Consulting and Clinical Psychology, 61,* 596–610.

Orlinsky, D., & Howard, K. (1986). Process and outcome in psychotherapy. In S. Garfield & A. Bergin (Eds.), *Handbook of psychotherapy and behavior change* (3rd ed.). New York: Wiley.

Orlinsky, D., & Tarragona, M. (1986). *Intersession Experience Questionnaire.* Chicago: University of Chicago Committee on Human Development.

Piaget, J. (1954). *The construction of reality in the child.* New York: Basic Books.

Rosenzweig, D., Farber, B. A., & Geller, J. D. (1996). Clients' representations of their therapists over the course of psychotherapy. *Journal of Clinical Psychology, 52,* 197–207.
Schafer, R. (1968). *Aspects of internalization.* Madison, CT: International Universities Press, Inc.
Schaffer, C., & Geller, J. D. (1995, June). *The role of attachment, alexithymia, and affect regulation in the internalization of the therapy relationship.* Paper presented at the Annual Meeting, Society for Psychotherapy Research, Vancouver, British Columbia, Canada.
Stern, D. N. (1985). *The interpersonal world of the human infant.* New York: Basic Books.
Summers, F. (1997). Transcending the self: An object-relations model of the therapeutic action of psychoanalysis. *Contemporary Psychoanalysis, 33,* 411–428.
Vygotsky, L. S. (1962). *Thought and language.* New York: Wiley.
Wzontek, N., Geller, J. D., & Farber, B. A. (1995). Patients' post-termination representations of their psychotherapists. *Journal of the American Academy of Psychoanalysis, 23,* 395–410.

CHAPTER

15

Measuring Clinically Significant Change

Michael J. Lambert
Brigham Young University

Ted P. Asay
Private Practice

The purpose of learning and practicing brief dynamic psychotherapy is to help people to improve their psychological functioning and make meaningful changes in their lives in a timely manner. How to most effectively evaluate the nature and degree of change that has occurred as a result of therapy is an important question for both therapists and researchers alike. It is no surprise to students and more seasoned psychotherapy practitioners that there is an increasing emphasis on the use of short-term psychotherapies, including brief dynamic psychotherapy (BDP), stemming from growing expectations from third-party payers, government agencies, and professional organizations for greater therapist accountability and demonstration of psychotherapeutic cost-effectiveness. To meet these demands, the systematic evaluation of psychotherapy outcomes is essential. Findings from outcome studies not only provide evidence regarding the effectiveness of therapy but also generate valuable information that can be used to improve and refine the treatment being offered.

Psychotherapy outcome studies have traditionally been conducted by investigators working in academic or research settings. More recently there has been an emphasis on studying therapy outcomes in routine clinical practice (Clement, 1996; Kazdin, 1996; Lambert, Hansen, & Finch, 2001), including outcome evaluation conducted by individual practitioners (Asay, Lambert, Gregersen, & Goates, 2002). In this chapter, we briefly review current approaches to evaluating treatment outcome and the results of selected outcome studies relevant to BDP. In addition, the use of patient-focused research to evaluate patient change is discussed with an emphasis on how this method can be used in routine clinical practice. Finally, an example of the use of this methodology to track patient progress and outcome by a psychodynamically oriented private practitioner is presented.

APPROACHES TO EVALUATING PSYCHOTHERAPY OUTCOME

The evaluation of psychotherapy outcomes has historically been conducted using a clinical trials methodology in which a sample of homogeneous patients are treated with a specific type of psychotherapy and then compared to a sample of similar patients who received a competing treatment, no treatment, or placebo. The emphasis of this efficacy research is on measuring the response of patients to a specific treatment in highly controlled experimental conditions. Results of this research has revealed that many types of psychotherapy are effective and, in general, one form of psychotherapy has not been shown to be consistently superior to another (Lambert & Bergin, 1994; Smith, Glass, & Miller, 1980). The effectiveness of psychoanalytic and psychodynamic psychotherapies has been specifically evaluated in large-scale meta-analytic studies of psychotherapy outcome. For example, Smith et al. (1980) reported average effect sizes (ESs) of .85 for psychotherapy in general (meaning that at the end of treatment the average person is doing better than 80% of those who did not receive treatment), .69 for psychoanalytic and Freudian therapies, and .89 for dynamic-eclectic therapies. Andrews and Harvey (1981) analyzed a subset of the Smith et al. (1980) data that focused on neurotic disorders and reported that dynamic therapies and psychotherapy in general produced average ESs of .72. The results of these reviews indicate that psychodynamic psychotherapy is more effective than no treatment and is just as effective as other forms of therapy.

The efficacy of BDP or short-term dynamic psychotherapy (STDP) has also been evaluated using meta-analytic techniques to summarize the results of outcome studies. In a meta-analysis of 19 comparative studies, Svartberg and Stiles (1991) reported a small average ES (.16) for STDP. They also found that at 6 months STDP was no more effective than a no-treatment waiting list and was significantly less effective than the alternative treatment to which it was compared. This latter finding was consistent at 1-year follow-up. In contrast to these results, Crits-Christoph (1992) reviewed 11 studies of STDP and reported an average ES of 1.10 in target symptoms, .82 in general symptoms, and .81 in the area of social adjustment. Crits-Christoph concluded that there were no significant differences between STDP and other forms of psychotherapy. The differing results of these two reviews are likely to be due primarily to methodological differences in the way the meta-analyses were conducted. Specifically, there was little overlap of studies reviewed most likely because Crits-Christoph only included studies that employed treatment manuals, used experienced therapists who were trained in STDP, and restricted his analysis to particular outcome measures.

In an attempt to shed additional light on the question of the efficacy of STDP, Anderson and Lambert (1995) conducted an updated meta-analysis of 26 studies of STDP with results indicating an ES of .71 in comparison to no treatment, .34 in comparison to minimal treatments, and no differential effectiveness in relation to alternative treatments. The authors concluded that STDP was not superior or inferior to other forms of psychotherapy.

The aforementioned studies not only provide empirical evidence for the effectiveness of STDP but highlight current methods and approaches to reviewing efficacy studies of psychotherapy outcome. Although efficacy research strives to conform to strict scientific guidelines, it has been criticized for often being irrelevant to actual clinical practice (Seligman, 1995).

Another type of psychotherapy outcome research concerns itself with evaluating treatment effectiveness in naturalistic settings. This effectiveness research (Seligman, 1995) seeks to understand patient change in psychotherapy as it is delivered in day-to-day clinical practice. Hence, traditional experimental conditions, such as randomization of participants and the use of control groups, do not apply. Results from one large-scale psychotherapy effectiveness study, the *Consumer Reports* study, were reported by Seligman (1995). In this study, data from a survey of *Consumer Reports* readers who had received treatment from a mental health professional ($n = 2,900$) were analyzed with results revealing that the majority of individuals who received treatment were doing better (87% to 92% reported feeling either very good, good, or so-so) at the time of the survey. In addition, no specific therapeutic modality performed better than any other for any problem, and people involved in long-term therapy improved more than those in short-term therapy.

In another example of effectiveness research, Freedman, Hoffenberg, Vorus, and Frosch (1999) evaluated the outcome of patients treated with traditional, long-term psychoanalytic psychotherapy in a community-oriented mental health center. Outcome was assessed using the Effectiveness Questionnaire, a measure adapted from the previously mentioned *Consumer Reports* study. The investigators reported that better treatment outcome was associated with longer treatment duration (e.g., patients who received 7–24 months of therapy did better than those who received 6 months or less) and greater session frequency (e.g., patients who received two or three sessions per week did better than those who were seen weekly). The advantage of effectiveness research over efficacy studies is that it is easier to generalize to actual clinical practice. However, it has been criticized because of a lack of experimental controls and the lengthy time required before results can be passed on to practitioners (Lambert, Hansen, & Finch, 2001).

PATIENT-FOCUSED RESEARCH AND PSYCHOTHERAPY OUTCOME

In addition to efficacy and effectiveness studies, a third psychotherapy research paradigm has recently emerged in the study of treatment outcomes. Introduced by Howard, Moras, Brill, Martinovich, and Lutz (1996), patient-focused research is aimed at monitoring an individual patient's progress over the course of therapy. Whereas efficacy and effectiveness studies focus on the average response of groups of patients to treatment in either controlled or naturalistic settings, patient-focused research attempts to answer the question, "Is this treatment working for this patient?" The information obtained can serve as valuable feedback to the practitioner, supervisor, or case manager who can make attendant treatment modifications in real time. This type of research is well suited to answering questions and addressing concerns of direct interest to the therapist because it focuses specifically on the ongoing treatment and progress of the individual patient.

Patient-focused research has received increasing attention in the professional literature as researchers and clinicians are looking more at the importance of assessing the outcomes of individual patients in routine clinical practice (Asay et al., 2002; Kazdin, 1996; Lambert, Hansen, & Finch, 2001). Accordingly, there is a growing body of research highlighting both the practicality and utility of this approach in clinical settings. For example, one type of patient-focused research attempts to assess the relation between the number of sessions received and the degree of patient improvement. This dose-response relation research is concerned with how much therapy is required to produce meaningful change. In a pioneering investigation, Howard, Kopta, Krause, and Orlinsky (1986) examined this issue in a study that used probit analysis to estimate recovery on a session-to-session basis. This analysis revealed very rapid improvement in the initial phase of treatment followed by smaller gains as the treatment progressed. It was also found that 53% of patients received a satisfactory benefit in just eight sessions. One shortcoming of this study, however, was that patient improvement was evaluated using pre-post estimates of change rather than session-by-session ratings of improvement. Kopta, Howard, Lowery, and Beutler (1994) also studied the dose-response effect using a sample of 854 clients suffering primarily from depression and anxiety. Therapists were 141 psychologists, psychiatrists, social workers, and trainees, and client change was assessed using an 18-item subset of the Symptom Checklist–90–Revised (Derogatis, 1983) items administered at several points during the course of treatment. Results revealed that patients with acute symptoms required 5 sessions, those with chronic symptoms required 14 sessions, and those with characterological symptoms required 104 sessions for 50% to receive clinically significant change.

In a similar study, Kadera, Lambert, and Andrews (1996) evaluated the course of 64 clients treated by trainees in a university outpatient clinic. Clients were suffering primarily from anxiety and depression and treatment progress was assessed weekly using the Outcome Questionnaire–45 (OQ-45; Lambert et al., 1996). Results revealed that 50% of clients were estimated to have attained clinically significant change by the 6th session and 75% by the 26th session. This study was replicated by Anderson and Lambert (2001) who combined the samples from both studies and found that 50% of patients needed 13 sessions of therapy before reaching criteria for clinically significant change. To reach a lesser standard of improvement (reliable change), 50% of clients needed 10 sessions and 75% of clients required 17 sessions. Using much larger and more diverse patient samples, Lambert, Hansen, and Finch (2001) reported that 50% of patients could be expected to reach clinically significant change following 21 sessions of therapy and 75% would be expected to reach this level after 45 sessions. Using the standard of reliable change, 50% of patients were estimated to improve after 7 sessions and 75% following 14 sessions.

The dose-response relation (i.e., the number of sessions necessary for a meaningful change to occur) has recently been expanded through the development of expected recovery curves and patient profiling (Howard et al., 1996; Lambert, Hansen, & Finch, 2001). These methods allow comparisons to be made between a particular individual's treatment progress and the rate and type of change that would be expected given his or her status on certain pretreatment variables such as initial distress levels. Patients who are not responding as expected to treatment can then be identified and the information used to make decisions about changes in the treatment approach. Lambert, Whipple, et al. (2001) described a system of coding patient progress and the positive effects of providing timely feedback to therapists regarding patients not responding well to treatment.

These examples of patient-focused research demonstrate the value of this method in assessing how much therapy is required to help patients change and how therapy progress can be monitored, leading to helpful changes in the treatment approach when necessary. This type of research is complimentary to efficacy and effectiveness studies and adds another important dimension to evaluating outcomes that can enhance clinicians' knowledge and improve methods of studying patient change.

CLINICALLY SIGNIFICANT CHANGE

In efficacy and effectiveness studies, the focus is generally on observing statistically significant differences between groups of individuals following treatment (e.g., between a treatment group and a control group). One problem with this methodology, however, is that statistically significant improvement does not necessarily translate into practical and meaningful improvements for the individual patient. For example, in psychotherapy outcome studies, statistically significant differences between treated and untreated groups may have very little practical significance in actual patient functioning. One advantage of patient-focused research is that it measures noticeable and clinically relevant changes that occur within each individual patient. It is, therefore, essential to have a clear definition of what constitutes significant change and a standard method of classifying the degree of change in each patient. The operationalizing of clinically significant change is central to patient-focused research because tracking patient responses to treatment requires a marker to make decisions about the degree of improvement (or deterioration) and whether continued treatment, a modified treatment approach, or termination would be in the best interest of the individual patient.

Although various methods have been proposed for measuring meaningful change (e.g., Kendall, 1999), the most commonly accepted method is the two-step marker proposed by Jacobson and Truax (1991). They operationalized clinically significant change as

1. Patient movement from the ranks of the dysfunctional into the ranks of the functional (based on normative comparisons).
2. Movement so large that it was not likely to be the result of measurement error (reliable change).

Patients who meet both criteria are classified as having reached clinically significant change or "recovery." Those whose change is reliable (meeting criteria only for the aforementioned Marker 2) are considered to be improved but not clinically significantly improved. An example of how clinically significant change is operationalized in patient-focused research is presented later in this chapter.

PATIENT-FOCUSED RESEARCH IN PRIVATE PRACTICE

In the studies cited previously, patient-focused research methods were used to evaluate the outcomes of large numbers of patients seen by multiple therapists using varying treatment methods. Although this is clearly a welcome addition to traditional psychotherapy research, an added value of patient-focused research is that it can be used by individual therapists to track patient progress and evaluate therapeutic outcomes. Currently, the vast majority of practitioners do not conduct any type of systematic or scientific evaluation of their own treatment effectiveness even though there have been several models proposed for conducting outcome research in private practice (Clement, 1996). There are many reasons for this including lack of funding, time constraints, lack of reinforcements for research activities, client resistance, lack of skill in research design and analysis, and resistance from therapists to looking at their own effectiveness (Clement, 1996; Morrison, 1984). At the same time, there are advantages for therapists to engage in outcome evaluation, such as enhancing treatment effectiveness, increasing patient satisfaction, and meeting the demands of third-party payers, professional organizations, and others for empirical demonstration of treatment effectiveness.

As an example of how patient-focused research methods can be utilized by private practitioners, we summarize the results of a study conducted by an individual psychologist in private practice (Asay et al., 2002) in which a particular type of patient-focused methodology, the dose-response relation, was used to track patient progress and outcome.

In the Asay et al. (2002) study, 29 adults and 40 youth (children and adolescents ages 5 to 17) were treated by a clinical psychologist in private practice. The adult patients were suffering primarily from mood and anxiety disorders and a majority (66%) also carried a personality disorder diagnosis. The children and adolescent patients were diagnosed with mood, anxiety, behavioral, and adjustment disorders with 13% diagnosed with personality disorders. The therapist had been in private practice for 14 years and was psychodynamically oriented, although other approaches and techniques (e.g., cognitive, behavioral, and family systems) were integrated and utilized as needed, particularly with the child and adolescent cases.

Patient progress was measured using the OQ-45 (Lambert et al., 1996) and the Youth Outcome Questionnaire (YOQ; Burlingame, Wells, & Lambert, 1996). The OQ-45 is a 45-item self-report questionnaire that measures three broad aspects of patient functioning: subjective discomfort, interpersonal relationships, and social role performance. The OQ-45 provides three subscale scores and a total score. The total score, which is a global assessment of patient functioning, was used in Asay et al. (2002). The YOQ is a 64-item parent report measure of treatment progress for children and adolescents receiving mental health treatment and provides six subscale scores and a total score, which is a measure of global functioning. As with the OQ-45, the total score was used in this study. Participants were asked to fill out an OQ-45 or YOQ before each session for the duration of treatment or until the study ended, whichever came first. The OQ-45 or YOQ that was administered before the first session served as the patient's baseline score. OQ–45 and YOQ data obtained before the second session reflected the effects of one session of therapy, data obtained before the third session reflected the effects of two sessions, and so forth.

Patient improvement in treatment was determined by using OQ–45 and YOQ cutoff scores for reliable change (RC) and clinically significant change (CS) based on recommendations by Jacobson and Truax (1991). RC, or improvement, occurred when patient scores on the OQ–45 changed by 14 points (13 points for the YOQ), and CS, or recovery, occurred when two criteria were met: the OQ–45 score changed by 14 points (13 points for the YOQ), and the patient began treatment in the dysfunctional range of scores, as compared to a normative group, and ended in the functional range. That is, their score at the end of treatment was 63 or below on the OQ–45 and 45 or below on the YOQ. The evaluation of patient progress was accomplished using survival analysis (Kaplan & Meier, 1958), a nonparametric procedure used to track patient functioning across several points in time. It is used in psychotherapy outcome research to predict the outcome status of patients at any point in time along the course of treatment (Lambert, Hansen, et al., 2001). In Asay et al. (2002) the procedure was used to predict the number of sessions required by adults and youth to reach RC and CS.

Results revealed that 25% of adult patients were expected to reach CS at 42 sessions, and 50% were expected to reach CS criteria in 54 sessions. In contrast, 25% of youth patients were predicted to achieve CS in 7 sessions and 50% in 14 sessions. Using the criteria for RC, a less stringent standard, 25% of adult patients were predicted to improve after 11 sessions, 50% after 42 sessions, and 75% after 56 sessions. At the same time, 25% of youth patients were expected to reach RC in 3 sessions, 50% in 7 sessions, and 75% in 12 sessions. Although statistically based modeling procedures estimate the likelihood of benefit following treatment sessions, patients often do not stay in treatment long enough to derive the full benefits of treatment. Thus, actual counts of the number of patients in a study who actually attain reliable change tend to be much lower.

In discussing their findings, Asay et al. (2002) concluded that using a standardized self-report measure for adults (OQ–45) and a parent report measure for youth (YOQ) was a feasible way for individual clinicians to study patient outcome using the dose-response relation. They also pointed out that even though survival analysis was used to predict patient recovery rates, it is not necessary to use this rather complex statistical procedure to evaluate patient progress using the dose-response methodology. In contrast, all that is required is that the clinician score the OQ–45 or the YOQ by hand or by computer and then compare the scores to the already established criteria for RC and CS. For example, using the OQ–45, RC is obtained when there is a 14-point change in the positive direction. Likewise, CS is obtained when there is a 14-point change and the patient's score has moved from the dysfunctional to the functional range, that is, scores at or below 63. The number of sessions for a patient to reach RC or CS can then be easily calculated and comparisons regarding the number of sessions required for 50% or 75% of patients to reach criteria can be made using previously published reports or other data sets from the therapist's own practice.

In regard to the results of the study, Asay et al. (2002) reported that the number of sessions required for patients to reach CS and RC were somewhat higher than those reported in other studies of the dose-effect relation. For example, Lambert, Hansen, et al. (2001) reported 50% of patients reached CS by the 21st session and 50% reached RC by the 7th session. As an explanation for the longer time frame required for patients to reach CS and RC, they suggested that the patients in their study had more severe levels of psychopathology than those in national samples and were, therefore, more difficult to treat. For example, whereas most of the patients in the national samples were diagnosed as having adjustment disorders and a variety of Axis I difficulties, a sizable majority (66%) of patients in this study received an Axis II personality disorder diagnosis. In addition, the authors suggested that the type of therapy being offered, open-ended psychodynamic psychotherapy, may have also contributed to longer treatment duration because the focus of therapy was directed more toward the underlying personality factors contributing to symptoms as opposed to focusing primarily on symptom reduction itself. It remains to be seen if this emphasis on personality has any demonstrable advantage to patients or if it reduces relapse.

Interestingly, even though the adult patients in the Asay et al. (2002) study required more treatment to reach RC and CS than those in national samples, the percentage of patients who actually reached CS before leaving treatment was higher (25%) than those reported in other naturalistic studies of the dose-response relation. For example, in a national health maintenance organization sample ($n = 936$), 16% of patients reached CS; in a national EAP sample ($n = 3,269$) 15% reached CS; in a state community mental health center sample ($n = 361$) 9% reached CS; in a university counseling center ($n = 1,188$) 13% reached CS; in a local health maintenance organization ($n = 595$) 11% reached CS; and in a university-based training clinic ($n = 123$) 20% reached CS (Hansen, Lambert, & Forman, 2002). Thus, the relatively longer treatment duration of adult patients in Asay et al. resulted in better treatment outcomes than those obtained in national samples. This finding is consistent with results of the *Consumer Reports* effectiveness study (Seligman, 1995), a recent effectiveness study of psychoanalytically oriented psychotherapy (Freedman et al., 1999), and a comprehensive review of psychotherapy process and outcome literature (Orlinsky, Grawe, & Parks, 1994), all of which found that longer treatment duration led to better patient improvement. It is somewhat disturbing to see the overall levels of CS change are so low. However, these low rates come from routine practice in which the actual number of sessions that patients attend is around three to five.

It was also noted that the youth group in the Asay et al. (2002) study improved at a significantly faster rate than the adults and required less therapy to reach RC and CS. The most likely explanation for this finding was that the youth group as a whole had lower initial levels of dysfunction and appeared to have less severe psychopathology. In addition, many patients in the youth sample were treated with behavioral and family systems approaches as well as psychodynamic interventions that may have contributed to faster rates of improvement.

The Asay et al. (2002) study just reviewed represents a preliminary effort by an individual clinician to utilize patient-focused research in evaluating treatment outcome. The methodology employed in that study appears to be a feasible, cost-effective, and meaningful way for individual clinicians to study patient outcomes. Although there is much more to be done in refining these procedures, the Asay et al. study provides a methodological foundation that practitioners can use to begin integrating evaluation methods into their clinical practice.

CONCLUSIONS AND RECOMMENDATIONS FOR PRACTITIONERS OF BDP

In this chapter we presented a methodology for measuring clinically significant change that can be used in brief dynamic psychotherapy using patient-focused research with an emphasis on how this method can be utilized by therapists in day-to-day clinical practice. Although conducting treatment outcome research requires some additional time on the part of the clinician, we believe that it does not have to be an overly cumbersome activity and is well worth the effort invested. Based on the research available and our own experience using patient-focused research methods, we offer the following conclusions and recommendations for therapists practicing BDP who are interested in evaluating treatment progress and outcome in daily practice.

1. Therapists' involvement in outcome research has several potentially valuable benefits, not the least of which is obtaining information that can contribute in a positive way to the psychotherapy process and ultimately enhance patient outcomes. Patient-focused research is especially well suited for BDP because it allows close, session-by-session monitoring of patient progress by the therapist. In addition, it can provide outcome data that is in-

creasingly required by third-party payers, government agencies, and professional organizations.

2. Conducting outcome research in clinical practice does not have to be a painstaking, time consuming, and overwhelming involvement. It will take some extra time initially to set up the evaluation protocol, but once the procedures are established it will probably take very little time and effort on a day-to-day basis. As mentioned previously, it is not necessary to use survival analysis and complex computer programs to evaluate the dose-response relation. In contrast, therapists simply need to use a measure in which criteria for CS and RC have been established. Once the measure has been scored, it is a relatively easy process to track patient progress and compare scores with already established criteria from other data sets.

3. The use of a standardized self-report measure, such as the OQ-45, is a feasible way to track patient progress that is reliable, valid, sensitive to change, inexpensive, and easy to manage by both the therapist and the patient. Although we have found the OQ-45 to have many advantages in measuring patient change, we also recognize that there are a number of measures that have been consistently used in evaluating treatment outcomes (Froyd, Lambert, & Froyd, 1996), such as the Symptom Checklist-90 (Derogatis, 1983), Beck Depression Inventory (Beck, Ward, Mendelson, Mock, & Erbaugh, 1961), and the State-Trait Anxiety Inventory (Spielberger, 1983) that could be used by the individual clinician. In addition, when therapists are working from a particular theoretical orientation, such as in BDP, it is helpful to use additional measures that are sensitive to patient change as conceptualized along theoretically determined dimensions. For instance, a therapist practicing brief psychodynamic psychotherapy could assess patient change using two types of measures: a general measure of outcome, such as the OQ-45, and a measure that is sensitive to change as conceptualized in psychodynamic theory.

An example of this type of measure is the scales developed by Hoglend et al. (2000), which were designed to assess change in brief psychodynamic psychotherapy in five specific areas: quality of friendships/family relationships, romantic/sexual relationships, tolerance for affects, insight and problem solving, and adaptive capacity. The scale format is similar to the Global Assessment Scale with 10 descriptive levels rated on scale points from 1 to 100. The scales are therapist rated and could easily be rated after each therapy session. There are several additional outcome measures that have been used in assessing patient outcome from a dynamic perspective (Froyd et al., 1996; Maruish, 1999) and could be adapted for use in studies by individual practitioners.

4. Data from therapist-conducted dose-response outcome research allows the therapist to compare the outcome of patients in his or her own practice with patients studied in large national samples. This can provide com-

parisons of outcome (benchmarks) from which to evaluate treatment effectiveness. Of course, there are important considerations to keep in mind in making such comparisons including the comparability of patient groups (e.g., initial level of maladjustment), the types of measures used to evaluate change, and the type of treatment being offered.

5. Outcome data obtained by a practicing clinician could be used to develop a database to be used as a comparison group for patients treated at a later date by the same therapist. This dose-response baseline would create an additional, perhaps more meaningful, perspective for assessing patient progress rather than relying solely on data sets from national samples. More specifically, for the therapists practicing BDP, comparisons with databases from other dynamically oriented practitioners, especially those using brief methods, would probably be more relevant and useful in evaluating treatment effectiveness.

6. Using the dose-response methodology, clinicians can receive immediate feedback (e.g., session to session) about the progress of a particular patient. If progress is slower than expected or if the patient is not changing or deteriorating, then the therapist can discuss this with the patient and possibly institute changes in the treatment approach that would lead to a better treatment response. This would be a helpful process in all psychotherapies, but is particularly relevant in brief approaches in which time constraints play a central role in the therapy process.

7. This methodology would also allow therapists to compare their own judgments of patient progress with statistical data obtained from outcome measures. For example, if a therapist makes a judgment that a patient has achieved CS, how does this compare with the level of patient change as measured by the OQ–45? It is possible in this regard that in some instances a therapist might believe that a patient is making progress, whereas the statistical data shows little or no improvement. In this case, sharing the statistical information with the patient could open an avenue for the patient and therapist to discuss the possible lack of progress and make any needed changes in the therapeutic approach accordingly.

8. It is also possible to use outcome measures to obtain important qualitative information about patient progress. By reviewing an individual OQ–45 completed just prior to a therapy session, for example, the therapist could become aware of important changes in functioning or areas of difficulty that might not be mentioned by the patient in the session. This is most likely to occur in the beginning phases of treatment when a strong treatment alliance has yet to be developed.

Although therapists may be hesitant to warm up to the idea of implementing outcome research in day-to-day practice, we believe that those who become involved will soon see the value of this enterprise in strengthening the therapeutic alliance, reducing patient dropout, enhancing treatment outcomes, and improving the quality of the therapeutic experience for both the patient and therapist.

REFERENCES

Anderson, E. M., & Lambert, M. J. (1995). Short-term dynamically oriented psychotherapy: A review and meta-analysis. *Clinical Psychology Review, 15,* 503–514.

Anderson, E. M., & Lambert, M. J. (2001). A survival analysis of clinically significant change in outpatient psychotherapy. *Journal of Clinical Psychology, 57,* 875–888.

Andrews, G., & Harvey, R. (1981). Does psychotherapy benefit neurotic patients? A reanalysis of the Smith, Glass, and Miller data. *Archives of General Psychiatry, 38,* 1203–1207.

Asay, T. P., Lambert, M. J., Gregersen, A. T., & Goates, M. K. (2002). Using patient-focused research in evaluating treatment outcome in private practice. *Journal of Clinical Psychology, 58,* 1199–1225.

Beck, A. T., Ward, C. H., Mendelson, M., Mock, J., & Erbaugh, J. (1961). An inventory for measuring depression. *Archives of General Psychiatry, 4,* 561–571.

Burlingame, G. M., Wells, M. G., & Lambert, M. J. (1996). *The Youth Outcome Questionnaire.* Stevenson, MD: American Professional Credentialing and Services.

Clement, P. W. (1996). Evaluation in private practice. *Clinical Psychology: Science and Practice, 3,* 146–159.

Crits-Christoph, P. (1992). The efficacy of brief dynamic psychotherapy: A meta-analysis. *American Journal of Psychiatry, 149,* 151–158.

Derogatis, L. R. (1983). *The SCL-90: Administration, scoring and procedures for the SC-90.* Baltimore, MD: Clinical Psychometric Research.

Freedman, N., Hoffenberg, J. D., Vorus, N., & Frosch, A. (1999). The effectiveness of psychoanalytic psychotherapy: The role of treatment duration, frequency of sessions, and the therapeutic relationship. *Journal of the American Psychoanalytic Association, 47,* 741–772.

Froyd, J. E., Lambert, M. J., & Froyd, J. D. (1996). A review of practices of psychotherapy outcome measurement. *Journal of Mental Health, 5,* 11–15.

Hansen, N., Lambert, M. J., & Forman, E. M. (2002). Comparison of clinically significant change in clinical trials and naturalistic practice settings: The dose-effect relationship and its implications for practice. *Clinical Psychology: Science and Practice, 9,* 329–343.

Hoglend, P., Bogwald, K. P., Amlo, S., Heyerdahl, O., Sorbye, O., Marble, A., Sjaastad, M. C., & Bentsen, H. (2000). Assessment of change in dynamic psychotherapy. *Journal of Psychotherapy Practice and Research, 9,* 190–199.

Howard, K. I., Kopta, S. M., Krause, M. S., & Orlinsky, D. E. (1986). The dose-effect relationship in psychotherapy. *American Psychologist, 41,* 159–164.

Howard, K. I., Moras, K., Brill, P. C., Martinovich, Z., & Lutz, W. (1996). Evaluation of psychotherapy: Efficacy, effectiveness, and patient progress. *American Psychologist, 51,* 1059–1064.

Jacobson, N. S., & Truax, P. (1991). Clinical significance: A statistical approach to defining meaningful change in psychotherapy research. *Journal of Consulting and Clinical Psychology, 59,* 12–19.

Kadera, S. W., Lambert, M. J., & Andrews, A. A. (1996). How much therapy is really enough?: A session-by-session analysis of the psychotherapy dose-effect relationship. *Journal of Psychotherapy Practice and Research, 5,* 1–22.

Kazdin, A. E. (1996). Evaluation in clinical practice: Introduction to the series. *Clinical Psychology: Science and Practice, 3,* 144–145.

Kendall, P. C. (1999). Clinical significance. *Journal of Consulting and Clinical Psychology, 67,* 383–384.

Kopta, S. M., Howard, K. I., Lowry, J. L., & Beutler, L. E. (1994). Patterns of symptomatic recovery in psychotherapy. *Journal of Consulting and Clinical Psychology, 62,* 1009–1016.

Lambert, M. J., & Bergin, A. E. (1994). The effectiveness of psychotherapy. In A. E. Bergin & S. L. Garfield (Eds.), *Handbook of psychotherapy and behavior change* (4th ed., pp. 143–189). New York: Wiley.

Lambert, M. J., Hansen, N. B., & Finch, A. E. (2001). Patient-focused research: Using patient outcome data to enhance treatment effects. *Journal of Consulting and Clinical Psychology, 69,* 159–172.

Lambert, M. J., Hansen, N. B., Umphress, V., Lunnen, K., Okiishi, J., Burlingame, G., Huefner, J. C., & Reisinger, C. W. (1996). *Administration and scoring manual for the Outcome Questionnaire (OQ-45.2).* Wilmington, DE: American Professional Credentialing Services.

Lambert, M. J., Whipple, J. L., Smart, D. W., Vermeersch, D. A., Nielsen, S. L., & Hawkins, E. J. (2001). The effects of providing therapists with feedback on patient progress during psychotherapy: Are outcomes enhanced? *Psychotherapy Research, 11,* 49–68.

Maruish, M. E. (Ed.). (1999). *The use of psychological testing for treatment planning and outcome assessment* (2nd ed.). Mahwah, NJ: Lawrence Erlbaum Associates.

Morrison, J. K. (1984). Crossing the research barrier in the private practice of psychotherapy. *Psychotherapy in Private Practice, 2,* 15–20.

Orlinsky, D. E., Grawe, K., & Parks, B. K. (1994). Process and outcome in psychotherapy: Noch einmal. In A. E. Bergin & S. L. Garfield (Eds.), *Handbook of psychotherapy and behavior change* (4th ed., pp. 270–376). New York: Wiley.

Seligman, M. E. P. (1995). The effectiveness of psychotherapy: The *Consumer Reports* study. *American Psychologist, 50,* 965–974.

Smith, M. L., Glass, G. V., & Miller, T. I. (1980). *The benefits of psychotherapy.* Baltimore, MD: Johns Hopkins University Press.

Spielberger, C. D. (1983). *Manual for the State-Trait Anxiety Inventory STAI (Form Y).* Palo Alto, CA: Consulting Psychologists Press.

Svartberg, M., & Stiles, T. C. (1991). Comparative effects of short-term psychodynamic psychotherapy: A meta-analysis. *Journal of Consulting and Clinical Psychology, 59,* 704–714.

PART
V

SPECIAL ISSUES

CHAPTER

16

Critical Factors in Supervision: The Patient, the Therapist, and the Supervisor

Susan Allstetter Neufeldt
University of California at Santa Barbara

To be certified or licensed, all mental health workers[1] must be supervised. In some countries, states, or provinces, supervision is required before licensure; in others, supervision continues throughout the licensed practitioner's professional career. *Supervision,* defined elegantly by Hess (1987), "is a relationship in which one person's skills in conducting psychotherapy and his or her identity as a therapist are intentionally and potentially enhanced by the interaction with another person" (pp. 255–256). I add that the interaction may occur in the context of a supervision group in which group members as well as a designated supervisor respond to the supervisee and the supervisee's cases, as well as in an interaction between two individuals working together without other participants in the room. Naturally, the relationship includes the supervisor, the supervisee, and sometimes the supervisee's colleagues, but also the client who, except in some forms of live or cotherapist supervision, is not physically present during supervision.

Psychotherapy and supervision take place in a context (Neufeldt, Karno, & Nelson, 1996). A given agency and opportunities or limits for care within that geographical area and client population affect the length of the relationship. How cases are assigned to therapists and how much supervision is provided under what conditions affect the delivery of care. Perhaps most important and often ignored, the demographic, political, socioeconomic,

---

[1]The terms *mental health worker, counselor, therapist,* and *psychotherapist* are used interchangeably. Likewise *counseling, therapy,* and *psychotherapy* are used interchangeably.

and cultural attributes that characterize the supervisor, therapist, and client are critical components of the therapeutic relationship (Arredondo, 1998; Brown & Landrum-Brown, 1995).

Based on published literature to that date, Carifio and Hess (1987) described the "ideal supervisor" as one who demonstrated high levels of empathy, respect, genuineness, flexibility, concern, investment, and openness. Good supervisors, they said, are knowledgeable, experienced, and clear in explaining their thoughts and expectations in supervision without generating a feeling of criticism and nonsupport. They provide appropriate teaching, goal setting, and feedback during their supervisory interactions. They are respectful and open to their supervisees. At the same time they maintain clear boundaries between their role as supervisor with the supervisee and their role as therapist with others.

In this chapter, general goals and intentions of supervision as well as related research findings are described first. These are followed with specific supervisory characteristics, interventions, and interactions and their effects. They are illustrated with references to the case provided earlier in the book. Because the supervisor and supervision process are not described, they are invented for the case.

GOALS AND INTENTIONS OF SUPERVISION

Before moving to the specific case provided in this book, I talk about general goals for supervision. Several goals are preeminent for supervisors: (a) development of the therapist, whether a novice student or a competent professional, into a psychotherapist with increased expertise and clinical wisdom (Jennings & Skovholt, 1999; Rønnestad & Skovholt, 1993; Skovholt & Jennings, in press; Skovholt & Rønnestad, 1992; Skovholt, Rønnestad, & Jennings, 1997); (b) the supervisee's acquisition of knowledge and understanding of the contextual factors operating in the therapy dyad as well as the supervision dyad (Neufeldt, 1999b; Neufeldt et al., 1996), particularly the cultural context (Brown & Landrum-Brown, 1995; D'Andrea & Daniels, 1997; Fong & Lease, 1997); (c) development of the supervisee's ability to form a good relationship with the client (Wampold, 2001), often described as the working alliance (Greenson, 1967; Horvath & Greenberg, 1989); (d) facilitation of the therapist's ability to conceptualize cases, both in terms of assessment of the client's characteristics and problem and selection of treatment (Beutler & Clarkin, 1990; Groth-Marnat, Roberts, & Beutler, 2001; Wampold, 2001); and (e) facilitation of the therapist's belief in the effectiveness of a given treatment approach and overall competence as a therapist, including the ability to carry out the planned treatment (Wampold, 2001). All of these goals, of course, improve the likelihood of increasing benefit to and protecting the welfare of the client whose case is under supervision—a primary intention and ethical requirement (Bernard & Goodyear, 1998; Falvey, 2002; Holloway, 1995) of supervision.

Development: Nature of Expertise, Development, and Reflexivity

After observing expert chess players, Chi, Glaser, and Farr (1988) described the ways in which experts functioned differently than did novices. Their work has been considered a model for the nature and development of expertise in a variety of areas, including psychotherapy and supervision (Binder, 1993; Dawes, 1994). Chi et al. elucidated several characteristics of experts. These principles follow, with examples that apply to psychotherapy.

- Experts excel mainly in their own domains, that is, an expert chemist cannot carry that expertise into work as a psychotherapist.
- Experts perceive large, meaningful patterns in their domain. Illustrative of this is an expert therapist who interviews a client and sees patterns in the client's behavior and relationships with family members and colleagues at work and is able to connect those patterns to the client's relationship with the therapist.
- Experts take more time to analyze a problem qualitatively, and they then can solve a problem fairly quickly. In psychotherapy, the expert's analysis of the client's characteristics, problem, history, and current functioning, once accomplished, is followed by a faster and more efficient decision about an appropriate treatment plan.
- Experts appear to have superior short-term and long-term memory because they have learned to do so many things automatically that their minds are freed up to concentrate on unique aspects of the situation at hand. They see and represent a problem in their domain at a deeper, more principled level than novices. Expert therapists pay attention to verbal, nonverbal, and paraverbal (pace, pitch, and tone) characteristics of the client's presentation, as well as to the client's history. They can then analyze these in a coherent, integrated manner before making treatment decisions, either moment by moment or in planning ahead. Novice therapists, on the other hand, frequently listen only to verbal content and then consider its discrete elements apart from one another.
- Experts have strong self-monitoring skills. Skovholt and his colleagues (Jennings & Skovholt, 1999; Skovholt & Rønnestad, 1992) reported that expert psychotherapists can supervise themselves because their ability to reflect on their interventions and the results of these interventions enables making adjustments in their perceptions and behavior both within sessions and between sessions.

How is it that some people develop as therapists (and often, concomitantly, as human beings) over 20 years of clinical experience, whereas others simply repeat 1 year 20 times? Many supervision theoreticians and researchers (Borders, Fong, & Neimeyer, 1986; Hill, Charles, & Reed, 1981; Loganbill, Hardy, & Delworth, 1982; Stoltenberg & Delworth, 1987; Stoltenberg, McNeill, & Delworth, 1998) have identified stages of counselor and therapist development, with development largely completed (or not studied) by the end of graduate study. However, in a large qualitative study of 100 counselors and therapists ranging in experience from individuals at the paraprofessional level to individuals with 40 years of clinical experience, Skovholt and Rønnestad (Rønnestad & Skovholt, 1993; Skovholt & Rønnestad, 1992) conducted extensive initial interviews and a follow-up with 60 of these 2 years later. On the basis of these interviews, they concluded that half of therapist professional development occurs before graduation and licensure, and half occurs in many subsequent years of practice. The same researchers with an additional colleague (Jennings & Skovholt, 1999; Skovholt et al., 1997) explored the qualities and length of practice of peer-nominated expert clinicians; the researchers determined that expertise in clinical practice takes an average of 15 years of experience to attain.

In addition to illuminating levels of psychotherapist development, Skovholt and Rønnestad (1992) determined that only some therapists reach expert status. These people demonstrated high levels of cognitive complexity, a tolerance for ambiguity, and a propensity to reflect on their work and change their understanding of clients or their interventions with clients as a result of their thinking about it. On the other hand, those who stagnated or left clinical work altogether tended to choose a theoretical approach early and then attempt to apply it to every client they saw; when it failed, they became discouraged and gave up, either on the ability of clients to change or on the general efficacy of psychotherapy. Holloway and colleagues likewise found that therapists who demonstrated higher levels of cognitive complexity formulated better clinical hypotheses (Holloway & Wolleat, 1980) and were more effective in counseling (Holloway & Wampold, 1986; Holloway & Wolleat, 1980).

Neufeldt et al. (1996) clarified the nature of reflectivity in a series of interviews with experts on reflectivity (Copeland, Holloway, Rønnestad, Schön, and Skovholt) in the fields of education, counseling, and architecture. They concluded that in clinical supervision (as well as alone or with colleagues between sessions of psychotherapy), therapists who take a reflective stance demonstrate specific characteristics and behaviors.

The reflective process is a search for understanding of the phenomena of the counseling session, with attention to the therapist's actions, emotions, and thoughts, as well as to the interaction between the therapist and the client. The intent to understand what has occurred, active inquiry, openness to that understanding, and vulnerability and risk-taking, rather than defensive self-protection, characterize the stance of the reflective supervisee. Supervisees use theory, their prior personal and professional experience, and their experience of themselves in the counseling session as sources of understanding. If they are to contribute to future development, reflections must be profound rather than superficial and must be meaningful to the supervisees. In our interview for this study, Schön told me that "a person can reflect back on tying his shoes" but questioned the depth, meaning, and importance of this reflection (personal communication, February 16, 1994). To complete the sequence, genuine reflectivity in supervision leads to changes in perception and counseling practice, and an increased capacity to make meaning of experiences.

Apparently, teaching therapists to reflect is as important in training and supervision as development of specific therapeutic competencies. After all, if they are to continue to develop as clinicians long after training ends, they will need that particular self-monitoring process.

Necessary Knowledge, Attitudes, and Skill With Multicultural Counseling and Supervision

Numerous experts have pointed out the necessity of considering the cultural context and cultural identity level of clients and counselors in the counseling relationship (Arredondo, 1998, 1999; Atkinson, Morten, & Sue, 1998; Constantine & Ladany, 2001; Sue & Sue, 1999). I add that, in my own experience, commitment to this idea is not the same as having a multicultural vision, such that no interaction can any longer be viewed outside of its cultural context. Again, as I have observed in myself and in others with little life experience outside of the European-based environment, this is a challenging cognitive and emotional shift for counselors or therapists who recognize their own commitment but fail to understand their inadequate vision or behavior. It is not, of course, as deep as the lived experience of culture and oppression (M. Ingram, personal communication, November 10, 2001). However, it is still a profound shift and is often precipitated by some long-term exposure and a painful emotional confrontation or experience. Likewise, Brown and Landrum-Brown (1995), Constantine (1997), D'Andrea and Daniels (1997), Fong and Lease (1997), Neufeldt (1999a), and others have all said that training in multicultural counseling is dependent on supervisors' multicultural knowledge, attitude, and skills in counseling, along with their application in the supervisory relationship. Although it sometimes occurs, the supervisee's job is not to teach the supervisor to hold a cultural view of supervision and therapy interactions anymore than clients should be expected to teach the therapist about the cultural worldviews, behaviors, and interactions of people like them.

Skill in Forming a Therapeutic Relationship

In an extensive meta-analysis, Wampold et al. (1997) showed that the beneficial outcome effect size associated with any given treatment approach over any other approach is .20; likewise, there is little effect due to specific ingredients of psychotherapy. In a subsequent book, Wampold (2001) pointed out that common factors in psychotherapy account for a larger percentage of outcome. In particular, the therapist must have a theoretical basis for conducting therapy and must believe in it. Allegiance to the approach was significantly more important than adherence to any specific ingredient of it. "When the therapist believes that the treatment is efficacious, he or she will enthusiastically communicate that belief to the client," Wampold (2001, p. 183) stated; on the other hand, "adherence to treatment protocols was generally not associated with outcome, although a few notable exceptions were found" (p. 183). This echoes the discovery of Strupp and his colleagues at Vanderbilt (Henry, Butler, Strupp, Schacht, & Binder, 1993) that the effort to adhere to a manual sometimes inadvertently causes therapists to be more hostile, that is, to have a poorer relationship, or working alliance, with the client.

Central to psychotherapeutic outcome, the working alliance (Bordin, 1979; Gelso & Carter, 1985, 1994; Greenson, 1967; Groth-Marnat et al., 2001; Horvath & Greenberg, 1989), comprised of agreement on task and goals and a bond between therapist and client, is a major predictor of psychotherapy outcome (Beutler, Machado, & Neufeldt, 1994; Wampold, 2001; Wampold et al., 1997). In training a therapist to work with clients, therefore, considerable attention must be given to formation of the working alliance, that is, attention to the basic relational skills usually taught early in mental health training. Facilitation of a therapist's skill at forming a working alliance with clients is a major goal of supervision. One way to do this is to consider the working alliance established between therapist and supervisor with the supervisor monitoring ruptures and undertaking repair where and when required. In a similar and related manner, the supervisor would monitor transference and countertransference issues as they become apparent and especially how they appear to manifest parallel processes between the therapist and the client.

Case Conceptualization and Therapist Competence

Wampold (2001) reported that client factors such as motivation, personality characteristics, social skills, support, and reactance account for much of the rest of the outcome. Client characteristics can facilitate a choice of treatment (Beutler & Clarkin, 1990) by matching client characteristics with an appropriate treatment. Further, the client's attribution of responsibility to self or others for both the problem and the solution can affect the success of treatment (Rabinowitz, Zevon, & Karuza, 1988). As Wampold (2001) stated, this is consistent with matching clients' worldviews to a therapeutic approach. Important indicators of clients' attitudes and worldviews are gender, race, ethnicity, culture, religion, and sexual orientation, among others.

Supervisors, then, need to make certain that their trainees conduct a careful and sometimes extensive intake to illuminate not only the problem but also the client and contextual variables. In this way, they increase the likelihood of selecting a treatment that is appropriate for the client. By recognizing the contextual variables, supervisors may also alert therapists to the power issues in supervision and psychotherapy.

Beyond encouraging therapists to make careful assessments of their clients' problems and personal and contextual characteristics, supervisors need to facilitate therapist competence in a broad sense, that is, in forming alliances and carrying out psychotherapy (Wampold, 2001). More competent therapists consistently produce better outcomes, even when they have been trained similarly and randomly assigned to clients with similar diagnoses (Blatt, Sanislow, Zuroff, & Pilkonis, 1996; Luborsky et al., 1986; Luborsky, McLellan, Diguer, Woody, & Seligman, 1997; Luborsky, McLellan, Woody, O'Brien, & Auerbach, 1975). Although precise adherence to a manual, for instance, is not required (Wampold, 2001), therapists need to know how to carry out the strategies consistent with the treatments, including integrated treatments, that they have chosen to use with a given client. To be effective with a variety of clients, they need to be competent in several approaches. This means that their supervisors likewise can be most effective if they are competent in several treatment modalities, particularly if they are supervising more than one case.

Given this important knowledge about effective therapy, how does the supervisor proceed? What characteristics of supervisors affect therapist competence, particularly the relation between the supervisory working alliance and particular supervisory outcomes? How are formative evaluations (continuing feedback) and summative evaluations best delivered and most easily received by supervisees and incorporated into their work? Likewise, how does the supervisor encourage supervisee reflectivity to encourage therapist development as a therapist? How well do supervisors facilitate incorporation of the contextual factors, particularly the cultural factors, in case conceptualization? Also, how do supervisors advance therapist competence?

Training and Supervision for Therapist Competence

Carrying out the treatment effectively is a matter of careful training and supervision. Binder (1993) underlined the importance of turning declarative (academic) knowledge into procedural (practice) knowledge. Declarative knowledge provides a guide for what is important to know, but such knowledge is insufficient without procedural knowledge, which serves as a guide for when and how to act, and the supervisor's task is to facilitate this transformation.

Two elements have been described as important in therapist training and supervision on the way to procedural competence. First, therapists need to learn principles behind the therapeutic approach and its fundamental strategies. This is part of becoming a competent therapist and probably also can increase the therapist's allegiance to the treatment as used with a particular client, both factors described by Wampold (2001) as important to outcome. However, Rounsaville, Chevron, and Weissman (1984) reported challenges they encountered in early efforts at training therapists to do Interpersonal Process Therapy (IPT), an approach similar to the cognitive analytic therapy approach described in the case exemplar provided for this book and most recently described in a current version of their manual (Klerman, Weissman, Rounsaville, & Chevron, 1999). Rounsaville et al. (1984) pointed out the pitfalls of a "cookbook" approach: "In regard to this point [avoiding a rigid, cookbook compliance with the manual]," they said, "the important thing is that although the manual defines the boundaries, the therapist is free to make use of individual variations in stance and timing. Some therapists missed the opportunity to find ways of forming a therapeutic alliance by spending too much energy going 'by the book' " (p. 166).

Rounsaville et al. (1984) reiterated that learning to do therapy is not a matter of simply acquiring declarative knowledge:

> Several therapists who, in reviews of videotape, were felt to be excellent had underrated their own work, whereas others, who could talk about IPT theories and techniques well and made a good presentation of their therapies, were rated less highly when actual sessions were viewed. . . . It is noteworthy that we dropped a written multiple-choice examination from the training and evaluation procedures because improvement on this instrument was found to be negatively correlated with ratings of therapists' skill in actually performing IPT. (p. 167)

SUPERVISION PRACTICES

If a cookbook approach is insufficient for training, supervision becomes considerably more complicated. Interventions become more complex, and as in psychotherapy, the relationship in which these interventions and interactions take place is central to its effectiveness. How might supervision look with a particular supervisee?

In the case presented in this book, we only have information about the therapist and the client. The therapist was a middle-class White English woman, pregnant with her first baby at the time of therapy, about mid-30s; for this chapter, I assume she was a psychologist. I give her a name, Amy. The client, June, was a working-class woman of 27 who dropped out of school early, was single and White, with no intimate relationships apparent in her life. I assume she has never had an intimate relationship. Also imagined for this case is a male 30-year-old, married, presently childless, Pakistani psychologist supervisor named Rashid.

The Supervision Relationship

Both Hess (1987, 1997) and Bordin (1983) believed in the importance of the working alliance, not only in psychotherapy but in the supervisory relationship between the supervisor and supervisee. At least two scales have been developed to measure the supervision working alliance. These include one specifically designed for supervision, the Supervision Working Alliance Inventory (Efstation, Patton, & Kardash, 1990), and one based on the original Working Alliance Inventory (Horvath & Greenberg, 1989) and adapted for supervision—the Working Alliance Inventory–Trainee version (Bahrick, 1990; Bahrick, Russell, & Salmi, 1991).

Ladany and his colleagues have demonstrated that the supervision working alliance is readily affected by behavior and traits of the supervisor. Ladany, Lehrman-Waterman, Molingaro, and Wolgast (1999) discovered that ethical lapses on the part of the supervisor were related to a poor working alliance and diminished supervisee satisfaction in supervision. Ladany, Brittan-Powell, and Pannu (1997) found that when supervisors and supervisees were poorly matched as to their level of ethnic identity development (whether or not they were of the same race), they had a weaker working alliance as well. Perceptions of Asian, Black, Hispanic, and Native American counseling and clinical supervisees were used to study the quality of cross-cultural individual therapist supervision (Cook & Helms, 1988). The authors found that when supervisees experienced their supervisors' unconditional interest, they were more likely to be satisfied with the quality of supervision. Subsequently, several authors (Brown & Landrum-Brown, 1995; Constantine, 1997; Constantine & Ladany, 2001; Cook, 1994) have recommended that the supervisor have a well-developed sense of ethnic-racial identity that matched or exceeded that of their supervisees. At that level, they suggested, supervisors need to learn to handle their discomfort and address supervisees' and their clients' racial and ethnic identities, along with their differences from the supervisee along other cultural dimensions, in supervision. I add that issues of gender, age, ability status, and sexual orientation are among the important factors to discuss as well.

Think then about the configuration of the client, therapist, and supervisor in our case example, as imagined previously. As a supervisor, Rashid, a male Pakistani, will need to address with his supervisee, Amy, the therapist in this case, the ways in which he and she differ along these various dimensions. It is important for the supervisor to address this first because the supervisee rarely will (Kleintjes & Swartz, 1996). As suggested by T. Parham (personal communication, April 12, 2000), a way for the supervisor to gain trust is simply to ask, "What do you need to know from me to believe I can help you?" In this case, Amy would then have the chance to ask Rashid questions she might have about his training and experience with clients, supervision, and the particular mode of therapy used here, along with questions about his feelings about pregnant therapists who continue to work, whether the supervisor has worked with English therapists and clients, how he might feel about a single, working-class woman, and so forth. Suppose further that there could be other value differences; for example, the client may be a lesbian, though that is not shown in the transcripts we have. Then Amy might also ask if Rashid has any negative feelings about lesbians, which she might imagine is a religious issue for him. All of these issues can be discussed openly, and if Rashid is candid and also willing to discuss how his experience and feelings could affect supervision, then Amy is more likely to trust in the relationship between her and Rashid, an element critical to the bond in the working alliance.

Supervision Focus

Although the bond facilitated through the previous discussion is significant, the focus of supervision assumes considerable importance. In a complex study of supervision within Interactional Social Work Theory, Harkness (1997) found that supervisees were most satisfied when the supervisor focused on the client and what to do with the client. This proved even more important than empathy, and in fact, whereas empathy enhanced supervisees' satisfaction when supervision was focused on the client, empathy without that focus detracted from supervisee satisfaction. Although supervisees might have not enjoyed the feedback at the time it was given, it proved valuable in their overall evaluations of supervision.

In a large psychotherapy project at Vanderbilt University in Tennessee, therapists were trained to use short-term psychodynamic therapy and supervised as they practiced (Henry, Butler, et al., 1993; Henry, Schacht, Strupp, Butler, & Binder, 1993). In these studies, which extended Harkness' (1997) finding to therapist performance, Henry, Schacht, et al. (1993) reported that the supervisor who asked therapists' intentions for their interventions and provided explicit feedback about specific aspects of therapist performance facilitated in-session performance in those areas. Trainees want that feedback, and their complaints in another study (Ladany et al., 1999), for example, "supervisor gives little feedback," reflect it. In fact, Ladany and his colleagues noted, failing to give explicit feedback is a supervisory ethical failure to protect the client's welfare.

Providing feedback as therapists carry out a specific mode of therapy is not the same as using a cookbook approach because it is directed to intentions and results of interventions in the session. In fact, asking about intentions and results is an important part of encouraging therapist reflection on their actions, an element of reflective supervision as well (Neufeldt, 1999b). It is then incumbent on our supervisor, Rashid, to watch or listen to Amy's tapes of her sessions with June and ask Amy about the intentions behind her interventions. After listening to the following exchange, for instance, Rashid could ask Amy to stop the tape. The segment from page 1 of the first transcript, which appears below, could be considered.

Q: 3-2: Did you blank out last week's session?
A: 3-3: Basically, yes, I think I did.
Q: 3-4: Any idea why all that happens?
A: 3-5: No.
Q: 3-6: No. So if I ask you to start keeping a diary soon about blanking things about, would you be able to do that, or would you blank that out as well?
A: I'd give it a go.

"Amy, how did you decide to ask June whether she'd blanked out last week's session?" Rashid might ask.[2] If she replied, "I wanted to see if she was continuing to blank out previous sessions and if we could do something about that," Rashid could then ask, "And what was the result?" Amy might reply, "She did acknowledge it and she also agreed to keep a diary about blanking things out. If she does that, we might learn when, how, and why she blanks out things, and perhaps then interrupt the blanking-out process." At this point Rashid might comment on his own perception of the effectiveness of the intervention and further present alternative interventions for Amy to consider if June fails to keep a diary. This avoids telling the therapist just what to do in a cookbook fashion and yet provides important possible interventions for Amy to choose or develop further to make the intervention her own.

---

[2] I have found as a supervisor that asking how the therapist decided to act produces less defensiveness than asking "Why did you do that?."

Supervisors' encouragement of therapists' attention to clients' nonverbal behaviors and response to them within a therapeutic session was correlated with increased client satisfaction in a session and a higher working alliance between the therapist and client in one study (Grace, Kivlighan, & Kunce, 1995). Although this one study is not conclusive, it would seem sensible for Rashid to direct Amy's attention to June's nonverbal behaviors and respond to them in session.

Important Factors in Supervision

Both Ladany et al. (1999) and Falvey (2002) emphasized the importance of supervisory ethics. Most explicitly defined by the Association for Counselor Education and Supervision (1995), there are ethical codes for supervision in most professional associations. Ladany et al. (1999) identified a number of supervisor violations of ethics described by supervisees and showed that these violations appeared to weaken the supervision working alliance. Further, of course, it is just good practice to follow ethical codes and can make lawsuits more unlikely (Falvey, 2002), at least in the United States, whose population is arguably more litigious than the population in many other countries. Rashid, therefore, should be careful to operate according to ethical codes in supervision.

In several qualitative studies, researchers investigated supervisees' experiences with one or more supervisors over an extended period of time. Worthen and McNeill (1996) explored good supervision experiences important to the supervisees' growth as therapists. These included experiencing the supervision relationship as empathic, nonjudgmental, and validating, with encouragement to explore and experiment, and in which struggle was normalized. As a result, supervisees felt freed of self-protectiveness and receptive to supervisory input, able to carry out a nondefensive analysis of their work and reexamine their assumptions and develop a metaperspective on their work. With this in mind, Rashid could demonstrate empathy, validation, and a nonjudgmental attitude with Amy that could enable reflection on her work and a modification of her behavior and thinking in a manner consistent with reflectivity.

In another vein, Gray, Ladany, Walker, and Ancis (2001) explored counterproductive events experienced by supervisees with their supervisors. Supervisors were described as unempathic, dismissive of supervisees' thoughts and feelings, and failing to understand supervisees. Supervisors appeared not to listen or respond to trainees and to push their own agenda. In reaction, supervisors reported feeling frustrated, irritated, angry, anxious, unsafe, confused, and undermined; they also experienced negative thoughts about themselves and the supervisory relationship. In a similar study, Nelson and Friedlander (2001) investigated conflictual supervisory relationships. Many supervisees felt unsupported from the beginning of the relationship and experienced a power struggle with the supervisor, sometimes because the supervisor was less experienced than the supervisee, or the supervisor appeared to feel threatened, or both. Beyond that, the two participants disagreed about what should take place in supervision. Several believed that supervisors misunderstood their or their clients' cultural worldviews or gender and sexual differences, and they disagreed with their supervisees' theoretical or technical approach to clients. In reaction, supervisees reported, supervisors criticized the supervisee in front of others, denied there were problems, or blamed the supervisee for problems. Most supervisors in this study were site supervisors, and some threatened to or did withhold evaluation or necessary letters to the department certifying completion of practicum. Clearly Rashid should demonstrate the behavior and attitudes described by Worthen and McNeill (1996) and avoid the appearance or presence of the negative attitudes and behavior (Gray et al., 2001; Nelson & Friedlander, 2001).

Case Conceptualization

Surprisingly, therapists, even if they have had courses in multicultural counseling and believe they are competent in that area, often fail to incorporate cultural factors into their case conceptualizations (Ladany, Inman, Constantine, & Hofheinz, 1997). Worthington, Mobley, Franks, and Tan (2000) found, however, that if supervisees were directed to attend to multicultural factors in a given case conceptualization, they would do so. In our case, Rashid could direct Amy's attention to June's working-class background. How might that context be an influence on June's behavior? Further, what values, beliefs, and other aspects of the worldview of English working-class people could be integrated into therapy to influence June's willingness to take care of her diabetes?

Several additional elements go into case conceptualization. Beutler and Clarkin (1990) proposed that clients' expectations, coping ability, and personality could be the basis of selection of treatments suited to particular clients. Groth-Marnat et al. (2001) recommended specific assessments, which could be given at intake and which would provide information about aspects of coping style and personality such as client reactance, avoidance, internalization or externalization of problems, and repression and denial. If Rashid had encouraged Amy to conduct these assessments at intake and had a choice about treatments, Amy might have determined that a short-term psychodynamic approach such as cognitive analytic therapy was or was not an appropriate approach for Amy to use with June. This would also provide Amy with reasons to be loyal to the approach with June, a factor associated with better outcome (Wampold, 2001).

CONCLUSION

Research in supervision has proliferated in the past 15 years (Bernard & Goodyear, 1998; Holloway & Gonzalez-Doupe, 1999). Careful quantitative and qualitative research studies can now inform supervisors and enable them to conduct themselves more effectively by displaying positive attitudes and behaviors conducive to forming good working alliances with supervisees. Likewise, supervisors can attend to and discuss cultural aspects of clients, supervisors, and themselves, facilitate case conceptualization, and make useful and timely interventions with supervisees.

There are still too few studies that link supervision to client outcome. This is made more difficult because, as Strupp stated in his discussion of supervision research at the American Psychological Association meeting in 1995, there are a number of mediators between the supervisor and the client. The personalities of the supervisor and therapist as well as the nature and severity of the disorder, the characteristics of the client, the context in which therapy takes place, and the length of time allowed for therapy, play a role in the outcome. Ways to overcome these obstacles in which treatment is selected systematically for a specific diagnosis and supervised by a number of therapists should be sought to facilitate a careful analysis of supervisors' effects on client outcomes. Without establishing such a controlled environment, investigators might co-vary the mediating variables to assess supervision effects on client outcome. Wampold and Holloway (1997) pointed out many additional questions that need to be answered by research and suggested ways to investigate them.

REFERENCES

Arredondo, P. (1998). Integrating multicultural counseling competencies and universal helping conditions in culture-specific contexts. *Counseling Psychologist, 26,* 592–601.

Arredondo, P. (1999). Multicultural counseling competencies as tools to address oppression and racism. *Journal of Counseling and Development, 77,* 102–108.

Association for Counselor Education and Supervision. (1995). Ethical guidelines for counseling supervisors. *Counselor Education and Supervision, 34,* 270–276.

Atkinson, D. R., Morten, G., & Sue, D. W. (1998). *Counseling American minorities.* Boston: McGraw-Hill.

Bahrick, A. S. (1990). Role induction for counselor trainees: Effects on the supervisory working alliance. *Dissertation Abstracts International, 51*(3), 1484B.

Bahrick, A. S., Russell, R. K., & Salmi, S. W. (1991). The effects of role induction on trainees' perceptions of supervision. *Journal of Counseling and Development, 69,* 434–438.

Bernard, J. M., & Goodyear, R. L. (1998). *Fundamentals of clinical supervision* (2nd ed.). Boston: Allyn & Bacon.

Beutler, L. E., & Clarkin, J. F. (1990). *Systematic treatment selection: Toward targeted therapeutic interventions.* New York: Brunner/Mazel.

Beutler, L. E., Machado, P. P. P., & Neufeldt, S. A. (1994). Therapist variables. In A. E. Bergin & S. L. Garfield (Eds.), *Handbook of psychotherapy and behavior change* (3rd ed., pp. 229–269). New York: Wiley.

Binder, J. L. (1993). Is it time to improve psychotherapy training? *Clinical Psychology Review, 13,* 301–318.

Blatt, S. J., Sanislow, C. A., Zuroff, D. C., & Pilkonis, P. A. (1996). Characteristics of effective therapists: Further analyses of data from the National Institute of Mental Health treatment. *Clinical Psychology, 64,* 162–171.

Borders, L. D., Fong, M. L., & Neimeyer, G. J. (1986). Counseling students' level of ego development and perceptions of clients. *Counselor Education and Supervision, 26,* 37–49.

Bordin, E. S. (1979). The generalizability of the psychodynamic concept of the working alliance. *Psychotherapy: Theory, Research, and Practice, 16,* 252–260.

Bordin, E. S. (1983). A working alliance model of supervision. *The Counseling Psychologist, 11,* 35–42.

Brown, M. T., & Landrum-Brown, J. (1995). Counselor supervision: Cross cultural perspectives. In J. G. Ponterotto, J. M. Casas, L. A. Suzuki, & C. M. Alexander (Eds.), *Handbook of multicultural counseling* (pp. 263–286). Thousand Oaks, CA: Sage.

Carifio, M. S., & Hess, A. K. (1987). Who is the ideal supervisor? *Professional Psychology: Research and Practice, 18,* 244–250.

Chi, M. T. H., Glaser, R., & Farr, M. J. (1988). *The nature of expertise.* Hillsdale, NJ: Lawrence Erlbaum Associates.

Constantine, M. G. (1997). Facilitating multicultural competency in counseling supervision: Operationalizing a practical framework. In D. B. Pope-Davis & H. L. K. Coleman (Eds.), *Multicultural counseling competencies: Assessment, education and training, and supervision* (pp. 310–324). Newbury Park, CA: Sage.

Constantine, M. G., & Ladany, N. (2001). New visions for defining and assessing multicultural competence. In J. G. Ponterotto, J. M. Casas, L. A. Suzuki, & C. M. Alexander (Eds.), *Handbook of multicultural counseling* (2nd ed., pp. 482–498). Thousand Oaks, CA: Sage.

Cook, D. A. (1994). Racial identity in supervision. *Counselor Education and Supervision, 34,* 132–141.

Cook, D. A., & Helms, J. E. (1988). Visible racial/ethnic group supervisees' satisfaction with cross-cultural supervision as predicted by relationship characteristics. *Journal of Counseling Psychology, 25,* 268–274.

D'Andrea, M., & Daniels, J. (1997). Multicultural counseling supervision: Central issues, theoretical considerations, and practical strategies. In D. B. Pope-Davis & H. L. K. Coleman (Eds.), *Multicultural counseling competencies: Assessment, education and training, and supervision* (pp. 290–309). Thousand Oaks, CA: Sage.

Dawes, R. M. (1994). *House of cards: Psychology and psychotherapy built on myth.* New York: Free Press.

Efstation, J. F., Patton, M. J., & Kardash, C. A. M. (1990). Measuring the working alliance in supervision. *Journal of Counseling Psychology, 37,* 322–329.

Falvey, J. E. (with Bray, T. E.). (2002). *Managing clinical supervision: Ethical practice and legal risk management.* Pacific Grove, CA: Brooks/Cole.

Fong, M. L., & Lease, S. (1997). Cross-cultural supervision: Issues for the White supervisor. In D. B. Pope-Davis & H. L. Coleman (Eds.), *Multicultural counseling competencies: Assessment, education and training, and supervision* (pp. 387–405). Thousand Oaks, CA: Sage.

Gelso, C. J., & Carter, J. A. (1985). The relationship in counseling and psychotherapy: Components, consequences, and theoretical antecedents. *The Counseling Psychologist, 13,* 155–243.

Gelso, C. J., & Carter, J. A. (1994). Components of the psychotherapy relationship: Their interaction and unfolding during treatment. *Journal of Counseling Psychology, 41,* 296–306.

Grace, M., Kivlighan, D. M., & Kunce, J. (1995). The effect of nonverbal skills training on counselor trainee nonverbal sensitivity and responsiveness and on session impact and working alliance ratings. *Journal of Counseling and Development, 73,* 547–552.

Gray, L. A., Ladany, N., Walker, J. A., & Ancis, J. R. (2001). Psychotherapy trainees experience of counterproductive events in supervision. *Journal of Counseling Psychology, 48,* 371–383.

Greenson, R. R. (1967). *The technique and practice of psychoanalysis.* New York: International Universities Press.

Groth-Marnat, G., Roberts, R. I., & Beutler, L. E. (2001). Client characteristics and psychotherapy: Perspectives, support, interactions, and implications for training. *Australian Psychologist, 36,* 115–121.

Harkness, D. (1997). Testing interactional social work theory: A panel analysis of supervised practice and outcomes. *Clinical Supervisor, 15,* 33–50.

Henry, W. P., Butler, S. F., Strupp, H. H., Schacht, T. E., & Binder, J. L. (1993). Effects of training in time-limited dynamic psychotherapy: Changes in therapist behavior. *Journal of Consulting and Clinical Psychology, 61,* 434–440.

Henry, W. P., Schacht, T. E., Strupp, H. H., Butler, S. F., & Binder, J. L. (1993). Effects of training in time-limited dynamic psychotherapy: Mediators of therapists' responses to training. *Journal of Consulting and Clinical Psychology, 61,* 441–447.

Hess, A. K. (1987). Psychotherapy supervision: Stages, Buber, and a theory of relationship. *Professional Psychology, 18,* 251–259.

Hess, A. K. (1997). The interpersonal approach to the supervision of psychotherapy. In C. E. Watkins, Jr. (Ed.), *Handbook of psychotherapy supervision* (pp. 63–83). New York: Wiley.

Hill, C. E., Charles, D., & Reed, K. G. (1981). A longitudinal analysis of changes in counseling skills during doctoral training in counseling psychology. *Journal of Counseling Psychology, 28,* 428–436.

Holloway, E. L. (1995). *Clinical supervision: A systems approach.* Thousand Oaks, CA: Sage.

Holloway, E. L., & Gonzalez-Doupe, P. (1999). *Empirically supported intervention programs: Implications for supervision as a training modality.* Unpublished manuscript. University of Wisconsin, Madison.

Holloway, E. L., & Wampold, B. E. (1986). Relationship between conceptual level and counseling-related tasks: A meta-analysis. *Journal of Counseling Psychology, 33,* 310–319.

Holloway, E. L., & Wolleat, P. L. (1980). Relationships of counselor conceptual level to clinical hypothesis formation. *Journal of Counseling & Psychology, 27,* 539–545.

Horvath, A. O., & Greenberg, L. S. (1989). The Working Alliance Inventory. *Journal of Counseling Psychology, 36,* 223–233.

Jennings, L., & Skovholt, T. M. (1999). The cognitive, emotional, and relational characteristics of master therapists. *Journal of Counseling Psychology, 46,* 3–11.

Kleintjes, S., & Swartz, L. (1996). Black clinical psychology trainees at a "white" South African university: Issues for clinical supervision. *Clinical Supervisor, 22,* 489–495.

Klerman, G. L., Weissman, M. M., Rounsaville, B. J., & Chevron, E. S. (1999). *Interpersonal psychotherapy for depression.* Northvale, NJ: Aronson.

Ladany, N., Brittan-Powell, C. S., & Pannu, R. K. (1997). The influence of supervisory racial identity interaction and racial matching on the supervisory working alliance and supervisee multicultural competence. *Counselor Education and Supervision, 36,* 189–202.

Ladany, N., Inman, A. G., Constantine, M. G., & Hofheinz, E. W. (1997). Supervisee multicultural case conceptualization ability and self-reported multicultural competence as functions of supervisee racial identity and supervisor focus. *Journal of Counseling Psychology, 44,* 284–293.

Ladany, N., Lehrman-Waterman, D., Molingaro, M., & Wolgast, B. (1999). Psychotherapy supervisor ethical practices: Adherence to guidelines, the supervisory working alliance, and supervisee satisfaction. *The Counseling Psychologist, 27,* 443–475.

Loganbill, C., Hardy, E., & Delworth, U. (1982). Supervision: A conceptual model. *The Counseling Psychologist, 10,* 3–42.

Luborsky, L., Crits-Christoph, P., McLellan, A. T., Diguer, L., Woody, G., O'Brien, P. W., Liberman, B., Imber, S., & Pilkonis, P. (1986). Do therapists vary much in their success? Findings from four outcome studies. *American Journal of Orthopsychiatry, 56,* 501–512.

Luborsky, L., McLellan, A. T., Diguer, L., Woody, G., & Seligman, D. A. (1997). The psychotherapist matters: Comparison of outcomes across twenty-two therapists and seven patient samples. *Clinical Psychology: Science and Practice, 4,* 53-65.

Luborsky, L., McLellan, A. T., Woody, G., O'Brien, C. P., & Auerbach, A. (1975). Therapist success and its determinants. *Archives of General Psychiatry, 43,* 602-611.

Nelson, M. L., & Friedlander, M. L. (2001). A close look at conflictual supervisory relationships: The trainee's perspective. *Journal of Counseling Psychology, 48,* 834-895.

Neufeldt, S. A. (1999a). *Supervision strategies for the first practicum* (2nd ed.). Alexandria, VA: American Counseling Association.

Neufeldt, S. A. (1999b). Training in reflective processes in supervision. In M. Carroll & E. L. Holloway (Eds.), *Training counselling supervisors: Strategies, methods and techniques* (pp. 92-105). London: Sage.

Neufeldt, S. A., Karno, M. P., & Nelson, M. L. (1996). A qualitative study of experts' conceptualization of supervisee reflectivity. *Journal of Counseling Psychology, 43,* 3-9.

Rabinowitz, R. C., Zevon, M. A., & Karuza, J., Jr. (1988). Psychotherapy as helping: An attributional analysis. In L. Y. Abramson (Ed.), *Social cognition and clinical psychology: A synthesis* (pp. 177-203). New York: Guilford.

Rønnestad, M. H., & Skovholt, T. M. (1993). Supervision of beginning and advanced graduate students of counseling and psychotherapy. *Journal of Counseling & Development, 71,* 396-405.

Rounsaville, B. J., Chevron, E. S., & Weissman, M. M. (1984). Specification of techniques in interpersonal psychotherapy. In J. R. W. Williams & R. L. Spitzer (Eds.), *Psychotherapy research: Where are we and where should we go?* (pp. 160-171). New York: Guilford.

Skovholt, T. M., & Jennings, L. (in press). *Master therapists.* Boston: Allyn & Bacon.

Skovholt, T. M., & Rønnestad, M. H. (1992). *The evolving professional self: Stages and themes in therapist and counselor development.* Chichester, England: Wiley.

Skovholt, T. M., Rønnestad, M. H., & Jennings, L. (1997). Searching for expertise in counseling, psychotherapy, and professional psychology. *Educational Psychology Review, 9,* 361-369.

Stoltenberg, C. D., & Delworth, C. D. (1987). *Supervising counselors and therapists.* San Francisco: Jossey-Bass.

Stoltenberg, C. D., McNeill, B., & Delworth, C. D. (1998). *IDM supervision: An integrated model for supervising therapists.* San Francisco: Jossey-Bass.

Strupp, H. (1995, August). Discussion. In C. E. Watkins (Chair), *Effectiveness of psychotherapy supervision.* Symposium conducted at the meeting of the American Psychological Association, New York.

Sue, D. W., & Sue, D. (1999). *Counseling the culturally different: Theory and practice* (3rd ed.). New York: Wiley.

Wampold, B. E. (2001). *The great psychotherapy debate: Models, methods, and findings.* Mahwah, NJ: Lawrence Erlbaum Associates.

Wampold, B. E., & Holloway, E. L. (1997). Methodology, design, and evaluation in psychotherapy supervision research. In C. E. Watkins, Jr. (Ed.), *Methodology, design, and evaluation in psychotherapy supervision research* (pp. 11-27). New York: Wiley.

Wampold, B. E., Mondin, G. W., Moody, M., Stich, F., Benson, K., & Ahn, H. (1997). A meta-analysis of outcome studies comparing bona-fide psychotherapies: Empirically, "All must have prizes." *Psychological Bulletin, 122,* 203-215.

Worthen, V., & McNeill, B. W. (1996). A phenomenological investigation of "good" supervision events. *Journal of Counseling Psychology, 43,* 25-34.

Worthington, R. L., Mobley, M., Franks, R. P., & Tan, J. A. (2000). Multicultural counseling competencies: Verbal content, counselor attributions, and social desirability. *Journal of Counseling Psychology, 47,* 460-468.

CHAPTER

17

The Ethical Challenges of Brief Therapy

Elizabeth Reynolds Welfel
Cleveland State University

Most people who come to outpatient psychotherapy are not interested in long-term treatment, psychoanalytic or otherwise, and at least half are able to profit from therapy in 10 sessions or less (Asay & Lambert, 1999; Lambert & Bergin, 1994). Of the remainder, approximately 15% to 30% are significantly more likely to benefit if therapy lasts more than 25 sessions (Asay & Lambert, 1999; Cummings & Cummings, 2000). Therefore, the first of many ethical challenges for psychotherapists is to competently differentiate between clients who may be helped by brief therapy and those for whom brief interventions are contraindicated. Once a reliable differential diagnosis is made, clinicians must also possess the necessary skills to administer therapies of varying lengths or have competent referral sources. To qualify as competent, brief therapy must rest on a foundation of education in the treatment modality and prior successful supervised experience. Too often, professionals trained in traditional therapies appear either to assume that this training is sufficient to allow them to use brief models effectively or to worry about incompetence in this modality without taking steps to remedy it. For example, Levenson and Davidovitz (2000) found that nearly all psychotherapists in their survey (89%) reported using time-limited interventions and that half of those offering such services had no formal brief therapy training at all. As one participant commented, "As a provider for a large health-maintenance organization I am required to do a lot of brief therapy. But I am ashamed to admit that I often don't know what I am doing, because I have never had any training in it" (Levenson & Davidovitz, 2000, p. 335).

Because practicing beyond the limits of one's competence is prohibited by the ethical standards (American Psychological Association [APA], 2002) and subject to discipline by licensing boards and because less skilled therapists who fail to maintain focus in sessions are more likely to produce negative outcomes (Lambert & Bergin, 1994), this deficit can be dangerous to client and therapist alike. Even if a therapist gains initial competence in brief interventions, continuing education in these models is essential as well because competence erodes quickly. According to Dubin (1972) and Jensen (1979), half of what a professional learns in graduate school is obsolete within 10 years of graduation.

The second major ethical challenge derives from the external pressures psychotherapists feel to select brief interventions for many clients. This pressure comes from insurance companies, health care employers, government funding sources, and from clients themselves. To borrow an adage a psychoanalyst friend learned while working in the restaurant business, this environment often leaves clinicians feeling compelled to "steak 'em and bake 'em and give 'em the check." In the United States, for example, where both governmental and private insurers reimburse self-employed professionals for providing care to qualifying patients, clinicians must follow strict reimbursement guidelines if they wish payment for services. These guidelines typically limit both the duration and the type of therapy acceptable for reimbursement. Some managed care companies pressure not just for brief treatment but also for ultrabrief treatment of 2 to 6 sessions (I. J. Miller, 1996). In the U.S. system, clinicians who do not play by the rules risk both denial of payment for current services and the opportunity to treat future clients from that reimburser (Acuff et al., 1999). Because third-party payors have made restraining the costs of outpatient psychotherapy a priority, U.S. psychologists report notable declines in incomes (Pingitore, Scheffler, Sentell, Haley, & Schwalm, 2001; Rothbaum, Bernstein, Haller, Phelps, & Kohout, 1998) and professional autonomy (Cooper & Gottlieb, 2000; Wright, 2000). In addition, clinicians frequently describe the quality of care under this system as substandard or mediocre (Benedict & Phelps, 1998; Phelps, Eisman, & Kohout, 1998; Russell et al., 2001) and their ability to comply with ethical standards as compromised (Murphy, DeBernardo, & Shoemaker, 1998). In countries with a nationalized health care system, psychotherapists also experience negative effects from fiscal restraints, but in addition, they are directly affected by high demand for limited services. In such systems offering one person long-term care can deprive several others of access to timely service for mental health problems. In other words, in the current global climate clinicians experience a conflict of interest in cases for which they judge brief interventions clinically inadvisable. If they succumb to these financial pressures, they are protecting their own welfare at the expense of the therapeutic benefit to the client, and if they rebel against these limitations, they are promoting the welfare of the client at substantial economic risk to themselves.

As a further complication, in systems in which reimbursers operate as for-profit businesses, they often require psychotherapists who seek to treat their members to sign contracts with language that is inconsistent with professional ethical standards. National health services and health maintenance organizations often have similarly problematic language in their employment contracts. For example, ethical standards identify a number of criteria for informed consent for treatment that are difficult for psychotherapists to carry out without violating their contractual agreements. For instance, the APA (2002) *Ethical Principles* specify that prospective clients should be informed about alternatives to the recommended treatment, but many managed care contracts discourage clinicians from discussing more costly alternatives to the reimbursable therapy. Clinicians are also often prohibited by contract from disclosing to clients the financial incentives they may have to keep care brief. Even if the language of the contract does not directly contradict existing codes and laws, clinicians are not free from the worry that adherence to the ethical ideals of the profession will cost them money.

This chapter elaborates on these and other ethical challenges and discusses recommendations to help clinicians to address them responsibly. These suggestions derive their authority from the ethical codes of the professions and the extensive scholarship on the ethics of practice in a managed-care world but carry no independent authority themselves. Specifically, the chapter addresses the following questions:

- How can I act responsibly in selecting clients for brief treatment?
- How can I maintain sufficient confidentiality of therapeutic interactions to keep client trust and yet still obtain the third-party reimbursements?
- How can I ethically handle informed consent for brief treatment?
- What are my ethical responsibilities related to the termination of treatment?
- What unique ethical issues arise when working with older adults, children, and adolescents?

SELECTING CLIENTS APPROPRIATE FOR BRIEF INTERVENTION

Differentiating those who are likely to benefit from brief psychotherapy is a difficult task for which no rigid rules exist. Some psychotherapists contend that virtually all prospective clients are suitable, but the preponderance of evidence and clinical experience suggest somewhat narrower selection criteria (Bloom, 1997). Three variables are consistently identified in the literature as influential in determining the prospects for benefit: the general attitude of the client toward psychotherapy, the severity and duration of symptoms, and the complexity of symptoms, especially the existence of multiple diagnoses (Asay & Lambert, 1999; Bloom, 1997).

First, clients need to be motivated for therapy. Those who are hostile, resistant, and whose expectations are to be passive recipients of care rather than active participants are probably poor candidates for brief interventions at least until their attitudes change (Asay & Lambert, 1999). Not surprisingly, individuals who have a history of unsatisfactory interpersonal connections are also unlikely to establish the requisite therapeutic alliance. Individuals with character disorders are frequently mentioned in this category, but such clients can be suitable for brief work if they have focused treatment goals to which they are committed (Bloom, 1997). Bauer and Kobos (1987) suggested that clients appropriate for brief psychoanalytic treatment should be psychologically minded, possess sufficient ego strength to tolerate the stress of therapy, and be able to make use of therapist interpretations.

Clients with multiple, complex, and longstanding problems are inappropriate for most brief interventions. For example, a client diagnosed with concurrent bipolar disorder, alcohol dependence, and an acute stress reaction to a recent trauma exemplifies the kind of client for whom treatment of short duration is contraindicated. Those with severe levels of acute problems commonly viewed as responsive to brief treatment may also be better served by lengthier interventions. According to research by Shapiro et al. (1996), those with severe levels of major depression were not helped by brief therapy and many of the severely depressed participants appeared worse off after eight sessions than they were at the start of the therapy. Seligman (1995) also found that consumers reported less satisfaction with treatment for depression when their therapy was restricted in length by managed care than when the length of therapy was unfettered by such rigid payment limits. In light of such findings, responsible clinicians, therefore, need to carefully evaluate not only whether brief treatment will benefit clients but also whether it avoids harm to them (Beauchamp & Childress, 1994). In short, the selection of clients for brief therapy must be based on competent diagnosis of client symptoms and capacity for therapeutic connection. Moreover, client progress must be carefully monitored so that treatment can be amended if progress is not occurring.

As Newman and Bricklin (1991) pointed out, most research supporting brief therapy models has not included significant numbers of culturally and ethnically diverse participants. Consequently, the scientific basis for the application of brief treatments to these populations is still largely unknown. Moreover, critics argue that by its very nature brief treatment allows very little room to modify treatment based on client culture or other unique client characteristics (Newman & Bricklin, 1991). Because cultural and social variables can also substantially affect motivation and expectations for therapy, the development of the therapeutic alliance, and response to treatment interventions (Sue, Zane, & Young, 1994), brief treatments may pose a risk of ineffectiveness or harm to culturally and ethnically diverse populations.

Some writers also wonder about the presence of gender bias in the use and efficacy of time-limited treatments. Edbril (1994) relayed anecdotal evidence that her female clients were more likely than male clients to express dissatisfaction with brief interventions. Similarly, Levenson and Davidovitz (2000) reported that male therapists were substantially more likely to use brief therapies than female professionals. However, little is really known about the role and function of gender in the selection or effectiveness of brief treatment. Until more credible research evidence becomes available regarding these variables, mental health professionals should exercise caution in using brief models with diverse populations and should adapt them to the unique cultural and social situation of the client. For example, when an Asian immigrant to a Western country presents for treatment because of social anxiety, the treatment protocol for this disorder recommended by the third-party payor (and by treatment manuals) may need to be substantially modified in favor of a more culturally sensitive approach. For example, if the standard protocol emphasizes behavior rehearsal and assertion training as central components of treatment for social anxiety, it is likely to be inconsistent with the cultural norms and values of an Asian immigrant. Without modification of the treatment, such clients may terminate prematurely, may fail to profit, or may engage in such behaviors at the risk of alienating others in their support system. As the need for effective treatment for diverse populations is so critical, and most people of any background prefer short-term treatment (Sue et al., 1994), the profession has an ethical obligation to obtain the necessary research evidence to identify appropriate and effective brief intervention models for these clients.

MAINTAINING CONFIDENTIALITY AMID PRESSURES TO DISCLOSE

Professional standards for confidentiality of client communications are not dependent on the length or type of psychotherapy provided. All professionals are obligated to guard client privacy to the fullest extent possible, allowing for disclosure of client information only with client consent, when mandated by law, or to protect the client's health and safety (APA, 2002).

Confidentiality is the cornerstone of the therapeutic alliance, which is in turn the cornerstone of effective treatment. Clients perceive confidentiality as crucial to honest communication and generally as all-inclusive (D. J. Miller & Thelen, 1986; VandeCreek, Miars, & Herzog, 1987). Clients tend to be unaware of the circumstances in which clinicians are obligated to breach confidentiality. If not forewarned about those circumstances, clients feel especially betrayed when therapists disclose information about them outside of sessions. When given reason to doubt the privacy of their therapeutic communications, clients are less likely to fully disclose relevant material (Kremer & Gesten, 1998; Nowell & Spruill, 1993). Consequently, the growing body of evidence that the confidentiality of client communications has been threatened by the current payment system is particularly troubling (Cooper & Gottlieb, 2000).

Typically, third-party payors will not assume the costs of treatment without information about the client's mental health status, psychiatric diagnosis, and their progress during therapy. Once that sensitive client information is released to third parties, both clinicians and clients lose control over it and the responsibility for maintenance of client privacy shifts to the payor. (Needless to say, mental health professionals are still obliged to keep client communications and records confidential from any other unauthorized access.) Governmental and private reimbursement organizations tend to have policies designed to safeguard confidentiality and many limit access to that data to employees with need for it (Frager, 2000). In spite of these protections, the privacy of client data in such systems is still at risk for several reasons. First, even at the most scrupulous third-party payor or governmental agency, multiple employees are likely to have access to client records. The more people with access, the greater is the potential for breach of privacy. Second, although the flagrant abuses of privacy by employees reported in the mid-1990s (e.g., Scarf, 1996) appear less frequently, clinicians' anecdotal reports suggest that payors' enforcement of privacy policies related to mental health data is still quite variable. Third, as efforts to contain costs have expanded from concern about duration and diagnosis into regulation of the type and structure of treatment itself (called *utilization review*), the volume and sensitivity of client data, which many reimbursers require, has also increased. Some managed care companies, for example, ask clinicians to send copies of all progress notes, assessment data, and client correspondence if they wish continued authorization for treatment. Cooper and Gottlieb (2000) cautioned strongly against compliance with this demand. They advised clinicians to develop a formal release-of-information policy that clarifies that they consider progress notes as a form of "raw test data" that are not subject to release (Cooper & Gottlieb, 2000, p. 195). Further, they recommended that this policy should substitute case summaries as evidence of appropriate diagnosis and treatment. Finally, they suggested that the policy be shared with the payment sources prior to entrance into a contractual arrangement with them.

The threats to confidentiality do not end there. During the last decade, reimbursers began to obtain and store client data electronically to reduce the volume of paper and speed communication. They have also initiated the development of a national computer database in the United States through which different reimbursers can share client data to reduce duplication of services and better detect client and clinician fraud (Appelbaum, 1996; Cooper & Gottlieb, 2000). Transmitting and storing sensitive client data in this medium is risky. The privacy of communications via computer is highly dependent on the adequacy of security measures in place in each computer in the network, the vigilance of each party in regularly updating those security measures, and the desirability of the material to hackers.

Thankfully, to date, few intrusions by hackers into mental health data have been reported. What are more common are inadvertent violations of the security of client data in electronic communications. Such an event happened in October 2001 when the psychological records of 62 children and adolescents were accidentally posted on the University of Montana Web site (Piller, 2001). The 400 pages of documents posted "described patient visits and offered diagnoses by therapists of mental retardation, depression, schizophrenia and other serious conditions" and provided the "patients' names, dates of birth, addresses and schools attended for most cases" (Piller, 2001, p. 1). In parallel fashion, Eli Lilly & Company, a drug manufacturer, inadvertently included the names of all Prozac® users in a bulk e-mail (Hayes, 2001) distributed to thousands. The U.S. Department of Health and Human Services accidentally posted on its Web site the names and addresses of people requesting brochures on substance abuse. These brochures had titles such as, "Moving forward with your life, leaving alcohol and other drugs behind" and "Learning to live drug free" (Sullivan, 2001).

Payers' uneven records of handling facsimile transmissions and regular mail communications containing client records weaken clinicians' confidence in the ability of third-party payors to safeguard electronic client data even more. Anecdotal reports of misdirected paper correspondence about clients, client case reports, and payment information abound in the professional literature (e.g., Davis & Meier, 2001).

These threats to confidentiality place two distinct responsibilities on the psychotherapist. The first is to understand the nature of the information that employers and third-party payors require to cover costs prior to signing any contracts and the second is to disclose to clients the limits of confidentiality related to third-party payment. Clinicians should read the language in their contracts carefully before signing them and seek modification of that language as necessary (Cooper & Gottlieb, 2000; Haas & Cummings, 1991; Koocher & Keith-Spiegel, 1998). They should obtain confidentiality policies of all organizations with access to client data and should seek to limit disclosure to the fullest extent possible. They should become familiar with the procedures institutions use to train and monitor employees who deal with confidential client information and the sanctions in place for violations. Finally, they need information on the inclusion of client data in any computer database and the privacy protections used for such data. When equipped with this knowledge, psychotherapists can make informed judgments about whether a professional connection with the institution or payor is ethically justifiable. They can then knowledgeably discuss these procedures with their clients.

CONDUCTING ADEQUATE INFORMED CONSENT

Frequently, clinicians view client consent as an unavoidable bureaucratic process that offers little therapeutic value to clients but that appeases employers, licensing boards, and risk managers (Welfel, 2002). Clients, on the other hand, want this information and react positively when it is provided (Braaten, Otto, & Handelsman, 1993). Moreover, research suggests that a well-conducted consent positively influences three variables associated with good outcomes from brief therapy—client motivation for therapy, attraction to the clinician, and positive opinion of the expertness of the therapist (Wagner, Davis, & Handelsman, 1998; Walter & Handelsman, 1996).

An adequate informed consent has two crucial components—disclosure of information the client needs to make a reasoned choice about participation in therapy and free consent to therapy without undue influence from others. Consent is grounded in the view that adult clients are fully autonomous human beings who deserve the freedom to make decisions about therapy that they exercise in other aspects of their lives. It involves frank conversations with clients about therapist credentials, recommended therapeutic activities, the benefits and risks of therapy, alternatives to it, costs and logistics of the process, and confidentiality of client records and disclosures. Usually, most of this material is discussed at the initiation of therapy, but informed consent is best regarded as a process that continues as needed throughout therapy, not as an isolated event (Appelbaum, Lidz, & Meisel, 1987). For example, if therapeutic direction changes in the midst of the process, professionals need to revisit the topic of risks and benefits of the new interventions. Similarly, if psychological testing is recommended while therapy is underway, clinicians are obligated to explain to clients the uses of the tests, the material that will be kept in their records, and their rights to feedback (APA, 2002; Pope, 1992).

The following strategies can increase the efficiency of consent procedures for brief therapy without compromising compliance with ethical standards. First, clinicians should develop written materials or taped explanations of therapy (or both) that can be given to clients prior to therapy. Research suggests that clinicians rely heavily on verbal discussion of consent issues (Handelsman, Kemper, Kesson-Craig, McLain, & Johnsrud, 1986), a cumbersome process that may compromise client recall of information (Handelsman, 2001) and limit clinicians' ability to document an adequate informed consent process in the event of a malpractice claim or ethics complaint (Bennett, Bryant, VanderBos, & Greenwood, 1990). Many models for consent documents exist in the literature; Handelsman and Galvin (1988) presented a particularly good one because it avoids a common problem in such consent forms—the use of language that is beyond the client's literacy skills. Very few professionals have availed themselves of taped materials (Somberg, Stone, & Claiborn, 1993), an oversight that seems inconsistent with the ease with which most people use recorded materials in other parts of their lives.

Second, clinicians should encourage frank discussion of the implications of using third-party payors to cover the costs of service. As mentioned in the prior discussion of confidentiality, clients have a right to understand what will happen to the therapeutic information they release to others and have a right to know how the use of such reimbursement mechanisms may affect the structure and duration of therapy. They have a right to basic information about the clinician's relationship with the payor and the financial incentives payors sometimes offer clinicians who follow standard protocols. Clinicians should aim for a balanced discussion of these issues, appreciating that clients often have little option but to use third-party payments or governmental systems and recognizing that some external funding systems aim for quality along with cost effectiveness.

Third, clinicians need to clarify to clients that both ethical and legal standards demand that their clinical recommendations regarding therapy be determined separate from payment considerations (Appelbaum, 1993). Indeed, virtually all managed care contracts include language that explicitly states that clinicians are responsible for making treatment decisions in the best interests of the client and that they not allow financial considerations to influence them to suggest treatments inconsistent with client welfare (Appelbaum, 1993; Welfel, 2001). Clients have the right to choose to accept or reject the protocols acceptable to payment sources and to know whether the therapist views those protocols as potentially helpful to the client.

Finally, clients should be informed about their options if they are not profiting from therapy or are dissatisfied with their therapeutic progress. They have the right to discuss their concerns with the therapist and to refuse to engage in treatments they believe unhelpful. Disclosure of this right is especially important in brief therapy in which client commitment to the process and honest communication about therapeutic impact is so essential to ultimate effectiveness.

TERMINATING THERAPY RESPONSIBLY

In contrast to traditional psychotherapy in which the point of termination is frequently uncertain at the initiation of service, in brief therapy a specific number of sessions are often planned for, either because that is the design of the model or because the client does not wish to continue beyond the point for which outside payment is available. The major ethical challenge of termination occurs when the planned treatment has not been successful, but additional sessions can occur only with unacceptable financial costs to the client or to the professional. Consider the following case.

> A client diagnosed with an episode of major depression (moderate severity) is allotted eight sessions of reimbursement for psychotherapy by his insurer. Both client and therapist agree to this schedule at the onset of service. At the end of the sessions, progress has been made but significant symptoms persist. The client no longer feels suicidal and has begun better self-care but has been unable to fully resume normal activities and still experiences frequent episodes of low mood, irritability, fatigue and insomnia. However, repeated appeals for additional reimbursable sessions to address the ongoing symptoms are denied and the client has little money to assume the costs of further sessions. Therapist and client are meeting today to discuss the situation.

The therapist has several options here: offer free or low-cost services, terminate therapy, or refer to another professional or agency within the client's budget. The ethical standards offer some direction here (e.g., APA, 2002, Section 4.09) by mandating professionals to discuss termination issues with clients and to arrange for referrals as needed. The ethical challenge embedded in this and similar cases is to make an objective judgment about whether continuing service is still needed and if so, who can competently provide it. If ending treatment at this point presents a reasonable risk of harm to the client or others, then the therapist is well advised to provide such service regardless of the financial cost or find the client competent service elsewhere. Clinicians may discontinue free or low-cost care at the point that clients no longer pose a risk to themselves or others even if the client refuses referrals to alternative low-cost service, provided that clinicians have discussed termination with the client and the client understands the options available.

This case reveals another important point related to the ethics of termination in brief therapy. Therapists risk noncompliance with ethical standards when they fail to appeal denials of additional reimbursement to third-party payors if they believe the judgments of the reimbursers to be inconsistent with adequate care for the client (Appelbaum, 1993). In some jurisdictions, a legal duty to appeal denials of reimbursement exists. Appelbaum (1993) suggested that therapists should always seek a reversal of the denial at the first level of appeal if they believe termination of care would not be in the client's best interests and recommended continued appeals at higher levels in circumstances that indicate substantial risk of harm to clients if care is ended. A client whose risk of suicide has not substantially abated or a client with an unresponsive eating disorder that is severely compromising health and functioning are two instances that seem to justify multiple appeals to a reimburser.

ADAPTING BRIEF THERAPY TO LEGAL MINORS AND VULNERABLE OLDER ADULTS

A professional's ethical duty to provide competent care in the best interests of the client does not waiver when the client is a legal minor or an older person incapacitated by a decline in mental functioning. However, the ethics of confidentiality and consent become more complex for both populations. For minors, the complications arise both from their limited legal rights to privacy and the rights of parents and guardians to make decisions on behalf of the minors for whom they are responsible. This circumstance does not impede therapy when parents make treatment decisions on the basis of the best interests of their children and when they recognize the developing maturity of adolescents approaching the age of majority. Unfortunately, parents do not always place their children's welfare as the highest priority and do not always acknowledge the increasing maturity of their adolescents. Nor do teenagers always accept the legal rights of their parents to make decisions for them. These realities are the source of thorny clinical and ethical challenges for psychotherapists. Current ethical standards offer professionals little specific guidance for working with minors except to require them to obtain consent appropriately from parents or guardians and to seek assent from clients unable to give consent (APA, 2002). The codes also remind professionals to differentiate the client from other interested family members and to disclose no treatment information to those without a legal right to it (APA, 2002).

Ethics scholars offer additional recommendations for responsible work with minors that are widely accepted (Gustafson & McNamara, 1987; Taylor & Adelman, 1989). First, Taylor and Adelman (1989) recommended that clinicians seek waivers from parents or guardians of their rights to all information from therapy because effective intervention is highly dependent on trust in the therapist, and trust cannot be established with teenagers without some assurance of confidentiality. Clinicians should view enlisting parental agreement to therapy for their child as their first agenda in treatment and should recognize that continuation of therapy is dependent on parental comfort with it. Therapists who reassure parents that they will be informed in the event that their child represents a danger to self or others and that their goals are similar to the parents' hopes for their children have a higher probability of successful treatment. The rules by which treatment will proceed should then be made clear to the minors. Second, when minor clients are close to the age of legal maturity, many jurisdictions allow for them to seek treatment independent of parental consent (Rozovsky, 2000; Taylor & Adelman, 1998). One of the justifications for this freedom is the fact that adolescents are sometimes capable of understanding the benefits and risks of treatment as well as adults (Gustafson & McNamara, 1987). Clinicians, therefore, need to be well informed about such statutes so that they can make appropriate decisions about care. Third, in the event that the best interests of a minor seem to conflict with the goals of the parents, clinicians' first duty is to protect the minor. When parental actions place a child at risk for harm, therapists must intervene to keep the child safe according to most statutes that define child abuse and neglect (Kalichman, 1999).

For older persons with declines in mental functioning the ethical challenges stem from their reduced capacity to make informed decisions about their treatment and from the extensive involvement of family members in their lives. Therapists cannot conduct consent or handle confidentiality matters without considering these realities. Therapists' first responsibility is to competently assess the client's capacity to consent to treatment and then to grant this population of older adults as full a measure of responsibility for making treatment decisions as possible. According to several research studies (e.g., Danzinger & Welfel, 2000; Gatz & Pearson, 1988; James & Haley, 1995), therapists are not immune from allowing age bias to impact diagnostic and treatment decisions. In fact, many professionals express disinterest in treating older adults (Busse, 1994) and mistakenly assume that they are unlikely to benefit from therapy when in fact they are more open to therapeutic change than many adults at midlife (Visser & Krosnick, 1998). Next, clinicians need to clarify their role with family members if individual therapy appears to be the treatment of choice. They may disclose confidential client data only with the consent of a competent client. When a client has cognitive deficits that make legal consent impossible, a legal representative (usually a family member) needs to provide substitute consent. Even in that circumstance, clinicians reveal client disclosures only to the extent necessary for effective treatment (APA, 2002). Older adults do not lose all their rights to privacy and dignity when their intellectual and physical functioning are compromised. An older adult's complaints about the behavior of his or her caregiver, for example, may be communicated to family only if such an action is likely to benefit the older adult and is directly related to the therapeutic goals. Finally, because many jurisdictions in the United States and other countries mandate reporting of elder abuse and neglect to the authorities (Quinn & Tomita, 1997; Welfel, Danzinger, & Santoro, 2000), therapists need to be alert to their legal responsibilities when treating older adults who may be vulnerable to such abuse.

SUMMARY

The central ethical challenge for therapists conducting brief therapy is to objectively assess their personal motives for choosing time-limited interventions so that they can overcome the influence of self-interested considerations in selecting this treatment and confirm that it is truly appropriate for the client's diagnosis. Once clinicians have resolved this issue, responsible care requires competence in the modality, careful attention to client progress, and the avoidance of the appearance of abandonment of clients when making decisions about termination. Consent procedures ought to be designed so the clients understand their rights and the benefits and risks of brief treatment. If confidentiality is limited by the involvement of third parties in payment for services, therapists are responsible for explaining these restrictions to clients and for advocating for as unobtrusive a role of third parties as possible.

When working with minors, their immaturity and limited rights to privacy affect every phase of individual treatment. As a result, clinicians must work proactively with parents to serve children's best interests and should grant adolescents as generous a portion of confidentiality and freedom of choice about treatment as possible. When the client is an older adult whose functioning is compromised by mental decline, clinicians should first clarify the degree to which the client can make independent decisions regarding treatment. When cognitive deficits require extensive family involvement and disclosure of client information, the client should be informed of that involvement. Moreover, clinicians should keep in mind that even when clients have cognitive impairments they do not lose all rights to privacy.

THE CASE OF JUNE

Questions are posed for discussion based on this chapter and the case study of June. Given what you have read in this chapter about responsible practice, what would the initial discussions with June on the topics of informed consent, confidentiality, and payment for services have been expected to include? June's need for psychotherapy is closely tied to her medical issues. Consequently, communication with her physician and other medical professionals is likely to be important to her continued health and progress in therapy. What ethical dimensions, if any, do you see to consultation with others on June's health care team? Sessions with this client were limited to nine. What client behaviors or comments that could have been made would signal to you that termination at this point might be adequate or inadequate? In this kind of short-term therapy that is focused on one major goal, many other important issues related to life satisfaction are often not explored or resolved. In this case, the client's readiness or willingness to find and keep meaningful work was not defined as a treatment goal. Should therapy have been extended to address such issues of life satisfaction even if it raised the immediate cost of treatment? Should the government (or insurance companies in other cases) take on the financial responsibility for such life satisfaction issues?

REFERENCES

Acuff, C., Bennett, B. E., Bricklin, P. M., Canter, M. B., Knapp, S. J., Moldawsky, S., & Phelps, R. (1999). Considerations for ethical practice in managed care. *Professional Psychology: Research and Practice, 30,* 563–575.

American Psychological Association. (2002). *Ethical principles of psychologists and code of conduct.* Washington, DC: Author. Retrieved November 1, 2002 from http://www.apa.org/ethics/

Appelbaum, P. S. (1993). Legal liability in managed care. *American Psychologist, 48,* 251–257.

Appelbaum, P. S. (1996). Managed care and the next generation of mental health law. *Psychiatric Services, 47,* 27–35.

Appelbaum, P. S., Lidz, C. W., & Meisel, A. (1987). *Informed consent: Legal theory and clinical practice.* New York: Oxford University Press.

Asay, T. P., & Lambert, M. J. (1999). The empirical case for the common factors in therapy: Quantitative findings. In M. A. Hubble, B. L. Duncan, & S. C. Miller (Eds.), *The heart and soul of change: What works in therapy* (pp. 33–56). Washington, DC: American Psychological Association.

Bauer, G. P., & Kobos, J. C. (1987). *Brief therapy: Short term psychodynamic intervention.* Northvale, NJ: Aronson.

Beauchamp, T. L., & Childress, J. F. (1994). *Principles of biomedical ethics* (4th ed.). New York: Oxford University Press.

Benedict, J. G., & Phelps, R. (1998). Introduction: Psychology's view of managed care. *Professional Psychology: Research and Practice, 29,* 29–30.

Bennett, B., Bryant, B., VanderBos, G., & Greenwood, A. (1990). *Professional liability and risk management.* Washington, DC: American Psychological Association.

Bloom, B. L. (1997). *Planned short-term psychotherapy: A clinical handbook* (2nd ed.). Boston: Allyn & Bacon.

Braaten, E. B., Otto, S., & Handelsman, M. M. (1993). What do people want to know about psychotherapy? *Psychotherapy, 30,* 565–570.

Busse, W. M. (1994). Age and gender bias among mental health professionals: The effect of therapist age, client age, and gender on clinical judgment. *Dissertation Abstracts International, 55*(4), 1662. (University Microfilms No. 9425004)

Cooper, C. C., & Gottlieb, M. C. (2000). Ethical issues with managed care: Challenges facing counseling psychology. *The Counseling Psychologist, 28,* 179–236.

Cummings, N. A., & Cummings, J. L. (2000). *The essence of psychotherapy: Reinventing the art in the new era of data.* San Diego: Academic.

Danzinger, P. R., & Welfel, E. R. (2000). Age, gender and health bias in counselors: An empirical analysis. *Journal of Mental Health Counseling, 22,* 135–149.

Davis, S. R., & Meier, S. T. (2001). *The elements of managed care: A guide for helping professionals.* Pacific Grove, CA: Brooks/Cole.

Dubin, S. (1972). Obsolescence or lifelong education: A choice for the professional. *American Psychologist, 27,* 486–496.

Edbril, S. D. (1994). Gender bias in short-term therapy: Towards a new model for working with women patients in managed care settings. *Psychotherapy: Theory, Research and Practice, 31,* 601–609.

Frager, S. (2000). *Managing managed care: Secrets of a former case manager.* New York: Wiley.

Gatz, M., & Pearson, C. G. (1988). Ageism revised and the provision of psychological services. *American Psychologist, 43,* 184–188.

Gustafson, K. E., & McNamara, J. R. (1987). Confidentiality with minor clients: Issues and guidelines for therapists. *Professional Psychology: Research and Practice, 18,* 503–508.

Haas, L. J., & Cummings, N. A. (1991). Managed outpatient mental health plans: Clinical, ethical, and practical guidelines for participation. *Professional Psychology: Research and Practice, 22,* 45–51.

Handelsman, M. M. (2001). Accurate and effective informed consent. In E. R. Welfel & R. E. Ingersoll (Eds.), *Mental health desk reference* (pp. 453–458). New York: Wiley.

Handelsman, M. M., & Galvin, M. D. (1988). Facilitating informed consent for outpatient psychotherapy: A suggested written format. *Professional Psychology: Research and Practice, 19,* 223–225.

Handelsman, M. M., Kemper, M. B., Kesson-Craig, P., McLain, J., & Johnsrud, C. (1986). Use, content and readability of written informed consent forms for treatment. *Professional Psychology: Research and Practice, 17,* 514–518.

Hayes, F. (2001, July 16). Damage control. *Computerworld.* Available online at: www.computerworld.com/securitytopics/security/privacy/story/0,10801,62222,00.html

James, J. W., & Haley, W. E. (1995). Age and health bias in practicing clinical psychologists. *Psychology and Aging, 10,* 610–616.

Jensen, R. E. (1979). Competent professional service in psychology: The real issue behind continuing education. *Professional Psychology: Research and Practice, 10,* 381–389.

Kalichman, S. C. (1999). *Mandated reporting of suspected child abuse: Ethics, law and policy* (2nd ed.). Washington, DC: American Psychological Association.

Koocher, G. P., & Keith-Spiegel, P. S. (1998). *Ethics in psychology* (2nd ed.). New York: Oxford University Press.

Kremer, T. G., & Gesten, E. L. (1998). Confidentiality limits on managed care and clients' willingness to self-disclose. *Professional Psychology: Research and Practice, 29,* 553–557.

Lambert, M. J., & Bergin, A. E. (1994). The effectiveness of psychotherapy. In A. E. Bergin & S. L. Garfield (Eds.), *Handbook of psychotherapy and behavior change* (4th ed., pp. 143–189). New York: Wiley.

Levenson, H., & Davidovitz, D. (2000). Brief therapy prevalence and training: A national survey of psychologists. *Psychotherapy: Theory, Research and Practice, 37,* 335–340.

Miller, D. J., & Thelen, M. H. (1986). Knowledge and beliefs about confidentiality in psychotherapy. *Professional Psychology: Research and Practice, 17,* 15–19.

Miller, I. J. (1996). Ethical and liability issues concerning invisible rationing. *Professional Psychology: Research and Practice, 27,* 583–587.

Murphy, M. J., DeBernardo, C. R., & Shoemaker, W. E. (1998). Impact of managed care on independent practice and professional ethics: A survey of independent practitioners. *Professional Psychology: Research and Practice, 29,* 43–51.

Newman, R., & Bricklin, P. M. (1991). Parameters of managed mental health care: Legal, ethical and professional guidelines. *Professional Psychology: Research and Practice, 22,* 26–35.

Nowell, D., & Spruill, J. (1993). If it's not absolutely confidential, will information be disclosed? *Professional Psychology: Research and Practice, 24,* 367–369.

Phelps, R., Eisman, E. J., & Kohout, J. (1998). Psychological practice and managed care: Results of the CAPP practitioner survey. *Professional Psychology: Research and Practice, 29,* 31–36.

Piller, C. (2001, November 7). Web mishap: Kids' psychological files posted. *Los Angeles Times,* p. 1.

Pingitore, D., Scheffler, R., Sentell, T., Haley, M., & Schwalm, D. (2001). Psychologist supply, managed care, and the effects of income: Fault lines beneath California psychologists. *Professional Psychology: Research and Practice, 32,* 597–606.

Pope, K. S. (1992). Responsibilities in providing psychological test feedback to clients. *Psychological Assessment, 4,* 268–271.

Quinn, M. J., & Tomita, S. K. (1997). *Elder abuse and neglect: Causes, diagnosis, and intervention strategies* (2nd ed.). New York: Springer.

Rothbaum, P. A., Bernstein, D. M., Haller, O., Phelps, R., & Kohout, J. (1998). New Jersey psychologists' report on managed mental health care. *Professional Psychology: Research and Practice, 29,* 37–42.

Rozovsky, F. A. (2000). *Consent to treatment: A practical guide* (3rd ed.). Boston: Little, Brown.

Russell, D. W., de la Mora, A., Trudeau, L. S., Scott, N. A., Norman, N. A., & Schmitz, M. F. (2001). Psychologists' reactions to Medicaid managed care: Opinion and practice change after one year. *Professional Psychology: Research and Practice, 31,* 547–553.

Scarf, M. (1996, June 16). Keeping secrets. *New York Times,* pp. 38–42, 50, 54.

Seligman, M. E. P. (1995). The effectiveness of psychotherapy: The *Consumer Reports* study. *The American Psychologist, 50,* 965–974.

Shapiro, D. A., Barkham, M., Hardy, G. E., Reynolds, S., Rees, A., & Startup, M. (1996). Effects of treatment duration and severity of depression on the maintenance of gains after cognitive-behavioral and psychodynamic-interpersonal psychotherapy. *Journal of Consulting and Clinical Psychology, 1995,* 378–387.

Sómberg, D. R., Stone, G. L., & Claiborn, C. D. (1993). Informed consent: Therapists' beliefs and practices. *Professional Psychology: Research and Practice, 24,* 153–159.

Sue, S., Zane, N., & Young, K. (1994). Research on psychotherapy with culturally diverse populations. In A. E. Bergin & S. L. Garfield (Eds.), *Handbook of psychotherapy and behavior change* (4th ed., pp. 783–820). New York: Wiley.

Sullivan, B. (2001, May 25). *Health site exposed consumer information.* Retrieved March 4, 2002 from MSNBC.com: http//www.msnbc.com/news/578476.asp

Taylor, L., & Adelman, H. S. (1989). Reframing the confidentiality dilemma to work in children's best interests. *Professional Psychology: Research and Practice, 20,* 79–83.

Taylor, L., & Adelman, H. (1998). Confidentiality: Competing principles, inevitable dilemmas. *Journal of Educational and Psychological Consultation, 9,* 267–275.

VandeCreek, L., Miars, R., & Herzog, C. (1987). Client anticipations and preferences for confidentiality of records. *Journal of Counseling Psychology, 34,* 62–67.

Visser, P. S., & Krosnick, J. (1998). Development of attitude strength over the life cycle: Surge and decline. *Journal of Personality and Social Psychology, 75,* 1389–1410.

Wagner, L., Davis, S., & Handelsman, M. M. (1998). In search of the abominable consent form: The impact of readability and personalization. *Journal of Clinical Psychology, 54,* 115–120.

Walter, M. I., & Handelsman, M. M. (1996). Informed consent for mental health counseling: Effects of information specificity on clients' ratings of counselors. *Journal of Mental Health Counseling, 18,* 253–262.

Welfel, E. R. (2001). Responsible interactions with managed care organizations. In E. R. Welfel & R. E. Ingersoll (Eds.), *Mental health desk reference* (pp. 496–502). New York: Wiley.

Welfel, E. R. (2002). *Ethics in counseling and psychotherapy: Standards, research and emerging issues.* Pacific Grove, CA: Brooks/Cole.

Welfel, E. R., Danzinger, P. R., & Santoro, S. (2000). Mandated reporting of maltreatment of older adults: A primer for counselors. *Journal of Counseling and Development, 78,* 284–292.

Wright, W. R. (2000). Managed care and the delivery of psychological services: An unmitigated disaster for quality mental health services. In R. D. Weitz (Ed.), *Managed care in mental health in the new millennium* (pp. 5–18). New York: Haworth.

CHAPTER

18

Curative Factors in Work With Older Adults

Michael Duffy
Texas A&M University

This will likely be the least documented chapter of this book. There is a dearth of research into therapeutic effectiveness with older adults or even documented discussions of clinical experience. Although there have been recent considerable gains in developing methods in psychological assessment with older adults, the field of geriatric psychotherapy has lagged far behind. This is particularly true of psychodynamic approaches to working with older adults, and by the same token, discussions of brief psychodynamic methods with older adults are almost nonexistent. Despite Freud's (1905/1953) classic opinion that older persons have very limited capacity for psychoanalytic exploration, most clinical gero-psychologists strongly challenge such a pessimistic view (Duffy, 1999b; Semel, 1996).

A more hopeful picture of the possibility of providing psychotherapy to older adults emerges when one considers that psychotherapy with older adults is much more the same than different from other age groups. Although there are important cohort, situational, and developmental differences, the fundamental dilemmas and strategies of human beings seem to be consistent across the wide span. Unfortunately, many therapists, especially prior to the incentives provided by Medicare reimbursement of psychological services, felt ill equipped to attempt psychotherapy with older adults. In particular, self-imposed limitations have led many experienced practitioners as well as trainees to shy away from doing psychodynamic psychotherapy with older adults.

The fact that there is relatively little psychotherapy, or indeed any psychological services, delivered to older adults is not entirely due to neglect by the professional community. Many contemporary older adults seem to be reluctant to seek out the services of counselors and psychotherapists. It seems likely that this reluctance is not so much based on the developmental nature of late life but is rather a feature of the current cohort of older adults for whom the notion of mental health and especially of psychotherapy is, at best, unknown and at worst a foreign and uncomfortable notion. Most referrals for psychotherapy come from religious pastors, physicians, and especially family members who are concerned about their own mental health and well-being in dealing with the stresses of living with and caring for impaired older family members. Consequently, one may expect that in the future the call for psychotherapy services for older adults will increase. Thus, cohorts like mine that have grown up with a concept of mental as well as physical health will seek service directly in that domain.

The body of the chapter addresses a series of psychodynamic themes that seem particularly pertinent in working with older adults in psychotherapy. However, many of these psychodynamic themes have easy application to psychodynamic therapy in other phases of life. I believe that fundamental psychological processes transcend age as well as gender, culture, ethnicity, and socioeconomic status. When the therapist has connected with the salient psychological themes in the client then there is a contact with universal human experiences that transcend, or lie beneath, these differences.

BRIEF PSYCHOTHERAPY WITH OLDER ADULTS

A factor in the length of psychotherapy must be the personality makeup of the client. I believe in some cases that my longer term clients are characterized not so much because of the seriousness of their concerns, but with their tolerance, appreciation, and need for the intensity of the psychotherapeutic relationship. It has been suggested that the reason why clients may choose long-term therapy is because of the satisfaction that they have felt in the initial short-term encounters. On the other hand, there are many clients who need therapeutic interaction but for whom such interaction poses an intolerable burden directly related to the nature of their disorder. This may be especially true for clients who manifest the schizoid quality in relationships. Such clients may reach for help in times of crisis or desperation but will be ambivalent and resistant in sustaining a commitment to a therapeutic relationship. Again, even if the therapeutic relationship is successful, these clients are likely to prefer periodic therapeutic interludes, adjusted to their felt need and tolerance rather than a sustained course of therapy.

It is possible to identify a situation that may apply specifically to older clients. There can be a sense of urgency that leads older clients to be uncomfortable with a long-term process (Gorsuch, 1998). Such older clients are frequently "timekeeping" in the sense that their level of comfort in the process of psychotherapy, which is already alien to them, is strained by a process that lasts more than 12 to 15 weeks. However, this is not intended to give the impression that only brief psychodynamic therapy, with brief sessions, is workable in later life. This is not the case. Stereotypic views of aging, rather than experience, lead to the impression that older adults are not inherently capable of extended therapeutic relationships. Many older adults have the same tolerance for long-term therapy as younger adults.

Finally, as older persons may be more likely to have limited incomes and opportunities, it is important to consider how cultural and socioeconomic factors may also impinge on the length of therapy. In my supervision of therapists in a clinic for low-income mental health patients, many of whom have significant dysfunctions related to impoverished life situations, there is discordance with the conventional culture of psychotherapy including the idea of regular appointments and multiple sessions. We as therapists encounter clients who live from day to day both economically and psychologically. They experience stress to such an extent that they contact a mental health professional but bring no expectation of ongoing process beyond the alleviation of the immediate need. In other words, if they felt helped and sufficiently changed by one or two therapy sessions, they had little sense of the need of continuity.

Therapists have grown up in a historical cohort, which is appreciative of psychological life and discussion. Older adults and those who have experienced very few of life's resources do not share such comfort or expectations. However, this does not imply that people who are old or poor or both have limited experience of the interior life. However long sessions last, if a therapist engages a client at a fundamental level of psychological experience in the world of intimacy, caring, love, trust, and so forth, then a psychotherapeutic bond can be effective and maintained. This is a universal language.

In work with older patients, therapists may need to reevaluate cultural and cohort expectations that psychotherapeutic change necessarily occurs in weekly, 50-min sessions that occur in the relative calm of a quiet office with soft lighting and comfortable chairs! It can be helpful in training to have therapists work in nontraditional settings such as community clinics and nursing homes so that they can appreciate what is most fundamental about therapeutic change as opposed to its more usual trappings. In providing psychotherapy training and supervision to doctoral students in the hurly-burly of nursing homes, I have found that the very difficulty in establishing the usual time frame, context, and client expectations helps enormously to break through to an understanding of the fundamental principles of psychotherapy as a naturalistic process that can occur in any environment in any period of time.

PSYCHODYNAMIC PROCESS

In this section, I articulate the psychodynamic approach and concepts that will inform the various psychodynamic themes that follow. In my view, the psychodynamic approach represents a process rather than a specific theoretical content (Duffy, 1999a). Within this approach, the psychodynamic interview takes on an inductive rather than a deductive posture. An inductive approach is not atheoretical, but rather theory is formulated on the basis of experience and observation. I believe that experienced psychotherapists who have practiced continuously for many years, despite their theoretical self-identity, will tend, often implicitly, to assume an inductive posture in psychotherapy. To do otherwise is to exclude many important data that do not fit within the parameters of a given, limited theory. This is especially important when working with older adults, as theories generally have been based on consideration of clinical experiences with younger or middle-aged adults.

Clinical experience also seems consonant with the current "common factors" approach, which is quickly overtaking theory-based approaches in explaining consistent equivalence data in recent psychotherapy research (Wampold, 2001). The results of the exploration into these common factors in psychotherapy have yielded many strands of therapeutic influence, which are clearly interpersonal and psychodynamic in nature. It can also be said with confidence that these factors focus on the process (the how) rather than the content (the what) of therapeutic interaction. This means that therapists who may designate themselves as behavioral, cognitive, or psychodynamic are having implicit effect on the psychotherapeutic process that is often beyond the explanatory capacity of their own theories.

However, research exploring the existence and effectiveness of common factors in psychotherapy, rather than the effectiveness of discrete theoretical approaches, does so from a nomothetic point of view. In other words, when the participants and data are aggregated (e.g., in medical and analytical research), it is correct to draw the conclusion that across the treatment groups there are no appreciable differences among theoretical approaches. However, if one approaches the data ideographically, and looks within an individual client or research participant, then one might likely see a different picture. In other words, at the ideographic level it is quite possible that a particular psychotherapeutic approach (e.g., cognitive, behavioral, psychodynamic) might be more effective in producing change in a particular client. This is reminiscent of a classic research in the 1960s suggesting an approach to client assignment, which asked the question "Which theoretical approach will work best with this client and with this problem?" (Truax & Carkhuff, 1967). Also, I might add, with this therapist. It is increasingly evident that the disposition of a therapist to choose a particular theoretical approach, and even choice of a patient group to work with, may very well be a function of his or her own temperament and personality style.

As mentioned earlier, an inductive stance allows the therapist to be open to a variety of explanations of behavior from the simple to the complex and to adopt a more parsimonious choice of therapeutic approach. This is particularly relevant in working with older clients who have a severe degree of cognitive impairment. As the higher cognitive processes of the brain become impaired, the pattern of behavior change moves from the complex to the simple. Complex psychodynamic explanations and interventions give way to the need for classical or operant conditioning techniques to provide assistance, for example, with retraining basic vegetative functions such as toileting and eating (Hussian, 1981).

PSYCHODYNAMIC THEMES

Transference and the Older Patient

Transference will occur in psychotherapy regardless of the age of the client or therapist. Two brief case illustrations will underline this process. Some years ago I was providing psychotherapy for an older woman in her home at the request of her adult daughter. Although within the litigious and somewhat formalized world of psychology home-based psychotherapy is rare (unlike the more flexible practice patterns of social work), it is often the case that therapists will not be able to provide psychotherapy services to older adults unless they are willing to provide them in nursing home or home-based formats. However, although the anxious concern of psychology may be overstated, it is important to remember that home-based services have some hazards. In this particular case I was providing short-term dynamic psychotherapy to a client who was perhaps 87 years old and I recall at a poignant moment in the therapeutic process the client asked if I would kiss her—and a passionate kiss was clearly implied! After hopefully sensitive management of the moment I was able to conclude the therapy session without the client feeling rejected and with my virtue intact! This was a sharp reminder to me both of the inevitable transferential elements in psychotherapy at any age as well as the importance of context in psychotherapy.

It may well be argued, of course, that this is an example of a dysfunctional real relationship rather than an example of transference. However, I believe that the following case will suggest the likelihood that such events in psychotherapy with older clients are of a transferential nature. In the second case, I was again providing home-based psychotherapy to a lady in her mid-80s who had lost her husband quite traumatically when he died in her arms as they waited for emergency medical services following a heart attack. She was referred to me because of a clinical depression associated with the complicated bereavement this experience had engendered and also because the family, on the death of her husband and their father, immediately sold her house, dispersed her belongings and furniture among the family, and moved her 300 miles away from home to be close to them. She had promptly gone into a significant depression that had led the family to seek help. Because I was already providing service to a wheelchair-bound patient in the same facility, I expressed my willingness to provide in-home service to this new client. This suggestion was also prompted by the fact that my new client was quite ambivalent about receiving psychotherapy and the prospect of leaving her home to go across town with marginal driving skills to a outpatient office would in all likelihood have convinced her to refuse therapy. During the course of the psychotherapy, it became clear to me, as I attended to interpersonal process signals, that my client had a distinctly childlike and hysteroid personality style, which was probably exacerbated by the loss of her husband. As expected, these dynamics played out in a transferential way in the therapeutic relationship and became an important vehicle for conducting therapy.

Transference enactment thus was associated with an increased intensity in the psychotherapy relationship and at the same time provided an opportunity for stabilizing and correcting this emotional relational experience. From an emotional and psychological point of view I, though much younger chronologically, was the "older" of the two as her behavior at times ranged from flirtatious to petulant in the manner of a young adolescent girl. Gradually over time the adult part of her personality, always implicitly present, began to take a prominent role in the management of her own affairs. She surprised her family members and me by expressing her determination to return to her hometown where she had lived with her husband and friends. She developed plans to register for a residential cottage community in that town and personally attended to details like wall color, painting, carpet, and so forth in her projected home. Strategically it was important not to dissuade her from these plans because any opposition would have likely reinforced them, although the family and I had doubts whether she would follow through. In fact she did follow through and made a successful and happy transition back to the home of her husband and marriage. The transference reflected her previous limited experience of intimacy and subsequent working through was a means of enabling her to establish a more mature relationship with me over time and allow her to make adult decisions and plans.

These factors indicate something of the challenge of tolerating and working with the countertransference with a client who is many years older than the therapist. It becomes a significant challenge both for trainee and experienced therapists to work with older adults in a manner that accepts these psychological positions even though they may engender some discomfort in the therapist. One of the most debilitating factors in therapists working with older clients is the tendency to handle the relationship in a way that either infantalizes or parentifies the older adult. In other words, the chronological distance between the two persons is sometimes handled by "talking down" to the older adult, coping with the disparity by diminishing their power and role so as to make the relationship manageable. Or, conversely, the discomfort with the older client might be handled by assuming the role of child-to-parent and positioning oneself in an overly submissive and compliant posture, which is not needed or desired by the older client.

This type of reaction to transferential feelings is very much a reciprocal process. The classic tradition in understanding transference is to assume that the transference predominately happens in the client and the therapist's countertransference is secondary to that. In inexperienced therapists working with older adults, it would be more accurate to suggest that the transference often occurs primarily in the therapist, and that the older client, in coping with the inappropriate posture, can be described as countertransferential. It is critical that the psychodynamic therapist read the transferential situation calmly and nonreactively and maintain a clear adult or parental posture toward the client even though they may be 50 years senior. When an older client accepts psychotherapy and brings psychological needs to the table, it is a disservice to the client to be immobilized by therapist transferential reactions, which either diminish or disempower the client.

If transference is a naturalistic phenomenon that occurs universally at the point in which a relationship becomes psychologically significant, then it will take place independent of the intended style or purpose of the therapist. In the traditional psychoanalytical view of transference, it is encouraged and assisted by a nondirective and somewhat obscured presence of the therapist. Indeed, it may be helpful in the initial phases of therapy for the therapist to be present in a somewhat "veiled" manner to not disturb the development of and emergence of transferential material (Kell & Mueller, 1966). Transference will occur vigorously, however, even despite a very directive style in the therapist. In other words, transference occurs through one's *need* as a person or client to construe the world as one needs it (or fears it) to be and people are very little dissuaded by the tolerance or reaction of those around them. Therapists and their clients are quite capable of construing the world and relationships in the way they see fit or can tolerate—despite evidence to the contrary! This means that the psychodynamic therapist with older clients, even in brief psychotherapy, will encounter transferential experiences whether he or she assumes a classic veiled posture or an active intervention posture. Understanding how the client is construing us as therapists—seeing ourselves through the client's eyes—will allow us to assume a corrective therapeutic posture that will enhance and correct the previous lived experience of the client.

Exploring Early Experiences

It is interesting that books written by gerontologists and even by psychologists providing psychotherapy for older adults tend to concentrate on psychotherapeutic issues that occur in late life itself. Therefore, for example, the topics often cover such issues as death and grieving and reaction to illness and so forth. Although these issues do have meaning in the lives of older adults, they most frequently constitute situational factors that can be stressful but are rarely core psychotherapeutic issues and themes for older adults. Generally, in the latter part of life we come to be quite well adjusted to the notions of death and dying and the decreases in function that foreshadow it. Somewhat humorously, it seems that death anxiety and fear of death are much more likely to be the concerns of middle-aged psychotherapists and authors than of their older clients. Generally, older people are quite competent in the domain of dying—it is younger adults, especially middle-aged adults who, recognizing the finality of life, begin to develop a greater or lesser degree of acute awareness of their own finality and death (Duffy, 1999b). Gradually, as mid-life extends into late life, these fears become reality tested and are taken in stride. In actual fact, for the older adult who accepts or seeks psychotherapy, it is much more common that the central therapeutic issues relate to unfinished issues in earlier life. Older clients turn not infrequently to early developmental experiences that may have been inadequately coped with and have been veiled in the hustle and bustle of adult life, parenting, and a professional work life. In other words, clients who are older adults are quite good at issues of late life and are more likely to be concerned with still prevailing developmental issues of youth and childhood even though they may be implicit and not be expressed in that manner.

Again, two brief psychotherapy cases help illustrate the concept of unfinished early life issues. In the first case, I was asked to see Veronica in the nursing home because of a series of acting out behaviors that had caused uproar among nursing home staff. Namely, she reportedly (being incontinent) had been hoarding soiled diapers (of both varieties) and storing them under the covers in her bed and on occasion wearing them as a hat walking down a corridor. Having strategically avoided the trap of opening my session with a discussion about her acting-out behavior, I worked on engaging Veronica in a hopefully pleasant and engaging therapeutic relationship to which she (surprised by my nonconfrontation on the presenting problem) had accepted with some surprise and good humor. Although she had objected to the therapy and was only convinced to agree by the staff's threat that she would otherwise be evicted from the nursing home, she was surprised to find herself enjoying our session. Her acting out behavior and the uproar that it had engendered in her family and nursing home staff (although not so much among residents) pointed to the presence of a pronounced personality disorder. As I opened the story of her life, and specifically her early life, she revealed an impoverished early life in which she had lost a father to an early death and experienced a relationship with her mother that was apparently nonnurturing and detached. Most painful to her was the sense that her mother had a warm and intimate relationship with her younger sister, all of which led to a childhood sense of aloneness and anger. During her subsequent married life to a man who clearly parented her through difficult times, she was relatively unassertive with adults and fairly punitive with her own children, three adult daughters (who I also saw from time to time in family sessions or through telephone consultations). In her early life she had been relatively submissive, although manipulative with her husband, and replayed with her own daughters the same detached relationship she had experienced with her own mother. It then seemed that in her late life, under the authoritative institutionalized conditions of a nursing home, her latent aggression at her mother and her life began to emerge, stimulated by the constraints and criticisms leveled by nursing home staff. It became critical to understand the early and psychologically still present dimensions of her life experience in explaining her current behavior. The psychotherapeutic relationship allowed her, even though not initially confronted about her behavior, to cease her acting out behavior and settle into a more constructive, although hypervigilant, relationship with nursing home staff.

A second case, which illustrates the importance of early, unfinished, and still psychologically present experiences, occurred in the case of my own mother. During her late 80s in her nursing home environment she gradually developed a typical dementia, which involved cognitive confusion, and considerable agitation, which was inconsolable without the assistance of major tranquilizers. In moments of lucidity in our conversations, my mother clearly expressed concern over whether her own mother loved her as a child. This anxiety had special poignancy for me because I knew that in her early teenage years growing up as the oldest girl in a large and poor Irish Catholic family, she was adopted out to a childless couple as a means of providing her with education and well-being. This custom, in which large families would be helped by childless families, was not unusual in that period and culture. However, not surprisingly, I found that my mother had at some level always wondered whether she was given away out of love or disinterest. This remaining anxiety-laden question of whether she was loved by her mother seemed to endure even during a period of cognitive confusion. This experience served for me as a powerful reminder of both the enduring presence of early life experiences and also of the continuity of emotional and psychological life even when logical and language life processes are disrupted through dementia.

These situations also help clarify a classic debate within psychodynamic theories and therapy systems. The seeming endless preoccupation with whether or not past history is necessary in the process of psychotherapy, in the light of these cases, becomes the wrong question and therefore a red herring. Any experience, whatever the chronology, which is psychologically significant now, is important within the psychotherapy process. Chronological time ceases to be important when one considers salient psychological material. In both of these cases it was because these early, unfinished experiences still held powerful emotional impact that they became important in understanding and (indirectly) dealing with in the psychotherapeutic process. Then and now becomes irrelevant in the world of the psychological present.

In coming to a thorough understanding of client dynamics, it is helpful to have a sense of psychological trajectory. In attempting to understand the meaning and the forces that shape current psychological and external behavior, and therefore developing accurate therapeutic strategies, the recounting and reexperiencing of early and late life experiences becomes critical. Encouraging older clients to tell their story, which, as is seen in the discussion of reminiscence, has implicit psychological benefits in and of itself, allows the therapist to gain an accurate sense of psychological processes, which assists in developing therapeutic strategy.

The recounting of early life history is not necessarily an extensive process and may take very little time in the psychotherapy process. It will likely be woven in and narrated as needed as the therapy progresses. Also, attention to early life experiences does not in all cases need to receive explicit discussion. In some cases the topic will be studiously avoided by the older client and will become noticeable and meaningful in its very absence. For example, in the atypical situation in which an older adult has a heightened anxiety about death, then this will be clinically meaningful. In such cases it may well be that a veiled anxiety masks an early history, which a client is unwilling to express. In this case the therapist, based hopefully on many parallel experiences, can make some accurate guesses about the early life experience of this patient. As the case described earlier of the older client who sought a "romantic" response, I was not surprised to find later from a family member that this client had been sexually abused as a young child. Even though this was not a topic of our discussion and had been masked during adult life, it was evidently a sign of symptomatic promiscuity that had resurfaced in late life, probably due to a lack of social constraint.

The Role of Interpretation and Insight

Interpretation and insight hold an honored and much deserved position in mainstream psychodynamic psychotherapy. The capacity of a client to gain insight through interpretation becomes an inclusion factor for appropriateness for psychotherapy.

In another scenario in which a client would be most willing to be given a diagnostic label and interpretation, the therapist should use caution. The very possession of a diagnostic label or interpretation can work against any further exploration of the problem and provide disincentive to take therapeutic action. If I can announce that I now understand my problems and recognize the importance of childhood trauma in the development of adult problems, I can handily forestall any need to make therapeutic change or take responsibility for my own behavior. In this way the therapist who prematurely interprets or diagnoses a problem can have the effect of "capping" or sealing off the emotional process that should be open to exploration (Mueller & Kell, 1972). Using interpretation to cap emotional experiences can also have a self-protective effect for any therapist who is ambivalent about exploring intense emotional feelings with the client. To give a diagnostic label, for example, depression, can prematurely close down the many different and powerful feelings that may be masked by the presence of depression.

The other question identified previously is, Is insight itself necessary for change? My answer to this question is no. I can think of many situations in which clients have been able to reshape their approach to life without any clear understanding of the dynamics of change. This is where the concept of reinforced behavior is pertinent. Certainly in the case of serious personality dynamics, such as borderline dynamics, clients will have a relative inability to understand the basis for their behavior. In these situations we can often make headway by behavior rehearsal of the desirable behavior so that our client can act "as if" and learn some new behaviors that can gradually become internalized.

Reexperiencing the problems in what has been called a "corrective emotional experience" can be another important dimension to therapeutic change. In the case of a cognitively incapacitated older client or a child client, for example, it is not reasonable to expect a clear insight into the dynamic basis of behavior problems. However, in the course of a significant therapeutic relationship, the older person or a child can come to trust, to feel safe, to learn to relate in ways other than manipulation, and so forth. In these cases change takes place because of a successful reexperiencing of fundamental psychological events.

How do we decide when interpretation, insight, and understanding are useful and effective in psychotherapy? I believe that insight is particularly important with clients with certain personality styles. Some people, including myself, have a strong need for "cognitive mastery." There is a felt need to make sense of one's life. This sense can lead to significant change. However, other personalities find little help or solace in understanding the problem areas. They seem to have a more pragmatic satisfaction with the effects of change strategies and seem untroubled by a desire for understanding psychological dynamics. In fact, cognitive mastery that some clients seek and find useful can be understood again as "constructive meaning making." Interpretation serves not only literal truth but also has a role in internal construction of meaning. Especially when given with authority by the therapist, an interpretation may be effective in making sense of a person's life and problems.

A final comment about interpretive process is relevant here. In the classical psychoanalytical tradition it seems that the interpretation is a product of the skill, insight, and ingenuity of the therapist. The therapist continues in an investigative mode asking questions, calculating critical angles, and developing an interpretive scenario, which eventually is presented to the client. Many of us as therapists and as clients have had the experience, however, of finding that this delivered interpretation is ill fitting rather like a suit of clothes that is almost but not quite an exact fit. The interpretation lacks idiosyncratic form and personal definition. In my experience, a much more effective way of reaching an interpretation is to proceed in a collaborative manner. Insights are shared in a tentative and provisional manner with the client as they take shape but before any final interpretive conclusion is reached. This incremental process allows the client to join in the process in a collaborative manner—changing a word here and there that better captures the inner experience and makes the "suit fit like a glove." It is the product of this kind of interpretive process that both therapist and client have a sense of mutually achieved understanding. In this scenario it is also more likely that the interpretation is viscerally understood and is not just an intellectual formula, which has little effect on behavior.

Working With Personality Problems

In recent years the advent of managed care constraints and the subsequent response of our profession to place emphasis on empirically supported treatments have led to an overemphasis on *Diagnostic and Statistical Manual of*

Mental Disorders–IV (DSM; 1994) Axis I symptomatic problems. Symptomatic problems such as anxiety and depression are relatively easily resolved through specific therapies or medication and thus have been the easiest sphere in which to demonstrate therapeutic effectiveness. *DSM* Axis II, personality problems, has been therefore eclipsed in recent years. Also, many public mental health programs, such as that in Texas, give little priority to personality disorders even though these constitute a large proportion of needed services. In the world of the nursing home and services to older adults, personality problems tend to consume a majority of the time and concern of staff members. It becomes important then to recognize the need for psychotherapy of the personality disorders, especially among older adults.

An important aspect of personality may be described as the "basic operating style"—usually interpersonal operating style—that a person has developed in coping with their life's situational, developmental, and interpersonal challenges. This may yield a dysfunctional adaptation as the person develops coping techniques such as developing a pattern of manipulation, distrust, or hypervigilance; or, in dealing with the world's lack of respect and compassion, the older adult may have developed a safer "good boy" posture in an often futile attempt to gain affirmation and self-esteem.

Gerontological research over many years has shown convincingly that there is a basic consistency of personality across the life span (Rowsowsky, Abrams, & Zweig, 1999). The characteristics that were observed in older clients demonstrate continuity with earlier parts of life. It may, however, be the case that these personality characteristics appear in a more extreme form in later life than existed in younger years in which social propriety demanded veiling more extreme features.

In working with older clients it becomes helpful to seek collateral impressions of adult children with regard to basic temperament and personality styles of our older clients. In many cases adult children will point to an essential continuity, although not initially obvious, in their experience of their parents across the life span. There is, however, some evidence of a mellowing of extreme personality characteristics in the course of aging. Forensic psychologists and those who work in the penal system, for example, point to the fact that there are relatively few "old" sociopaths in prison. This may be the result of a strengthening of the ego or self-concept that happens naturalistically over the course of development. However, some therapists see this as a diminishing of the acting out aspect of the disorder while leaving the internal personality problem relatively intact. In other words, there may be decrease of antisocial behavior, but the internal sociopath's lack of altruistic regard remains. Both views are relevant, but my perspective on self psychology leads me to seriously consider the more optimistic viewpoint that as the self strengthens over the life span then personality dysfunction becomes redundant and lessens.

However, any therapist who works in the nursing home context will be aware of the resilience of narcissism in later life in the nursing home. I was also reminded of the resilience of narcissism in the life of Mark Twain. In attending his daughter's wedding ceremony, Mark Twain could not resist the temptation to wear his bright red Cambridge University academic robes, recently awarded to him in an honorary doctorate. Even at this late, and ostensibly mature, point of his life, Mark Twain apparently could not resist upstaging his son-in-law groom and making himself the center of attention! Working in an institutional context like a nursing home will repeat this kind of experience; it is difficult to stage a group activity without happening on several nursing home residents who seem bent on being the center of attention and dominating all group processes.

Developmental Readiness

It is interesting that although a developmental perspective is highly consonant with a psychoanalytic viewpoint, the classic works of psychoanalysis are relatively impoverished in a sensitive understanding of developmental process (Messer & Warren, 1995). The developmental milestones that exist in the work of Freud, for example, are relatively static and reified (e.g., the Oedipal conflict) rather than dynamic. They can restrict a therapist who pays attention to developmental processes in a more idiosyncratic and inductive manner. In the work of Klein and Mahler (1967) one can begin to get a sense of developmental sensitivity that can truly guide the therapist.

Understanding the client's position in the developmental trajectory is helpful to the therapist in anticipating future behavior and experiences for the client. Armed with this developmental sense, the therapist can anticipate not only the next developmental hurdles but also the likely reaction of the client to these challenges. As a specific example, a developmental sense of trajectory is extremely important in the use of suggestion as a psychological intervention. It is important to avoid making suggestions that are outside the scope of a client's developmental capacity at a given moment. Thus, to suggest to a socially immature adolescent that they are likely to overcome their shyness and meet friends easily in the near future, would be developmentally insensitive and produce a failure experience that could produce regression.

Some aspects of the concept of development and developmental readiness need clarification. First, there is the difference between the client's actual and perceived development. There can be a significant difference between the observed external level of development as indicated through the clients behavior and the client's own self-perceived level of psychological development in the internal forum. A case will clarify here. Some years ago, Olive's family and physician referred her to me with a severe depression resulting from a complicated bereavement. At age 65 she had lost her husband of 40 years to a heart attack. It became clear that they had a codependent relationship in which she had essentially given over her life in his care and he covertly received emotional support by being the giver. She came from a parental environment in which her schoolteacher mother was very emotionally detached from her (while being regarded by other local children as warm and loving!). Not surprisingly, Olive has a highly anxious temperament, which was best described as a generalized anxiety disorder. Her marriage represented a haven and through it she received a significant amount of parenting from a Middle Eastern man who provided a gentle mantle of authority. When he died suddenly, even though the heart condition was well known, she experienced a "parental" loss that threw her into a complicated bereavement. From Olive's point of view she experienced herself as totally bereft of any capacity to survive or thrive independently. Certainly her self-perception and external symptoms would have led to an agreement with this portrayal. However, over time it became clear to me that this client had far more resources available to her than initially apparent to herself or to me. I became aware that my client, although seemingly developmentally delayed, actually had a developmental potential beyond the external facts. In fact she had experienced a "successful maternal parenting" (fathers are often "mothers") in the marital relationship and for the past many years and was actually more able to manage an independent life than she realized. Marriage, as it often does, had compensated for impoverished parenting. The evidence for these internal resources became clear over time, and even though she continued to see herself as a child in need of an adult protector, her life took on a shape that suggested she had indeed more resources and resilience than she or I had credited initially. She eventually began to make friends and travel internationally including to the Middle East to reconnect with her husband's family. This case reminded me of a developmental phenomenon that has impressed me throughout my therapeutic career, namely to pay attention to the actual internal developmental level as well as to the external chronological markers of development.

Another important distinction in understanding human development is between overall life span development and the developmental trajectory that occurs within many discrete human experiences such as bereavement, divorce, trauma recovery, and so forth. Indeed, much of what appears in a typical psychology syllabus and texts as developmental psychology would be better described as developmental behavior. It is often only in the chapter discussing Erik Erikson's developmental stages (Erikson, 1950/1963), for example, that we begin to get a discussion of truly psychological development, namely, the internal developmental trajectory. Recent emphasis on life-span development has helped emphasize this area, but even here the focus is on the client's position in the overall or total life span. There is, however, as indicated earlier, another critical meaning of development that occurs within discrete human experiences. Thus, the therapist can recognize in Olive a predictable sequence of psychological experiences associated with the complicated bereavement. By complicated bereavement we refer to a bereavement that is out of the normal course of events, such as a death "out of due season," or that the circumstances, as in this case, were traumatic in and of themselves. We know that the resolution of this experience follows a predictable trajectory that has a defined roadmap and possible conclusion. Understanding this process allows the therapist to work with the client as the experience unfolds over time. This can help the client feel supported, not rushed or pressured to reach resolution.

Thus, in the process of grieving, whether it is the loss of person or the sudden loss of autonomy after admission to a nursing home, the therapist will be helped by close attention to the developmental markers in the course of treatment. For example, such markers include the initial reluctance to accept the loss, the anger, denial, depression, and the variety of ways the client deals with the loss, either by removing all reminders of the person in their life—clothes, books, photos—or by avoiding entering the marital bedroom or dealing with the closet full of papers and clothes. A developmentally sensitive therapist will not push a person to a level beyond their current capacity.

The development perspective not only applies to the client's life but also to the process of therapy itself. Meta-analytic psychotherapy research has found a uniform pattern within the process of brief psychotherapy that starts with an initial experience of a large improvement in well being occurring in the first several sessions (Messer & Warren, 1995). This progresses to symptom reduction and finally to the overall improvement in current life functioning over 1 to 15 sessions. Thus, the developmentally oriented therapist moves in a harmonious way down the therapeutic road with the client. If a time-limited structure is used in brief psychotherapy, it should be sensitive to and in accord with the individual tempo and needs of the client. To assume a fixed, time-limited schedule across different problems and different clients and different personalities is inadvisable.

Finally, developmental unfolding occurs not just in the clients' life or in the process of psychotherapy but also is a dominant element in professional training itself. It is not possible to speed up the development of therapeutic skill by a short or even intensive practicum experience. Time, as the vehicle of change, is needed. The various skills necessary for the therapist unfold on a developmental trajectory that can certainly be brief but cannot be rushed. As the trainer works with students, it again becomes helpful to "look down the road ahead of them," to anticipate and recognize the issues that will confront them. Clearly, these issues will differ among students, but the overall process will be characterized by a gradual unfolding of professional skill. A poignant example of this development is the task of the new therapist in his or her mid-20s learning to work powerfully and effectively with a client in their mid-80s. Gradually counteracting the transferential temptation to either infantilize or aggrandize their older client, coming to recognize their own inner resources, avoiding the frequent stereotypic assumption that late life experience is psychologically inert, all take a gradual process that rewards close, developmentally oriented supervision. In my own work in training doctoral students to work as psychotherapists with older adults I consider that the major milestone is to develop a comfort level and self-acceptance in working with adults who are 50 years their senior (Duffy & Morales, 1997). There is a gradual recognition, as mentioned earlier, that when a person asks for help then chronological age drops away. Frequently, young therapists disempower themselves and deprive the older client of much needed assistance.

Counterintuitive Dynamics

Many effective strategies follow a counterintuitive direction. An important early strategy, for example, is to avoid premature reassurance but to accept and understand the patient's situation, even accepting a worst case scenario. The effect on the client is paradoxical; they actually feel more supported than if reassurance had been offered directly. Another common example of counterintuitive dynamics in therapy is the manner of dealing with resistance in our clients. In the classical psychoanalytic tradition and in several of the structurally oriented brief therapies such as that of Davanloo (1980), the task of the therapist is to overcome and counteract resistance of the client to the interpretation and required necessary changed behavior. In the experience of many therapists, however, such battling to overcome the resistance has the reverse effect. Even though it would seem intuitively reasonable to engage the client in a confrontation about their resistant behavior, in fact such confrontation produces and increases resistance. A counterintuitive position, now accepted among therapists, is to develop empathy for the resistance—to "go around rather than through the mountain."

Especially important in working with debilitated older adults is the manner in which therapists handle dependency needs of their clients. When a client exhibits inappropriate dependency, even experienced therapists may tend to intuitively push back and demand autonomy of the client. A wiser, counterintuitive, approach is to accept the dependency needs of the client. What transpires is that the urgency of felt need of the client often diminishes, and, thus comforted, their actual autonomous (although not felt) resources become available to them. Olive, quite passive dependent, asked that I promise her that I would always see her in therapy if she needed and requested it. After a moment's anxious hesitation I answered yes! The effect of this counterintuitive response was that she was able to feel calm and approach therapy termination. It was 5 years before she requested to see me again, and then for only three sessions following an anxiety reaction to the September 11, 2001, disaster (her husband had been an Arab).

The following case will help elucidate the importance of counterintuitive strategy in working with a patient with hypochondria in a nursing home. Some time ago I was asked to work with John, an older parent who had been recently admitted into a retirement community and had quickly become symptomatic with acute anxiety alternating with extreme psychosomatic self-preoccupation. The first few sessions established an overall sense of well-being and comfort in the client and controlled the anxiety, and the next task was to deal with the psychosomatic symptoms. The general posture of physicians, nursing staff, and even mental health professionals involves an initial stage of taking the medical complaints seriously and finding no medical cause. This is followed by intuitively reasonable attempts to persuade the patient they do not have the medical symptoms that disturb them and they need no further medical attention. What follows is an increasingly frustrating sequence of events in which the more the health professional attempts to dissuade the patient, the more the patient grasps for evidence that the disorders actually exist. At an earlier point in my work as a psychotherapist, I learned, from others, the counterintuitive approach to working with hypochondriasis. This involves a counterintuitive strategy of not dissuading the client from the belief of their symptoms. It involves not arguing against the various medical conditions but accepting them as phenomenologically real for the client. Most importantly, it involves not pushing the person away from treatment. Conversely, the most effective strategy involves welcoming the person to make regular contacts, which are encouraged. This, in fact, reverses the polarity of the relationship. Instead of feeling pursued, the therapist is now in control of the relationship, which can then be controlled to the tolerance level of the therapist but enables the patients to have a sense of security and attentiveness. Given this strategy, after about 12 weeks John's psychosomatic symptoms begin to drop out of the therapeutic picture. He began to be less self-preoccupied and began to integrate into the life of the facility.

Interiority and Religious Themes

Although it is not true that older adults in general fear death, there is considerable evidence from clinical experience and research that as we age we tend to move more toward interiority: As we age, there is a capacity to go within, to seek life's meaning within our internal world, to become more introspective and introverted, and therefore to tolerate aloneness in a way that would have been uncomfortable in earlier life. Even though, for example, the introversion–extroversion personality parameter tends to be fairly fixed and consistent across the life span, it does seem that as we age we tend to become more interior or introverted.

The very significant clinical and research work that has been done on the process of reminiscence and life review in late life has found that this interior reflection seems to characterize later life (Haight & Webster, 1995). Reminiscence serves the purpose of reviewing and evaluating life's achievement, successes, and failures with the general purpose of putting one's house in order. During this period of life, increased interiority also suggests an increase in religious interest and observance and it seems that this tendency is driven by both developmental and pragmatic considerations; as life begins to reach closure it is understandable that we might ask the pragmatic question of our disposition beyond death!

Through my own life and clinical experiences, which has involved working with children as well as older adults, I believe that the tendency to reminisce is not exclusive to late life but can also be found in children and in other phases of the life cycle. However, the tendency to reminisce and recapitulate on life does seem to have a special place in the later parts of life. The narratives and life stories provided by older clients are a valuable opportunity for the new therapist to learn about the idiosyncratic experiences of the older clients, which counteract the generic stereotypes of aging. The beginning therapist quickly learns that the inner life of an older adult is no less interesting and indeed is usually more complex psychologically than that of younger persons. They learn soon that this older adult has developed a resilience and life experience that allows them to survive trauma that would overtax a younger person (Duffy & Iscoe, 1990). The experience of hearing of an older adult recounting of early life traumata and abuse can quickly dispel the idea that working with older adults is a lesser form of psychotherapy. In my experience many beginning trainees and experienced therapists who start to work with older adults may be attempted to leave the field with a sense of disillusionment assuming that psychotherapy with older adults is not as challenging and interesting as with younger adults. This is simply the result of not reaching a psychologically intimate position in therapy with older adults. Because of the difference in age, transferential factors can impede the necessary intimacy that must exist in any therapeutic relationship. A key contribution of close supervision is to ensure that the novice therapist moves beyond the external relationship into a close and intimate connection with the older client, at which point chronological age fades into the background.

Although fear of death and death anxiety is not normative in late life, there are numerous clinical situations in which death anxiety is present in older adults. In the case of my own mother who had experienced ambivalence about the love of her mother throughout her life, I sensed a distinct anxiety about death that went beyond the agitation incurred by the dementia process. The essential nurturance and comfort that had eluded her in her relationship with her mother remained a troubling internal representation throughout life and made dying an anxiety-provoking experience. There is a distinction between fear of death and fear of dying. In some cases the prospect of nonexistence is accepted with some degree of comfort. It is the prospect of dying, being buried, and decomposing that is alarming to some older persons. Working with the patient's death anxiety will involve the same intensive therapeutic relationship that can have a compensatory effect with regard to the loss of significant intimacy in the older adult's life.

This sense of relational loss may have been veiled in the busy task-oriented episode of earlier life only to become more visible in the last moments of life in which activity slows and the mind turns inward. This may particularly occur when cognitive impairment strips the older adult of the defensive structure that it had provided. There has been considerable debate about the usefulness of intensive psychotherapy with older adults who have a dementia disorder. Clearly, psychotherapy is not a simple rational process and also involves intensive emotional and affective connections with the client. A psychotherapeutic relationship is even more imperative at this point of life in which cognition is clouded and a person is on the edge of the unknown with fear and a great sense of aloneness. Such moments, understood in this way, are both powerful and satisfying for the therapist.

SUMMARY

There is little documentary evidence for the relevance of brief dynamic approaches to psychotherapy with older adults. Accumulating and consensual clinical experience, however, suggests that these approaches are relevant. Indeed, the last section on the increase of interiority in late life would suggest the importance of psychotherapy methods that attend to and involve the inner, dynamic psychological life. Therapists know that working with older adults is much more the same than different from younger adults; therefore, much of the rich literature on dynamic psychotherapy is quite appropriate. Our lives remain as rich, psychologically complex, as eccentric, and as problematic during our later years.

Questions for the therapist who is considering working therapeutically with older adults include, how does one feel about working with an older adult?: more cautious?, overly respectful?, patronizing? In the therapists' personal family life, do they have a warm and intimate relationship with an older relative? Could you use confrontation with an older client if necessary? I suggest that readers arrange a visit with an older person in a personal home or nursing home to interview them about their greatest satisfaction, what in their lives would they change, who is the person they have been closest to, what worries them most in life, and if they have any unfinished issues with family members.

REFERENCES

American Psychiatric Association. (1994). *Diagnostic and statistical manual of mental disorders* (4th ed.). Washington, DC: American Psychiatric Association.
Davanloo, H. (1980). *Short-term dynamic psychotherapy.* New York: Jason Aronson.
Duffy, M. (Ed.). (1999a). *Handbook of counseling and psychotherapy with older adults.* New York: Wiley.
Duffy, M. (1999b). Individual therapy in long-term care settings. In V. Molinari (Ed.), *Providing psychological services to older adults* (pp. 73–112). New York: Hatherleigh.
Duffy, M., & Iscoe, I. (1990). Crisis theory and management: The case of the older adult. *Journal of Mental Health Counseling, 12,* 303–313.
Duffy, M., & Morales, P. (1997). Supervision of psychotherapy with older patients. In C. E. Watkins, Jr. (Ed.), *Handbook of psychotherapy supervision* (pp. 366–380). New York: Wiley.
Erikson, E. H. (1950/1963). *Childhood and society.* New York: Norton.
Freud, S. (1905/1953). *On psychotherapy: Standard edition* (Vol. 7). Toronto, Canada: Hogarth Press.
Gorsuch, N. (1998). Time's winged chariot: Short-term psychotherapy late life. *Psychodynamic Counselling, 4,* 192–202.
Haight, B. K., & Webster, J. D. (1995). *The art and science of reminiscing: Theory, research, methods and applications.* Philadelphia: Taylor & Francis.
Hussian, R. A. (1981). *Geriatric psychology: A behavioral perspective.* New York: Van Nostrand Reinhold.
Kell, B. L., & Mueller, W. J. (1966). *Impact and change: A study of counseling relationships.* New York: Appleton-Century-Crofts.
Mahler, M. S. (1967). On human symbiosis and vicissitudes of individuation. *Journal of the American Psychoanalytic Association, 15,* 740–763.
Messer, S. B., & Warren, C. S. (1995). *Models of brief dynamic therapy.* New York: Guilford.
Mueller, W. J., & Kell, W. L. (1972). *Coping with conflict: Supervising counselors and psychotherapists.* Englewood Cliffs, NJ: Prentice Hall.
Rosowsky, E., Abrams, R., & Zweig, R. (Eds.). (1999). *Personality disorders in late life: Emerging issues in diagnosis and treatment.* Mahwah, NJ: Lawrence Erlbaum Associates.
Semel, V. G. (1996). Modern psychoanalytic treatment of the older adult. In S. H. Zarit & B. G. Knight (Eds.), *A guide to psychotherapy and aging: Effective clinical interventions in a life-stage context* (pp. 101–120). Washington, DC: American Psychological Association.
Truax, C. B., & Carkhuff, R. R. (1967). *Toward effective counseling and therapy.* Chicago: Aldine.
Wampold, B. E. (2001). *The great psychotherapy debate: Models, methods and findings.* Mahwah, NJ: Lawrence Erlbaum Associates.

APPENDIX
The Case Study: The Therapy, the Patient, and the Therapist

Jackie Fosbury
St. Thomas' Hospital

This is the case of "June" who received 9 sessions of a 16-session cognitive analytic therapy (CAT). CAT formed part of the clinical service to people with poorly controlled diabetes in a major teaching hospital. The service had been set up after the results of a clinical trial of CAT with poorly controlled patients (Fosbury, Bosley, Ryle, Sonksen, & Judd, 1997).

CAT has been developed and researched by Ryle (1990). It is a time-limited, focused psychotherapy combining techniques and understandings from both psychoanalytic and cognitive behavioral therapy. A central feature of the approach is the emphasis on the reformulation of the patient's problems. Over the first three sessions the patient and therapist work together to achieve the clearest possible description of the patient's harmful or ineffective procedures derived from early experiences and relationships. The term *procedure* refers to an individual's way of organizing their lives and relationships in destructive and harmful ways.

The emphasis of CAT is placed on the therapy relationship. In nearly all cases, procedures responsible for damaging an individual's life will be reenacted in the therapeutic relationship and interpreted by the therapist. Many patients with poor diabetes control in this service had received long-term diabetes education and previous forms of psychological help. However, an approach that demands the rational cooperation of the patient in the treatment process will often fail because the patient is uncooperative, that is, the patient behaves in a way (with their carers and their diabetes) that is typical of their central difficulties (Ryle, Boa, & Fosbury, 1993). June is very typical of this description. As noncooperation or resistance is a central feature of these patients and central to the work of psychotherapy, a more psychoanalytically orientated approach to treatment was felt to be more appropriate to these patients and difficulties.

THE PATIENT: JUNE

Biography

June was 25 when she was referred to a major teaching hospital. She was diagnosed as having diabetes at the age of 10. She lived alone in a rented housing association flat 50 miles from the hospital. Her mother and father lived locally to her and she had a married sister 4 years older who also lived nearby and a brother who was 38 years who lived abroad.

Referral

Her local hospital consultant who had looked after her diabetes since childhood referred June. He described her as an "unfortunate young girl" with poor control, recurrent Diabetic Ketoacidosis (DKA), microvascular complications, and severe retinopathy. Her HbAlc on referral was 12.2%. The normal HbAlc range is 5–7.6%. June had a history of psychiatric intervention for depression and local community psychiatric nurses and an art therapist had also been involved in her care since diagnosis. She was described as "unmotivated" with a history of "considerable interpersonal and family difficulties." Her consultant had heard a talk I had given about CAT with poorly controlled patients with diabetes and wondered if I could accept a referral for assessment.

Assessment

On assessment June described herself as "not being bothered" about her diabetes or herself and generally felt "in limbo." She sometimes took her insulin, never blood glucose monitored, and ate what she wanted. She had constant pain in her feet and permanent headaches. She broke down in tears and didn't know why. Her past medical and psychological carers were spoken about disparagingly. They all reminded her of teachers who made her feel "stroppy," and as a result she didn't listen to them. This made her wonder why they bothered with her. The more they bothered, the less she did.

June had worked as a shop assistant since leaving school but had been off sick for a year due to depression and poor diabetes control. She had a lot of contact with her parents. She was particularly close to her mother but felt that her sister Cathy was the favorite and "takes precedence." When this happened, June felt "blanked out." Mum was like June however; she always got "walked all over." June felt that her father loved her mother but treated her badly. He fixed things to show his love but never completed anything and their house was a terrible mess. She believed her mother had lost friends because of this, as no one could ever come to the house—it was "in a state." June felt "real hate" toward her father because of her mum's feelings. Father and June had a temper, although June "bottles things up." June's sister felt that the brother was the favorite and June was low down on the list of care priorities. June's mother and father were described as devastated by her diabetes. She suddenly received a lot of attention. This attention turned sour at the age of 14 or 15 when she felt (as if) all their attention was only about her diabetes. This "drove me crazy." She felt she was "spoilt" only because of her diabetes and this did not feel "good enough."

I asked why June wanted to attend this assessment. She said she had gotten to a point in which she never saw herself as being happy until she was sorted out and was willing to "give it a go." The art therapist treated her as a "four year old" and if I did this she would not attend. I had been warned.

THE THERAPIST

My initial impressions were of concern about June's ability to commit to the therapy given the history outlined in her referral letter together with the journey she would have to undertake. However, June arrived early for her appointment and I set out the terms and conditions of attendance and immediately predicted the difficulties in attending both in journey times and potential psychological barriers. In my work with poorly controlled patients it seems to have always been helpful to outline ways in which people might find it difficult to attend from the outset. This predictive work has prevented a lot of dropout in therapy, as poorly controlled patients with diabetes are often notoriously poor attenders, reflecting their poor self-care (Ryle et al., 1993). It also, as in June's case, reflected a central psychological difficulty "if I must, then I won't." As I was saying "you might not," she was saying, although not overtly, "then I will." Thus her attendance seemed assured.

Although June was due to have 16 sessions of CAT, she in fact received 9 because I was going on maternity leave. The tight time limit of June's therapy did cause me some anxiety, although we both knew that after my maternity leave she was coming back for a review with the possibility of more sessions.

My initial countertransference on assessing June for CAT was slightly one of futility: "How can I do anything in this time with these difficulties," and "She is virtually catatonic." However, we both decided to proceed, June on the basis of rebellion—that is, after I made a transference interpretation on assessment and suggested that her attendance would be erratic and blanking out (as a reflection of her poor self-care and anger and resentment toward others)—and me on the basis that she was in a very dangerous mental and physical situation.

As for my countertransference, June made me feel very sad and challenged. I did not want to let her go but didn't want to give her attention just because of her diabetes! I was also aware that although I wanted to have her with me in therapy, she was a slippery customer. Therefore, I had decided to take all the opportunities I could to reflect on her resistance as a challenge to her to keep with me. I also decided to focus on her "core pain" about not being someone who mattered—hence not bothering with herself. Would bothering with her actually feel like negative attention?

THE THERAPY

The key or focus of June's therapy was on her relationship to self and others, including her therapist via her blanking out state. Blanking out served a number of functions. It represented her core pain insofar as she was blanked out by her family, it represented a reflection of self-care in terms of her diabetes management and general presentation, and enabled her to elicit anger and resentment of others (also experienced in herself) when she felt let down, resentful, jealous, and responsible for them.

A cognitive behavioral therapy (CBT) approach to collaborative work with June would most likely agree on the goals of the therapy and this would include the elimination of blanking out. Goals, like "taking time out" without blanking out would not be used in CAT, as it is primarily an analytic relational therapy and thus the meaning of blanking out and its primary cause and effect on others (in this respect me, the therapist) would be discussed at length. It has been argued that once therapists using cognitive behavioral therapy take on the work of goals, they are often, as Milton (2001) stated, "more paternalistic in assuming the therapist knows best about relationships" (Milton, 2001, p. 5). This approach is also reflected by Eeells and Lombart in chapter 6, this volume who state that "we would work on learning more appropriate ways of expressing anger." This cognitive behavioral goal-orientated approach to treatment can "avoid painful aspects of the work and deprives the patient of an opportunity to work in the negative transference, thereby limiting the scope of the work" (Milton, 2001, p. 5).

The therapy with June revolved around her blanking out, which was interpreted and analyzed in the transference in terms of how it made her feel and how blanking out made others reject her. As usual the therapist was offered a very strong "invitation" to confirm this early patterning but declined that offer. In so doing, June experienced not being blanked out. This started her on a road to working out her own ways of being within the safety of the therapeutic relationship, which involved not blanking out her self-care. This fundamental change was not based on June having compassion for herself but occurred within the experience of compassion in the therapy. Thus, by the end of therapy, June felt that she mattered.

My personal circumstances particularly limited her CAT and made me work at consolidating a lot of the transference work, particularly at the last sessions, in a much more cognitive, pragmatic way. Perhaps, this came across as "dissuasion" outlined by Gelso in chapter 11, of some of the transference work. This also included some need to reality check when June was in fact worried that she would start blanking out the sessions after termination, that is, forget everything and go back to square one, particularly as I could have put words into her mouth or mind. Thus, she was reminded that it was her words that created her reformulation, her diagrams, and the construction of the therapy.

In the therapy it quickly emerged that her father modeled forms of incomplete care and was the one who started something and couldn't be bothered to finish it. The house was in a state; then June began to complain that her body was in a state. This incomplete and "not bothered" theme affected June's ability to care for herself appropriately and adequately and affected her ability to work consistently and find boyfriends who would treat her respectfully. After all, if she didn't, why should they?

June also began to see some connections and paradoxes with her feelings toward her mother and her diabetes management. This involved the feeling that her mother blanked her out in relation to her brother and sister but spoilt her only when she was diagnosed. This not good enough care brought the greatest distress to June and rebellion against her diabetes. By session three, June realized for the first time why she resisted her self-care.

By session four we worked on a diagram together to plot and monitor June's feelings in relation to herself, her diabetes, her family and friends, and her therapist. We also included her medical and nursing carers. She always kept her diagram with her. The central procedure was "feel blanked out (worthless and rejected) so don't matter, rejects self (care) and others, others don't care for me, which confirmed I don't matter."

The reenactments of June's procedures in the therapy were monitored closely. During her treatment, June oscillated between blanking out (attending in a semicatatonic state) and angry rebellious resentment. I focused increasingly on providing good enough care that was to do with her as a loveable, likeable human being. I felt very close to her. On two occasions she actually laughed—at herself. Toward the end of our contact, she described herself as feeling "more human," that she was "very open," did not feel "numb," and that we had dealt with her problems "together." June's HbAlc at the end of therapy was 10.1%.

FOLLOW-UP AND REVIEW

We had decided to complete our work on my return 6 months later. When I saw June again she described some flat and negative times but she now had a boyfriend and they were thinking of living together. She had very few arguments with her parents and was looking after a friend's child until she felt ready to go back to work full-time. She had described feeling "shocked" at how little she discovered she knew about her diabetes in this period. Her resistance had therefore also resulted in ignorance. She was taking her insulin and blood glucose monitoring and described her consultant as a "nice bloke" for the first time. I saw June to consolidate and complete our work for a further six sessions and 3 months after that date her HbAlc was 8.2%.

REFERENCES

Fosbury, J. A., Bosley, C. M., Ryle, A., Sonksen, P. H., & Judd, S. L. (1997). A trial of cognitive analytic therapy in poorly controlled type 1 patients. *Diabetes Care, 20,* 959–964.
Ryle, A. (Ed.). (1990). *Cognitive analytic therapy—Active participation in change.* London: Wiley.
Ryle, A., Boa, C., & Fosbury, J. A. (1993). Identifying the causes of poor self-management in insulin dependent diabetics: The use of cognitive analytic therapy techniques. In M. Hodes & S. Moorey (Eds.), *Psychological treatment in disease and illness* (pp. 157–165). London: Gaskell.
Milton, J. (2001, November). *Integration in psychotherapy, Is it possible?* Association for Psychoanalytic Psychotherapy in the NHS (APPN Newsletter). No. 26, pp. 4–5.

TRANSCRIPT OF SESSION 3

Q: 3–1: We're on session 3 aren't we, and I wrote some notes from our last session, and that said we needed to start working on the [Cognitive Analytic Sequential] diagram about how everything linked together really. So how are you anyway, generally? Did you blank out last week's session?

A: 3–3: Basically, yes, I think I did.

Q: 3–4: Any idea why all that happens?

A: 3–5: No.

APPENDIX 389

Q: 3-6: No. So if I ask you to start keeping a diary soon about blanking things about, would you be able to do that, or would you blank that out as well?

A: I'd give it a go. A bit of an argument about coming here today, last night.

Q: Right. With whom? With your Dad? [nota bene: June's father often gave June a lift to her therapy sessions.]

A: 3-7: No. No. My sister. Basically my sister, and Mum was in the middle as well. He'd been in bed all day and I just felt that the argument she was having was basically about somebody looking after Debbi (June's niece) rather than being concerned about how Dad was or me having to get up here. And basically what she was saying was, you know, well he's probably willing so don't even ask him whether he wants to come or not, just say that he's going and then has to get out of bed to look after Debbi sort of thing. Because she was of the mind that if I came on my own, she'd be leaving Debbi with him but Debbi would be downstairs on her own all day while he was being ill in bed. And she seemed to find ... I felt that she was saying, that's not good enough. She wanted him to be looking after Debbi rather than being ill. Umm ... my Mum's got this attitude that Dad always gets ill around Christmas and that it's more in his head than it's anything else. And I said, well, hold on a minute, we've all had it, and he's gone through without getting it, for the past ... well, I've forgotten now how many months I've had it. And he's looked after us you know. I've been there, I was literally in bed for three days solid or something, and he was basically nursemaiding me. And I said, just give him a bit of leeway, after all it was a Sunday, it wasn't as if he had to go to work or anything like that. He wasn't sort of bunking off from anything. Umm, and just basically Cathy and Mum seemed so put out by the fact he was ill, and I just sort of ... you know, give ... the thing is, I do think this sometimes, I think give the poor bloke a break, because I can see two sides to the argument the whole time. I mean, my Mum's ... basically she's admitted she's not in love with him any more, and they're just living together really because they couldn't sell the house even if they wanted to and split up or anything. It's just ... you know, it wouldn't be practical.

Q: But your Dad's illness doesn't suit them?

A: 3-8: I think she ... the way it sounded was as if he was doing it on purpose. And I just thought, you know, basically, Cathy's and Mum's attitude was, well everyone else gets up and goes to work and things like that, well, yeah, fair enough, but why on a Sunday if he's not feeling well, if he wants to stay in bed all day, then let him, as far as I can see. But they weren't having that, you know. And all . . . as I say, with Cathy, all I felt was that it was just so Debbi could be looked after. And basically, Debbi was not particularly well either, and I sort of said, I basically said to Cathy, well wouldn't it be better for the both of them to stay here in the warm, rather than have to get on buses and trains and things to get up to London, you know. I ended up getting her dressed and everything, she stayed at Mum's last night, and I stayed there as well. Because that seemed to suit everybody else. So I get her dressed and everything, and she's as white as a sheet, and I saw she wasn't well, and I said to Dad, if you're not feeling well, I can see she's not feeling well, why don't you just stay here. Oh, no, no, no. Then of course, when we're trying to get her coat on and that she's just getting genuinely upset. She really didn't want to come out. And he's literally dragging her into the car screaming, and I just thought, I don't want this. I'd rather come up here in peace, I don't want screaming kids and that on the train. Anyway, when we got to the station she'd calmed down, but . . . the train was running 10 minutes late, so that sort of put me back a bit.

Q: 3-9: Why do you think your Dad is so insistent on bringing you here, when you could have done it on your own, he could have stayed at home even with Debbi, if he wanted to, that's up to him, isn't it?

A: 3-10: I think he may feel that I feel I need someone here. And I don't know, perhaps if was my friend Gail coming with me, I'd feel fine about it. But it's the fact that it is dragging Debbi out all the time . . . I mean, I don't know, I don't know if he feels some sense of responsibility or just the case that if he does, it's letting go again. I know he took me moving out really hard, it's like, you know, I'm the youngest, I was the last one there and when I moved out it was like, I suppose it was like, he was losing his baby or something.

Q: 3-11: It's just that it's interesting, how you and your Dad have this really acute sense of responsibility for others. And you describe him as someone who starts a job and never finishes it, incomplete. So people he actually lets down, like your Mum, and you might start a bit of diabetes management, but you certainly never finish that, you don't go all the way on that, and it's quite a flip isn't it?

A: 3-12: I have come to the conclusion that I am very like my Dad in a lot of ways. Physically and mentally.

Q: 3-13: Your Dad, yes. When we first met and it was much more about you and your Mum, it's a lot to do now with your Dad isn't it?

A: 3-14: Yeah, we're very . . . we've never been a particularly affectionate family, but we are very alike. But see, I can still feel how my Mum feels. I can still see that. But I seem to get criticised when I stand up for my Dad. And I must admit I do *fight** a fair bit.

Q: 3-15: But you're standing up for the bits in your Dad that are like you. Aren't you?

A: Yes.

Q: 3-16: Because there's a side of him that's irresponsible, and there's obviously definitely in terms of your self care, definitely a side of you that's very irresponsible.

A: Yes.

Q: 3-17: I put irresponsible up there on this list, but we'll link it all together soon.

A: 3-18: Cathy and my Mum do get on very well together. But Cathy also gets on with my Dad.... I personally see Cathy ... like last night, she wasn't taking Debbi's feelings into consideration, she wasn't taking my Dad's feelings into consideration. I know she's got to out and work. But I just feel that sometimes ... you know, Debbi wasn't well. She said, well I can't take the day off because I'll get sacked. Well to me, that wouldn't be a priority. I think if Debbi really wasn't well, I would rather make sure that she's all right. I mean, she's left ... my Dad's taking her to the doctors, like Debbi to the doctor's before now, rather than give up an hour to take her. I find ... I find that ... I mean she says I'm selfish, she's told me to my face that she thinks I'm selfish, umm ... but I find her in some ways very selfish. Whether she is or not, I don't know, it's just how I feel.

Q: It certainly ... there's certainly another thread of irresponsibility going on with Cathy, isn't there. That, O.K., it's this flip again, she's very responsible about going to work and will lose her job if she takes time off, but she also is able to be irresponsible to Debbi for example, because she maneuvers everyone else to look after her.

A: Yeah.

Q: Yeah?

A: Yeah.

Q: So everyone in your family, it's not so clear with your Mum, but certainly with you, and certainly with your Dad, and actually certainly with Cathy, it's pretty ... you have these sort of flip things ... don't you?

A: Yeah.

Q: 3-19: I don't know whether selfish could be .... I mean I put selfish onto Cathy, selfish ... you could be described as selfish, it's more ...

---

*In this June refers to heated verbal arguments.

I don't know, it's ... you said you were spoilt because of your diabetes.

A: 3-20: I was definitely spoilt you know, as far as Dad goes.

Q: 3-21: Sure. And I think this thing about you either feel blanked out (excluding and rejected) or you feel invaded and others are totally involved. And when you get in both those positions as you say, you become abusive to others, shouting, temper, you're more like your Dad and have a temper. So that could be seen as selfish. But generally you are sort of, almost like inappropriately responsible towards others, aren't you? Which is not quite the same as being selfish.

A: 3-22: No. No, I mean I suppose I can see how she'd say that with regards to me not looking after myself, that's selfish because if I were to die, then she sees that as being completely selfish because of every one I'm leaving behind. She also says that anyone that tries to commit suicide is completely selfish and has no feelings for others, but the fact is, I've been in the position when I've wanted to do something like that, and I feel that if you're that low that you can do something like that, you're not thinking of anybody else. The reason you're doing it is to put an end to all your troubles, you're not considering anybody else, so yeah, maybe that it is selfish, but you don't actually think of yourself as being, you don't think of anybody else when you're in that position.

Q: No, you're in too much suffering to worry about that.

A: Exactly.

Q: 3-23: But if you think, June if you don't think you matter the 90% of the time, which is what you've spoken about, then generally you're not being selfish, are you?

A: No, no.

Q: 3-24: Anyway, it's just interesting how all of you seem to have these issues that manifest themselves in you, is very self destructive, very abusive to yourself. Cathy may be abusive to other people, for example, but your Mum might feel that your Dad's being abusive towards her because he starts a job and never finishes it, but the point is your manifestation has had very dangerous results. Much more dangerous than anything that Paul's come across, Cathy's come across, or your Mum's come across, isn't it?

A: Yes.

Q: That's the point. And I think that's the thing on a day-to-day level at the moment, that you just have to try and remind yourself of.

A: Yes.

Q: And your Dad probably does get really ill, but your Mum and Cathy think of it as like a bit of a fantasy, in the way that they think about

your ... you know, like it's self induced flu or something. In the way that they understand your diabetes management will be self induced, the problems with it. Which it is of course, but they don't understand what causes it.
A: Yeah.
Q: Does that make sense?
A: Yeah.
Q: So you get ill and your Dad gets ill, your Dad just doesn't have diabetes and he doesn't get as ill as you. So there's something in that configuration that both you and your Dad turn in against yourself. Mum and Cathy might ... the word's a bit extreme, but Mum and Cathy might abuse other people, but you and your Dad abuse yourself.
A: Yeah.
Q: An one of the ways in which you might do that, there's a lot of similarities between you and Dad really, it's by rebelling. And breaking things up.
A: Yeah.
[Long period of silence.]
Q: 3-25: And when you're blanked out, you think, why should I look after myself, why should I do what I'm told, so that rebellion flips again, doesn't it.
A: 3-26: I just don't seem to think though a lot of the time. I don't sit there and think, why aren't I doing it particularly, when I say blanked out, I mean blank where I'm just nothing.
Q: 3-27: That's your ... numb, that's what you describe as being numb.
A: 3-28: And most of the time I don't think about anything I should be thinking about. If I sit and do a crossword, then I read the clues, I do the crossword and that's it. I don't think about anything else. That doesn't make me think of something else, or watching the telly. I literally, if I'm watching the telly, I just stare at the ... I'm basically just staring at the screen I'm not really listening to what's going on. It's a long time since I've actually paid much attention to what's really going on, on the screen.
Q: 3-29: This piece of paper, with some diagrams for you, so this is what I think's going on for you, and what goes on in your every day life, and it's pretty devastating. What would you ... and you didn't blank it out, because it was with you all the time, what do you think you're reaction would be?
A: 3-30: I think I'd either be in tears a lot of the time, I'd be thinking about things that either make me want to cry, or there's just ... there'd be too much feeling for me to cope with.

Q: 3-31: Ok.

A: 3-32: Too many emotions to . . . I think that's what I blank out, these feelings.

Q: 3-33: Exactly.

A: 3-34: If I don't feel, I don't get hurt.

Q: So how would you feel eventually if we were to take you into that bit, for you to come out the other side?

A: I just don't know. Umm . . . if it means that I have some sort of normal life, then the way I feel at the moment, I'd do most anything I think. I know it's me that stops myself from feeling anything, but I do get sick of not being able to . . . it's not that I'm not able to, I can, but not wanting to feel anything.

Q: It's probably going to be terribly, terribly painful, at first. And maybe it might feel very dangerous and out of control, but this is dangerous and out of control isn't it? Bleeding at the back of the eyes is pretty dangerous and out of control, isn't it?

A: Yep. And every other little twinge of pain I get I think, is this something else, you know.

Q: Yes. Exactly.

A: Then I think if my feet hurt, or even if just my big toe hurts, then I do think, but I still can't do anything about it. I still can't make myself think, feeling like this and do something about it.

Q: 3-35: Hang on a minute, you just said, if you don't feel like you matter for 90% of the time and you blank your own self out, and that you blank most feeling things out, and you've got to take a lot of responsibility for others, it's mainly volunteered even though you might feel exploited and abused, and there's another part of you that thinks, why should I do IT when you're not blanking out and you're going into this rebellion thing. And when you're doing that you think why should I look after myself. Of course it doesn't matter that you get these twinges. You might think to yourself, Oh there's something else, but why would you expect yourself to do something about it?

A: I suppose it's because it's what every body tells you.

Q: Yes, but this is going on, isn't it [pointing at diagram]. So how can you adjust your insulin? . . . Move your injection sites away from your stomach because there are injection pads there, or eat properly. But this is going on, and you're blanking it out . . .

A: 3-36: Yes. I suppose for 15 years all I've been listening to is, you should be doing this, you should be doing that. It's doctors, nurses, parents or whatever. There's always someone telling you, should you be eating that? And you just think, go away. There's always that someone that is there, it doesn't matter if I switch myself off or not, it still goes in. If someone is telling you something you'll still ... very halfheartedly, but you do listen.

Q: 3-37: Then you blank it out.

A: 3-38: I do blank it out. A lot of the time, but there are those, I suppose that 10% of the time that I do perhaps think something of myself. It makes you think, well hold on a minute, try and buckle down. I mean I can think that perhaps of an evening, when I think, I'm going to wake up tomorrow and I'm going to be a different person. And I wake up the next day, I put the kettle on, I light up a fag and I think, sod it. And it's just down the drain. Before the day's practically even started, it's down the drain.

Q: 3-39: Right. But do you know why? Given what we've spoken about so far, do you have an inkling why that would be the case?

A: 3-40: In all honestly, no. That's why I want to find out, because I think, if I find that out, then I might be able to start doing something about it.

Q: 3-41: O.K. So perhaps even all the things I've said so far, about what's gone on in your family, and how and why you don't feel like you matter, about being blanked out, it still doesn't ... sink in, in terms of how they all configurate around why you do what you do. Where does it come from. Yes?

A: Yes.

Q: 3-42: So we will have to do all this work I've just described on getting a diagram together, and getting you to monitor things. To bring it all to the fore basically.

A: O.K.

Q: O.K. Shall we start looking at it now, in diagram form? Yes?

A: Yeah ...

Q: Are you up to that? Do you want to say anything else about anything else that's happened during the week before we do that?

A: Nothing's happening that's any different to any other week really.

Q: And this little argument about you coming here and everything, that's actually a different manifestation of the same problem, isn't it?

A: Yeah.

Q: 3-43: ... so to start then, if we just look at all the things that you've described, how you described yourself ... I'll give you a copy, I'll just write it now. "I'm numb, I don't matter 90% of the time. I've got very poor self-care. Irresponsible. I've got very responsible care towards others which then makes me feel exploited and resentful." This isn't in any sort of order. "I reduce insulin to keep my weight down. I think about my body shape. I'm abusive to myself. I can be abusive to others, shouting, temper, like that, or quite unkind. I feel blanked out, excluded and rejected, or I can feel totally invaded by others. When I'm alone in my flat, I feel in control." Stop me if I say something that's incorrect. "I feel abused by others." That comes into the exploitative and resentful thing. "I bottle things up. I was spoilt because of my diagnosis. I feel easily replaceable as a person. I feel like a child in front of my parents. I'm rebellious and I hate being told what to do. Why should I if I'm blanked out, I only get attention if I have diabetes." Anything else to add to that? Not very nice list is it?

A: No. I don't think so. ... Cathy is someone who can take my friends away.

Q: ... she gets attention. Is it the same sort of feeling that you're being excluded?

A: Maybe not quite as strongly but the same sort of thing, yeah.

Q: The same thing. So it's transferring, like from your parents onto other people, that ... is that right?

A: Could do, yeah.

Q: O.K. And your Dad's list then, key things about your Dad, are very similar to your things. "That he starts a job and never finishes it. Incomplete. Irresponsible with regard to the home. Very responsible with regard to Cathy, June. Has a temper.... Can blank out mum. Volunteers for things." And I've got a question mark, does he feel taken advantage of, and easily replaceable. Is that when he gets sick I'm just wondering. And that's your Dad really.

A: So I said, starting jobs and not finishing them. Around his home, that is definitely true.... But being at home, as you say, he doesn't particularly seem to care much really about home. You know, the extension was started 7 years ago, and it's still isn't completed.

Q: Right.

A: He's very stubborn as well, which in a way, is like me I suppose.

Q: Right. So, why should he be told what to do in relation to the house?

A: He, I think, he sees things as he wants to do them, and he's going to stick to that.... Mum feels very strongly about it. She wants the dryer in the extension. ... Now I can understand her point of view there. What's the point in having a utility room if you're not going to make the use of it? And I ... in some ways I'm surprised he doesn't want to do that. Because then that would give him more space in his garage, it would be his.

Q: Yes, but you're looking at your Dad's behavior in a rational way in the way that people look at your behavior. Why doesn't she do this, because if she did this she'd feel better. You know what I mean?

A: Yes.
Q: You're doing to him, or your Mum's doing to him, and probably Cathy's doing, what people do to you.
A: Yeah.
Q: Do you see that all start linking up?
A: Mm.
Q: What about that final bit on your Dad, do you think he feels taken advantage of and easily replaceable? Thinking about what you just said.
A: I honestly don't know. He's so easy to get on with, I don't really know. Maybe he does. I suppose ...
Q: You could ask him.
A: I know what he'd say to me.
Q: He doesn't feel it with you, I'm not saying he feels it with you June.
A: No, if I asked him in general, I know he'd say, No, and he would just tell me xxx, he'd avoid actually answering it truthfully. He'd say, you know I don't mind doing anything for you or Cathy, or Paul. That's exactly what he'd say.
Q: I think both of you have poor self-care for reasons.
A: He doesn't ... his poor self-care isn't physical on himself. Because he eats a healthy diet all the time, he's fit, he takes generally good care of himself.
Q: But he gets ill. Yours is much more acute, much more extreme.
A: I know he gets very tired ... he's going to be 67 in March.
Q: But he's carrying on as if he's not that age, you're carrying on as if you don't have diabetes.
A: Yeah.
Q: As if.
A: Yeah.
Q: And that's like the denying isn't it?
A: Yeah.
Q: 3-44: O.K. Just finally, let's just go through the Mum list. ... "Your Mum feels let down, disappointed by Dad with the state of the house. Your Mum definitely blanks you out. You're very close to your Mum."
A: 3-45: I'm a lot closer to my Mum than I'm sure a lot of other people are. But I don't feel as close as Cathy is. Which is perhaps another thing that I'm jealous of. She's very kind and everybody would say it, she is, she's a genuinely kind person.
Q: Quiet and kind like you, or just kind?

A: No, I think she's quiet. I suppose ... again, Cathy says, Can you have the kids Friday? Oh yes, of course I can. Which is the same as I am with Cathy. It's like ... it's like there's almost a fear I suppose of refusing her.

Q: Because?

A: 3-46: I don't know. I don't know. One day, I mean I did ... I've tried to explain to Mum and Dad how I feel about having the kids, but it's just.

Q: Yes, but aren't having the same feelings and problems, are they, so they're going to find it difficult to understand what you're getting at.

A: 3-47: I actually mentioned to Cathy the fact that I wasn't too happy about having both kids together, which I think I mentioned last week. And she turned round and she said, Well, Monday you're having ... you'll be going up to London anyway, so you might as well take Sally with you. know, I don't know ... the thing is ... I still love her as my sister. But I also feel that sometimes there's quite a bit of hate there. I don't know, and that makes it a bit hard for me. The thing is, I don't ... you see when Mum does this thing, with the hovering [vacuuming], you know, I feel really pissed off about it, but I don't feel hate for her. But as soon as Cathy comes in, it's ... there you go. Stop the hoovering ...

Q: Do you feel hate for Cathy at that time?

A: I mean yes, I'd say slightly. Not as much as I have other times, but ... I don't know if I feel hate or if I just feel completely jealous of her, which, you know, usually turns into hate. I just don't know.

Q: 3-48: So jealousy goes into hate and that might fuel the feeling that you don't matter. Yes? Which then leaves you to not bothering about yourself, yes?

A: Yeah.

Q: O.K. So in a way, all your relationships at home with your Mum, and with your Dad and with Cathy, all fuel self destructive behavior, don't they?

A: Yeah.

Q: Actually they make you take acute responsibility for every body else.

A: Yeah.

Q: And it looks like Cathy is the antithesis of that, she takes very little responsibility for anybody else, in fact, total responsibility for herself. The flip of you isn't it?

A: Yeah.

Q: Yeah.

A: I mean, if she ever heard that, she'd completely say ... I'm sure she'd say she's totally the opposite.

Q: But this is your feeling, and this is your experience?
A: Yeah.
Q: Your perspective may be a bit distorted, of course it may, it's your perspective. But this is how you feel . . . Cathy walks into the room, your Mum's hoovering with a walkman on, she's ignoring you, and Cathy walks in and she blanks you out.
A: Yes.
Q: Cathy would say, you're at the hospital tomorrow, you might as well take Sally up, Mum's not working Christmas Eve so she can have the kids, de da de da de da, and you start to hate her, because you would never conceive being important enough to arrange your life in that way.
A: Yes.
Q: 3-49: Before we come to a close today, any worries or concerns about what's going to happen to you and how you deal with it, or what I might think of you, or . . . thoughts like that?
A: 3-50: As long as they never hear any of it.
Q: 3-51: No. Who is they?
A: 3-52: My family in general, I don't . . .
Q: 3-53: How would they hear about it?
A: 3-54: I don't know. . . . I've tried saying things before. And I've basically been told, how stupid I am to think that. And then of course I get all het up and nothing ever gets said. But I've thought in the past, wouldn't it be lovely just to sit round the table, and for everyone to have their say, without interruption, but with my sister there it never happens. She can't help herself.
Q: Well this is your place for that.
A: Yeah. No, they're my only fears. If I decide one day that I'm strong enough to tell them exactly what I think of them well . . . some day I hope I can say that to them.
Q: Tell me first, that's the first step. You might not even feel like you want to tell them what you think of them by the end of the therapy, you might just decide that you know what you think of them, it's a lot more clearer in your mind what you think of them and what's gone on and that you just need to move away from letting them influence you so much that you are destroying yourself.
A: Yes.
Q: We'll see what happens. O.K. well we'll stop there. Another quick hour.

Author Index

A

Abrams, R., 373, 381
Ackerman, S. J., 114, 117
Acuff, C., 344, 356
Adams, J., 51, 65
Addis, M. E., 253, 269, 272
Adelman, H. S., 353, 354, 358
Agnew, R. M., 106, 112, 116, 257, 269
Ahn, H., 330, 341
Albani, C., 128, 140
Alexander, D. A., 280, 288
Alexander, F., 51, 65, 251, 270
Alexander, K., 149, 163
Allen, J. G., 167, 173, 181, 183, 190, 212
Amlo, S., 113, 117, 170, 180, 183, 319, 321
Ancis, J. R., 336, 337, 340
Anderson, E. E., 9, 21, 23, 33, 44
Anderson, E. M., 23, 24, 25, 26, 27, 28, 30, 31, 40, 42, 43, 104, 105, 114, 115, 116, 117, 311, 312, 321
Andrews, A. A., 26, 43, 114, 117, 312, 321
Andrews, C., 301, 307
Andrews, G., 310, 321
Andrusyna, T. P., 105, 106, 117
Appelbaum, P. S., 349, 350, 351, 353, 356
Applebaum, H., 71, 99
Arnold, E. G., 293, 294, 299, 300, 301, 302, 303, 305
Aron, L., 233, 234, 235, 248
Arredondo, P., 326, 329, 338
Asay, T. P., 309, 312, 315, 316, 317, 318, 321, 343, 346, 365

Asay, T., 3, 18, 19
Atkinson, D. R., 329, 338
Atwood, G., 188, 214, 289, 290, 291, 306
Audin, K., 4, 11, 19, 21, 23, 33, 42
Auerbach, A., 29, 43, 331, 341
Aveline, M. O., 253, 270
Azarian, K., 149, 150, 162
Azim, H. E., 28, 29, 44
Azim, H. F. A., 76, 77, 78, 79, 93, 94, 95, 98, 99, 100, 105, 107, 109, 110, 118, 152, 153, 154, 163, 168, 169, 170, 171, 172, 173, 174, 175, 176, 178, 180, 182, 183, 184

B

Bachrach, H. M., 171, 183
Bahrick, A. S., 333, 338
Baird, B. N., 282, 287
Bakeman, R., 127, 140
Baker, H. S., 29, 29, 42
Banon, E., 181, 182
Baranackie, K., 14, 19, 149, 162
Barber, J. P., 4, 8, 15, 16, 17, 19, 21, 24, 25, 42, 51, 60, 66, 107, 113, 116, 127, 133, 137, 140, 142, 148, 149, 152, 153, 162, 171, 172, 174, 189, 183
Barchat, D., 294, 306
Barkham, M., 4, 11, 19, 21, 23, 33, 42, 105, 106, 112, 113, 116, 117, 118, 257, 269, 346, 358
Bartholomew, K., 8, 20
Batchelder, S. T., 8, 21, 198, 208, 209, 210, 213, 214
Bauer, G. P., 51, 65, 346, 356
Bauer, P. B., 24, 25, 27, 28, 29, 30, 42

Bearden, C., 252, 270
Beauchamp, T. L., 346, 356
Beck, A. T., 14, 19, 40, 42, 115, 116, 319, 321
Beerup, C., 51, 62, 67
Behrends, R., 289, 290, 291, 292, 301, 306, 307
Bellak, L., 51, 65
Bender, D., 294, 295, 301, 303, 306, 307
Benedict, J. G., 344, 356
Benjamin, A., 51, 62, 65
Benjamin, L. S., 8, 19, 26, 42, 190, 201, 212
Bennett, B. E., 344, 351, 356
Bennett, D., 123, 142, 255, 260, 267, 268, 270
Benninghoven, D., 128, 140
Benson, K., 330, 341
Benson, L., 11, 19, 23, 33, 42
Bentsen, H., 319, 321
Bergin, A. E., 29, 37, 39, 42, 43, 47, 65, 310, 322, 343, 344, 357
Bergman, A., 291, 307
Bergmann, M., 290, 298, 306
Berman, J. S., 37, 44, 105, 106, 117
Bernard, H., 290, 294, 306
Bernard, J. M.,
Bernstein, D. M., 344, 358
Bers, S., 292, 293, 306
Beutler, L. E., 4, 5, 8, 10, 16, 19, 20, 23, 33, 42, 50, 65, 269, 270, 312, 322, 326, 330, 337, 338, 339, 340
Bienvenu, J. P., 78, 100, 106, 118, 148, 151, 163, 166, 169, 183
Binder, J. L., 25, 30, 42, 51, 67, 106, 112, 116, 118, 126, 130, 142, 143, 146, 163, 192, 194, 212, 327, 331, 334, 339, 340
Blacker, K., 293, 307
Blagys, M. D., 114, 117
Blaser, G., 128, 140
Blass, R. B., 292, 293, 306
Blatt, S. J., 5, 11, 14, 19, 22, 289, 290, 291, 292, 293, 295, 306, 307, 331, 339

Bloch, S., 70, 98
Blok, G., 52, 63, 65
Bloom, B. L., 51, 59, 65, 346, 356
Blotcky, M. J., 253, 269, 272
Boa, C., 383, 388
Boddy, G., 115, 117
Bogels, S. M., 52, 63, 65
Bogwald, K. P., 319, 321
Bohart, A. C., 3, 16, 19, 22
Bond, M., 181, 182
Borden, E., 54, 60, 65
Borders, L. D., 328, 339
Bordin, E. S., 192, 212, 251, 252, 270, 330, 333, 339
Boroto, D. R., 95, 99
Bosley, C. M., 383, 388
Bostic, J. Q., 253, 269, 272
Bower, G. H., 124, 140
Boyer, S. P., 277, 288
Braaten, E. B., 350, 356
Bradley, C., 3, 19
Brandchaft, B., 188, 214
Bricklin, P. M., 344, 346, 347, 356, 358
Brill, P. C., 312, 321
Brill, P. L., 4, 5, 9, 10, 20, 281, 288
Brittan-Powell, C. S., 333, 340
Brown, G. K., 115, 116
Brown, M. T., 326, 333, 339
Brownlow, A., 301, 307
Bruner, J. S., 291, 296, 301, 306
Bryant, B., 351, 356
Bucci, W., 123, 123, 129, 140, 141
Budman, S. H., 51, 65, 275, 278, 280, 288
Burge-Callaway, K., 127, 140
Burlingame, G., 26, 31, 43, 313, 315, 321, 322
Burstein, E., 71, 99
Busch, F. N., 121, 142
Buss, A. H., 71, 98
Busse, W. M., 354, 356
Butcher, J. N., 34, 42
Butler, S. F., 3, 14, 19, 22, 187, 193, 212, 234, 248, 334, 340
Buysse, D., 252, 270

C

Canter, M. B., 344, 356
Cardella, H., 51, 53, 67
Carifio, M. S., 326, 339
Carkhuff, R. R., 365, 381
Carozzoni, P., 242, 249
Carpenter, D., 37, 39, 44
Carroll, K. M., 26, 42
Carter, J. A., 330, 339
Case, R., 71, 99
Caston, J., 129, 140
Castonguay, L. G., 6, 20, 266, 270
Chambless, D. L., 112, 116
Chance, S. E., 127, 140
Charles, D., 328, 340
Charman, D. P., 4, 19
Cheavers, J. S., 8, 22
Chevron, E. S., 51, 66, 292, 295, 306, 332, 340
Chew-Graham, C., 115, 117
Chi, M. T. H., 327, 339
Childress, A., 149, 163
Childress, J. F., 346, 356
Chittams, J., 113, 116, 149, 150, 162
Christensen, E. R., 33, 39, 43
Ciarlo, J. A., 36, 37, 39, 44
Cierpka, M., 128, 140
Claiborn, C. D., 351, 358
Clark, J. M., 4, 21
Clarkin, J. F., 326, 330, 337, 338
Clement, P. W., 309, 315, 321
Cohen, K. D., 149, 163
Collins, J. F., 28, 45
Collins, J. L., 29, 43
Collins, W. D., 111, 116
Colson, D. B., 167, 173, 181, 183, 190, 212
Connell, J., 4, 11, 19, 21, 23, 33, 42
Connolly, M. B., 148, 149, 150, 152, 153, 162, 171, 172, 174, 189, 183
Constantine, M. G., 329, 333, 337, 339, 340
Cook, D. A., 333, 339
Cooley, R. S., 292, 293, 294, 295, 296, 297, 301, 302, 303, 307

Coonerty, S., 292, 306
Cooper, A., 127, 140, 154, 162
Cooper, C. C., 344, 348, 349, 357
Copper, A. M., 121, 142
Cornell, W. F., 51, 66
Coyne, L., 71, 99, 167, 173, 181, 183, 190, 212
Crago, M., 6, 16, 19, 20
Craig, R., 47, 51, 52, 53, 62, 63, 66, 67
Cristol, A. H., 56, 67
Crits-Christoph, P., 4, 8, 15, 16, 17, 18, 19, 20, 21, 24, 25, 29, 42, 43, 51, 60, 66, 104, 105, 107, 113, 116, 117, 126, 127, 137, 140, 142, 146, 148, 149, 150, 152, 153, 154, 162, 163, 171, 172, 174, 189, 183, 196, 213, 252, 271, 310, 321, 331, 340
Crocker, P., 188, 195, 214, 253, 257, 271
Culverwell, A., 106, 112, 116
Cummings, J. L., 343, 357
Cummings, N. A., 343, 349, 357
Curtis, D., 129, 141
Curtis, J. T., 107, 1101, 116, 118, 123, 126, 129, 130, 140, 141, 142, 143, 153, 163
Cusack, A., 51, 62, 67

D

D'Andrea, M., 326, 329, 339
Dahl, A. A., 112, 118
Dahl, L., 127, 140
Dahlbender, R., 128, 140
Daigle, D., 128, 141
Daniels, J., 326, 329, 339
Danzinger, P. R., 354, 355, 357, 359
Datz, J., 51, 53, 67
Datz-Weems, H., 51, 62, 67, 377, 381
Davanloo, H., 51, 58, 66, 112, 116, 166, 183
Davanloo, I. I., 25, 29, 30, 42
Davidovitz, D., 343, 347, 357
Davies, J. M., 188, 212
Davis, M. K., 187, 213

Davis, S. R., 36, 44, 349, 350, 357, 358
Dawes, R. M., 327, 339
De Bosset, F., 276, 281, 283, 288
De Carufel, F. L., 78, 98, 148, 151, 163, 166, 169, 183
de la Mora, A., 344, 358
Debbane, E. G., 78, 100, 106, 118, 148, 151, 163, 166, 169, 183
DeBernardo, C. R., 344, 358
DeCarufel, F. L., 27, 28, 29, 30, 44, 78, 100
DeJulio, S. S., 33, 39, 43
Delaney, M. K., 127, 142
Delworth, C. D., 328, 341
Delworth, U., 328, 340
Demorest, A., 149, 150, 162
Derogatis, L. R., 299, 306, 313, 319, 321
DeRubeis, R. J., 31, 45, 95, 99, 108, 117
Diamond, D., 292, 306
Diemer, R., 238, 250
Diguer, L., 6, 9, 11, 21, 105, 106, 117, 127, 140, 142, 331, 340, 341
Dixon, W. J., 78, 99
Docherty, J. P., 9, 19
Dorpat, T., 16, 19
Drob, S., 290, 294, 306
Dubin, S., 344, 357
Duffy, M., 361, 364, 368, 375, 379, 381
Duncan, S. C., 13, 18, 21, 78, 79, 93, 98, 100, 169, 173, 182, 183

E

Eagle, M., 72, 98
Eagles, J. M., 280, 288
Eaves, L. J., 121, 141
Edbril, S. D., 347, 357
Edelson, M., 289, 306
Eells, T. D., 107, 116, 122, 123, 128, 129, 141
Efstation, J. F., 333, 339
Ehrenberg, D. B., 188, 212

Einstein, D. A., 114, 117
Eisenthal, S., 51, 66
Eisman, E. J., 344, 358
Elkin, I., 9, 11, 13, 14, 19, 28, 37, 38, 39, 43, 45
Ellenberger, H. F., 6, 20
Elliott, R., 4, 22, 37, 42, 195, 208, 212, 214
Enggelstad, V., 170, 180, 183
Epstein, L., 234, 237, 248
Epstein, M., 206, 212
Erbaugh, J., 40, 42, 319, 321
Erikson, E. H., 132, 133, 141, 375, 381
Evans, C., 11, 4, 19, 21, 23, 33, 42
Ewert, M., 128, 129, 141
Eysenck, H. J., 33, 42

F

Falvey, J. E., 327, 336, 339
Farber, B. A., 290, 293, 294, 295, 297, 298, 299, 301, 302, 303, 305, 306, 307, 308
Farber, E., 127, 140
Farr, M. J., 327, 339
Fassinger, R. E., 241, 249
Faude, J., 127, 142
Feiner, A. H., 234, 237, 248
Fenigstein, A., 71, 98
Fiegenheimer, W. V., 50, 59, 66
Finch, A. E., 10, 11, 21, 23, 33, 43, 114, 117, 309, 312, 313, 317, 322
Firth-Cozens, J. A., 12, 22, 148, 163
Flasher, L. V., 234, 248
Flegenagimer, W., 25. 26, 44, 45, 52, 67
Fonagy, P., 4, 16, 20, 22
Fong, M. L., 326, 328, 329, 339
Foreman, S. A., 151, 162, 192, 212, 253, 270
Forman, E. M., 317, 321
Fortune, A. E., 278, 282, 285, 288
Fosbury, J. A., 383, 388
Fossum, A., 170, 180, 183
Fox, R., 56, 67

Frager, S., 348, 357
Frances, A., 167, 183
Frank, E., 252, 267, 270
Frank, J., 62, 66
Franks, R. P., 337, 341
Freedman, N., 311, 317, 321
French, T. M., 51, 65, 251, 270
Fretter, P. B., 110, 118, 130, 143, 153, 163
Freud, S., 72, 98, 127, 141, 145, 162, 231, 232, 238, 243, 248, 290, 291, 293, 294, 306
Frevert, G., 128, 140
Fridhandler, B., 129, 141
Fried, D., 18, 20, 149, 162
Friedlander, M. L., 336, 337, 341
Friedman, S. H., 51, 65, 120, 142
Frieswyk., S., 167, 173, 181, 183, 190, 212
Frosch, A., 311, 317, 321
Froyd, J. D., 35, 36, 42, 319, 321
Froyd, J. E., 36, 42

G

Gabbard, G. O., 167, 173, 181, 183, 190, 212, 233, 235, 248, 249
Gaines, R., 304, 307
Galvain, M. D., 351, 357
Garant, J., 78, 100, 106, 118, 148, 151, 163, 166, 169, 183
Garb, H. N., 122, 141
Garfield, S. L., 15, 20, 25, 27, 42, 47, 65, 251, 270
Garske, J. P., 187, 213
Gaston, L., 12, 13, 20, 192, 212
Gatt, C., 292, 306
Gatz, M., 354, 357
Gawin, F. H., 26, 42
Geller, J. D., 290, 291, 292, 293, 294, 295, 296, 298, 298, 299, 301, 302, 303, 305, 306, 307, 308
Gelso, C. J., 191, 212, 233, 235, 236, 238, 239, 240, 241, 242, 243, 249, 250, 275, 276, 277, 279, 282, 286, 287, 288, 330, 339

Gendlin, E. T., 110, 117, 209, 213
Gesten, E. L., 348, 357
Geyer, M., 128, 140
Gill, M. M., 166, 183
Glaser, R., 327, 339
Glass, D., 28, 45
Glass, G. V., 10, 11, 12, 22, 281, 288, 310, 322
Goates, M. K., 31, 34, 43, 309, 312, 315, 316, 317, 318, 321
Goldfried, M. R., 6, 20
Goldman, R., 120, 141, 279, 288
Goldrfied, M. R., 253, 266, 268, 270
Gomez, M. J., 241, 249
Goodyear, R. L., 327, 338
Gorkin, M., 238, 249
Gorman, B. S., 210, 213, 214
Gorman, J. M., 4, 21
Gorsuch, N., 363, 381
Gottlieb, M. C., 344, 348, 349, 357
Gough, H. G., 76, 98
Grace, M., 336, 339
Grawe, K., 27, 28, 29, 44, 252, 271, 317, 322
Grawe-Gerber, M., 201, 212
Gray, L. A., 336, 337, 340
Greenberg, J. R., 78, 98, 187, 192, 212, 213, 234, 249
Greenberg, L. S., 9, 18, 20, 54, 63, 66, 120, 141, 194, 214, 252, 257, 260, 268, 270, 271, 326, 330, 333, 340
Greenson, R. R., 190, 191, 212, 326, 330, 340
Greenwood, A., 351, 356
Gregersen, A. T., 309, 312, 315, 316, 317, 318, 321
Grenier, M., 181, 182
Grenyer, B. F. S., 127, 141
Grissom, G., 9, 21, 23, 33, 44, 105, 114, 115, 116, 117
Groth-Marnat, G., 326, 330, 337, 340
Gruen, R., 292, 307
Gunderson, J. G., 253, 272
Gurman, A. S., 275, 278, 280, 288
Gustafson, J. P., 279, 288

Gustafson, K. E., 353, 354, 357
Guthrie, E., 115, 117
Guyatt, G., 34, 35, 43

H

Haas, E., 31, 40, 42
Haas, L. J., 349, 357
Haight, B. K., 379, 381
Hales, R. E., 25, 45
Haley, M., 344, 358
Haley, W. E., 354, 357
Haller, O., 344, 358
Halstead, J., 106, 112, 116
Handelsman, M. M., 350, 351, 356, 357, 358
Hannöver, W., 23, 33, 43
Hansen, N. B., 10, 11, 21, 26, 31, 43, 114, 117, 309, 312, 313, 315, 317, 321, 322
Harady, G. E., 113, 117
Hardy, E., 328, 340
Hardy, G. E., 105, 106, 112, 118, 346, 358
Harkness, D., 334, 340
Harp, J. S., 242, 249
Harper, H., 200, 212, 257, 269
Harrie, S., 51, 62, 67
Harrington, V. M. G., 106, 112, 116
Hartkamp, N., 112, 117
Hartley, D., 129, 141, 292, 293, 294, 295, 296, 297, 301, 302, 303, 307
Hartmann, K., 131, 141
Harvey, R., 310, 321
Harwood, T. M., 4, 19
Hathaway, S. R., 34, 42
Hawkins, E. J., 31, 34, 43, 313, 322
Hayes, A. M., 266, 270
Hayes, F., 349, 357
Hayes, J. A., 233, 235, 236, 238, 240, 241, 242, 249, 250
Haynes, S. N., 120, 142
Heath, A. C., 121, 141
Heimann, P., 233, 249
Helms, J. E., 147, 151, 162, 333, 339

Henry, W. P., 8, 9, 14, 18, 20, 189, 190, 192, 202, 212, 213, 252, 253, 270, 334, 340
Hensen, N. B., 23, 33, 43
Herron, W. G., 10, 22
Hersen, M., 51, 53, 66
Herzog, C., 348, 358
Hess, A. K., 326, 333, 339, 340
Heyerdahl, O., 113, 117, 170, 180, 183, 319, 321
Hill, C. E., 15, 20, 51, 53, 62, 66, 147, 151, 162, 195, 214, 242, 249, 328, 340
Hill, R. D., 31, 40, 42
Hilliard, R. B., 8, 9, 14, 18, 20, 190, 213
Hillis, G., 280, 288
Hilsenroth, M. J., 114, 117
Hoeglend, P., 25, 27, 28, 42
Hoffenberg, J. D., 311, 317, 321
Hofheinz, E. W., 337, 340
Hogland, P., 95, 98, 108, 109, 113, 117, 152, 163, 167, 170, 171, 172, 180, 183, 319, 321
Holahan, W., 276, 279, 288
Hole, A. V., 149, 163
Holland, S. J., 111, 117
Holloway, E. L., 327, 328, 338, 340, 341
Honig, M., 294, 295, 297, 307
Horney, K., 189, 213
Horowitz, L. M., 8, 20, 27, 28, 29, 32, 36, 37, 38, 39, 43, 71, 99, 167, 173, 181, 183, 190, 212
Horowitz, M. J., 51, 66, 95, 99, 108, 117, 126, 128, 129, 141
Horvath, A. O., 9, 12, 13, 18, 20, 54, 66, 187, 213, 252, 270, 290, 307, 326, 330, 333, 340
Howard, K. I., 4, 5, 8, 9, 10, 11, 12, 20, 21, 23, 33, 44, 57, 67, 114, 115, 117, 281, 288, 290, 307, 312, 321, 322
Hoyt, M., 51, 65
Huefner, J. C., 26, 31, 43, 313, 315, 322

AUTHOR INDEX

Hulse, S. H., 71, 99
Hussian, R. A., 365, 381

I

Imber, S., 252, 271, 331, 340
Imbers, S. D., 28, 45
Imboden, J. B., 71, 99
Ingram, R. E., 29, 43
Inman, A. G., 337, 340
Iscoe, I., 379, 381
Ivey, A., 51, 52, 66

J

Jackson, P. R., 256, 270
Jacobs, M., 286, 288
Jacobson, N. S., 253, 256, 269, 271, 272, 314, 316, 321
James, J. W., 354, 357
Javier, R. A., 10, 22
Jenkins, W. W., 51, 66
Jennings, L., 326, 327, 328, 340, 341
Jensen, R. E., 344, 357
Jersell, J., 49, 67
Jilton, R., 8, 21, 209, 210, 213
Jochem, J., 51, 53, 67
Johnson, D. H., 243, 249
Johnson, M. E., 131, 141
Johnson, S., 127, 142
Johnsrud, C., 351, 357
Johnston, R., 292, 293, 306
Jollkovsky, M. P., 239, 249
Joyce, A. S., 18, 22, 28, 29, 44, 76, 77, 79, 82, 93, 94, 95, 99, 100, 105, 107, 109, 110, 117, 118, 152, 153, 154, 163, 168, 169, 170, 171, 172, 173, 174, 175, 176, 178, 180, 183, 184, 266, 271
Judd, S. L., 383, 388
Junkert-Tress, B., 112, 117
Jurich, J., 51, 65

K

Kachele, H., 128, 140

Kadera, S. W., 26, 43, 114, 117, 312, 321
Kadlec, M., 51, 53, 67
Kalichman, S. C., 354, 357
Kamas, N., 25, 43
Kanfer, F. H., 51, 62, 66
Kapur, N., 115, 117
Kardash, C. A. M., 333, 339
Karno, M. P., 325, 326, 328, 341
Karp, J. F., 252, 270
Karuza, J., Jr., 331, 341
Kaslow, N. J., 127, 140, 292, 306
Kavanagh, G., 292, 307
Kazdin, A. E., 15, 20, 309, 312, 321
Keisler, D. J., 110, 117
Keith-Spiegel, P. S., 349, 357
Kell, B. L., 367, 381
Kell, W. L., 371, 381
Kemper, M. B., 351, 357
Kendall, P. C., 314, 322
Kendler, K. S., 121, 141
Kernberg, O., 71, 99, 233, 249
Kerr, G. P., 209, 214
Kerr, I. B., 254, 271
Kessler, R. C., 121, 141
Kesson-Craig, P., 351, 357
Kestenbaum, R., 26, 45
Kiel, S., 51, 62, 67
Kiesler, D. J., 202, 206, 209, 213, 233, 234, 235, 249, 253, 271
King, R., 4, 20
Kirshner, B., 34, 35, 43
Kivlinghan, D. M., 192, 213, 253, 271, 336, 339
Klein, M. H., 16, 20, 110, 117, 192, 213
Klein, R., 25, 28, 43
Kleintjes, S., 334, 340
Klerman, G. L., 51, 66, 121, 142, 332, 340
Knapp, S. J., 344, 356
Kobos, J. C., 24, 25, 27, 28, 29, 30, 42, 63, 65, 346, 356
Koerner, K., 120, 142, 253, 269, 272
Kohout, J., 344, 358
Kohut, H., 73, 99, 192, 213

Koocher, G. P., 349, 357
Kopta, S. M., 114, 117, 312, 321, 322
Kordon, M., 48, 51, 66, 67
Kordy, H., 23, 33, 43
Korner, A., 128, 140
Krakauer, I. D., 113, 116
Kramer, S. A., 278, 288
Krause, E. D., 105, 106, 117
Krause, M. S., 114, 117, 312, 321
Kremer, T. G., 348, 357
Kreutzkamp, R., 52, 63, 65
Krosnick, J., 354, 358
Krupnick, J. L., 11, 22
Kuhn, T., 216, 230
Kunce, J., 336, 339
Kurcias, J. S., 14, 19

L

Ladany, N., 329, 333, 335, 336, 337, 339, 340
Lafferty, P., 8, 20
Laikin, M., 113, 118, 167, 168, 180, 184
Lambert, M. J., 3, 8, 10, 11, 12, 19, 21, 22, 23, 24, 25, 26, 27, 28, 29, 30, 31, 33, 34, 36, 37, 38, 39, 40, 41, 42, 43, 44, 104, 105, 114, 116, 117, 309, 310, 311, 312, 313, 315, 316, 317, 318, 319, 321, 322, 343, 344, 346, 356, 357
Lampropoulos, G. K., 4, 21
Landrum-Brown, J., 326, 329, 333, 339
Langs, R., 16, 21, 204, 213, 215, 216, 217, 218, 220, 222, 228, 230, 280, 288
Lansford, E., 192, 213
Latts, M. G., 239, 241, 249
Lavelle, N., 252, 270
Lazare, A., 51, 66
Leach, C., 11, 19, 23, 33, 42
Lease, S., 326, 329, 339
Leber, W. R., 28, 45
Lebowitz, B. D., 4, 21
Lee, R. R., 277, 288

Lehrman-Waterman, D., 333, 335, 336, 340
Leifer, M., 47, 52, 53, 63, 67
Leonardi, F., 51, 66
Lessler, K., 56, 67
Levenson, H., 126, 130, 131, 142, 234, 249, 347, 357
Levenson, L., 131, 141
Levine, F. J., 149, 163
Levitt, J. T., 105, 106, 117
Liberman, B., 252, 271, 331, 340
Lidz, C. W., 350, 356
Ligiero, D. P., 241, 249
Linehan, M. M., 26, 45, 120, 142, 253, 271
Liton, C., 49, 67
Littlel, M., 233, 249
Loewald, H. W., 289, 290, 293, 307
Loganbill, C., 328, 340
Lowry, J. L., 114, 117, 312, 322
Luborsky, E., 240, 243, 249
Luborsky, L., 4, 6, 8, 9, 11, 12, 13, 15, 17, 18, 20, 21, 29, 43, 51, 58, 60, 66, 78, 100, 105, 106, 107, 112, 117, 123, 126, 127, 128, 133, 137, 140, 141, 142, 146, 148, 149, 152, 153, 154, 162, 163, 167, 171, 172, 173, 174, 183, 190, 191, 196, 213, 240, 241, 243, 249, 250, 252, 271, 290, 307, 331, 340, 341
Lucock, M., 11, 19, 23, 33, 42
Lueger, R. J., 8, 9, 10, 20, 21, 23, 33, 44, 114, 115, 117
Lunnen, K., 26, 31, 43, 313, 315, 322
Lutz, W., 4, 5, 9, 10, 20, 21, 23, 33, 44, 114, 115, 117, 281, 288, 312, 321
Lutz, Z., 4, 5, 9, 10, 20

M

Machado, P. P., 50, 65, 269, 270, 330, 339
Mackway-Jones, K., 115, 117
Mahlelr, M., 291, 307

Malan, D. H., 10, 16, 21, 25, 27, 28, 29, 30, 44, 51, 66, 71, 99, 106, 107, 113, 117, 151, 163, 166, 183, 275, 278, 279, 282, 288
Maling, M., 114, 117
Mann, E., 51, 53, 67
Mann, J., 25, 44, 279, 288
Marax, J. A., 276, 277, 279, 286, 287, 288
Marble, A., 319, 321
Marciano, P., 301, 307
Marginson, F. R., 4, 11, 19, 21, 23, 33, 42
Marini, Z., 71, 99
Marino-Francis, F., 115, 117
Mark, D., 51, 66, 127, 140, 240, 243, 249
Marmar, C. R., 27, 29, 32, 43, 60, 66, 95, 99, 108, 117, 151, 162, 192, 212, 253, 270
Marmor, J., 26, 29, 44
Martin, D. J., 11, 22, 187, 213
Martinovich, Z., 4, 5, 9, 10, 20, 21, 23, 33, 44, 114, 115, 117, 281, 288, 312, 321
Maruish, M. E., 319, 322
Marziali, E. A., 166, 183
Masters, K. S., 37, 39, 40, 41, 43, 44
Masterton, J. F., 6, 21
Matarazzo, J. D., 51, 66, 68
Mathieu, P. L., 110, 117
Mathieu-Coughlan, P. L., 192, 213
May, P. R. A., 78, 99
Mayer, J., 28, 45
McCallum, M., 18, 22, 28, 29, 44, 71, 74, 76, 77, 79, 82, 93, 94, 95, 99, 100, 105, 107, 109, 110, 118, 152, 153, 154, 163, 168, 169, 170, 171, 172, 173, 174, 175, 176, 178, 180, 183, 184, 266, 271
McClanahan, M. K., 242, 249
McCracken, J. E., 242, 249
McCullough, L., 26, 45, 51, 67, 113, 118, 167, 168, 180, 184
McGlynn, E. A., 37, 44
McGrath, G., 4, 11, 19, 21, 23, 33, 42

McKinley, J. C., 34, 42
McLain, J., 351, 357
McLaughlin, J. T., 252, 271
McLean, P., 26, 44
McLellan, A. T., 6, 9, 11, 21, 252, 271, 331, 340, 341
McMain, S., 198, 195, 214, 253, 257, 271
McNamara, J. R., 353, 354, 357
McNeill, B. W., 328, 336, 337, 341
McWhirter, J. J., 127, 142
Meier, S. T., 36, 44, 349, 357
Meisel, A., 350, 356
Meissner, W. W., 290, 307
Melles, R., 52, 63, 65
Mellon, J., 127, 131, 140, 141, 149, 163
Mellor-Clark, J., 11, 19, 23, 33, 42
Meloy, J. R., 48, 67
Mendel, E., 115, 117
Mendelson, M., 40, 42, 319, 321
Menninger, K., 107, 118
Mergenthaler, E., 129, 141
Messer, S. B., 17, 21, 104, 105, 106, 111, 112, 114, 116, 117, 118, 130, 142, 374, 376, 381
Meuller, W. J., 367, 371, 381
Miars, R., 348, 358
Michael, S. T., 8, 22
Millbrath, C., 128, 129, 141
Miller, D. J., 348, 357
Miller, R. C., 37, 44
Miller, T. I., 10, 11, 12, 22, 281, 288, 310, 322
Milner, J., 34, 44
Milton, J., 386, 388
Ming, S., 149, 163
Mintz, J., 29, 43
Mitchell, S. A., 17, 21, 78, 98, 192, 212, 234, 238, 249
Mobley, M., 337, 341
Mock, J., 40, 42, 319, 321
Mohr, D. C., 6, 8, 11, 13, 21, 279, 288
Moldawsky, S., 344, 356
Molingaro, M., 333, 335, 336, 340
Mondin, G. W., 330, 341

Moody, M., 330, 341
Moorey, J., 115, 117
Moos, R. H., 28, 44
Morales, P., 375, 381
Moran, G., 16, 20
Moras, K., 4, 5, 9, 10, 20, 281, 288, 312, 321
Morrell, B., 31, 40, 42
Morris, M., 127, 142
Morris, W., 260, 271
Morrison, J. K., 315, 322
Morrow, D. G., 124, 140
Morse, J. O., 113, 116
Morten, G., 329, 338
Muenz, L., 149, 150, 162
Muran, J. C., 8, 21, 113, 118, 187, 188, 193, 198, 291, 206, 207, 208, 209, 210, 213, 214, 251, 253, 257, 271
Murphy, M. J., 344, 358
Murray, P., 188, 195, 214, 253, 257, 271

N

Najavits, L. M., 6, 7, 8, 12, 13, 14, 21
Nathan, P. E., 4, 21
Nathans, S., 130, 142
Neale, M. C., 121, 141
Neimeyer, G. J., 328, 339
Nelson, M. L., 325, 326, 328, 336, 337, 341
Neufeldt, S. A., 50, 65, 269, 270, 330, 325, 326, 328, 329, 335, 339, 341
Newman, F. L., 36, 37, 39, 44, 260, 270
Newman, R., 346, 347, 358
Newsom, G., 167, 173, 181, 183, 190, 212
Nezu, A. M., 120, 142
Nezu, C. M., 120, 142
Niedeerehe, G., 4, 21
Nielsen, S. L., 31, 34, 43, 313, 322
Nixon, G. W. H., 78, 79, 93, 98, 99, 169, 173, 182

Norman, H., 293, 307
Norman, N. A., 344, 358
Norville, R., 153, 163
Nowell, D., 348, 358
Nuland, S. B., 124, 142

O

O'Brien, P. W., 331, 340, 341
O'Kelly, J. G., 18, 22, 178, 180, 184, 266, 271
Ogles, B. M., 37, 39, 40, 41, 43, 44
Ogrodniczuk, J. S., 18, 22, 76, 77, 79, 82, 93, 94, 99, 100, 105, 118, 173, 174, 175, 180, 183, 266, 271
Okey, J. L., 127, 142
Okiishi, J., 26, 31, 43, 313, 315, 322
Oliveri, M. E., 28, 45
Oremland, J., 293, 307
Orlinsky, D. E., 6, 8, 9, 10, 11, 12, 15, 20, 21, 27, 28, 29, 44, 57, 67, 114, 117, 252, 271, 290, 291, 292, 295, 307, 312, 317, 321, 322
Osimo, F., 25, 29, 30, 44
Otto, S., 350, 356

P

Pannu, R. K., 333, 340
Park, L. C., 71, 99
Park, T. J., 71, 99
Parks, B. K., 27, 28, 29, 44, 252, 271, 317, 322
Parloff, M. B., 37, 45
Parry, G., 255, 267, 268, 270
Patalano, F., 10, 22
Paterniti, A., 210, 214
Patton, M. J., 333, 339
Peabody, S. A., 239, 249
Pearlingi, B., 278, 282, 285, 288
Pearson, C. G., 354, 357
Peircy, F., 51, 65
Pekarik, G., 276, 280, 288
Perry, J. C., 126, 131, 132, 133, 142
Perry, S., 167, 183
Phelps, R., 344, 356, 358

Piaget, J., 291, 307
Pilkonis, P. A., 5, 14, 19, 28, 35, 44, 45, 331, 339, 340
Piller, C., 349, 358
Pine, F., 231, 249, 291, 307
Pingitore, D., 344, 358
Pinsker, H., 51, 67
Pinsof, W. M., 63, 66
Piper, W. E., 13, 18, 21, 22, 27, 28, 29, 30, 44, 71, 74, 76, 77, 78, 79, 82, 93, 94, 95, 98, 99, 100, 105, 106, 107, 109, 110, 117, 118, 148, 151, 152, 153, 154, 163, 166, 168, 169, 170, 171, 172, 173, 174, 175, 176, 178, 180, 182, 183, 184, 252, 266, 271, 280, 283, 288,
Pokomy, D., 128, 140
Polkinghorne, D. E., 123, 142
Pollack, J., 25, 26, 44, 45, 52, 67, 113, 118
Popp, C., 127, 131, 133, 140, 141, 142, 240, 243, 249
Primavera, L. H. H., 10, 22
Prince-Gibson, E., 292, 306

Q

Quinlan, D. M., 292, 295, 306
Quinn, M. J., 355, 358
Quintana, S. M., 276, 277, 279, 288

R

Rabinowitz, R. C., 331, 341
Racker, H., 234, 249
Raney, J., 216, 230
Raue, P. J., 6, 20, 266, 270
Redington, D., 129, 141
Reed, K. G., 328, 340
Rees, A., 105, 106, 112, 113, 116, 117, 118, 346, 358
Reich, A., 236, 239, 249
Reisinger, C. W., 26, 31, 43, 313, 315, 322
Revenstorf, D., 256, 271

Reynolds, S., 105, 106, 112, 113, 117, 118, 346, 358
Reznikoff, M., 71, 76, 100
Rhodes, R. H., 195, 214
Rice, L. N., 194, 209, 214, 260, 268, 271
Richard, M., 23, 33, 43
Ricks, D. F., 7, 13, 22
Ritzler, B., 293, 306
Robbins, L. L., 78, 100
Robbins, S. B., 239, 249
Roberts, N. E., 111, 117
Roberts, R. I., 326, 330, 337, 340
Rochelle, C. D., 278, 282, 285, 288
Rogers, C., 50, 62, 67
Ronnestad, M. H. 326, 328, 341
Rosenbaum, D. N., 48, 67
Rosenbaum, R., 27, 29, 32, 43, 95, 99, 108, 117
Rosenberg, S. E., 8, 20, 107, 116
Rosenberger, E. W., 241, 250
Rosenthal, R., 51, 67, 105, 106, 117
Rosenzweig, D., 294, 295, 308
Rosie, J. S., 18, 22, 76, 77, 79, 82, 92, 100, 178, 180, 184, 266, 271
Rosowsky, E., 373, 381
Roth, A., 4, 16, 22
Rothbaum, P. A., 344, 358
Rounsaville, B. J., 26, 42, 51, 66, 332, 340
Rozovsky, F. A., 354, 358
Rubin, N., 47, 52, 53, 63, 67
Rudolph, B., 47, 48, 51, 52, 53, 62, 63, 67
Russell, D. W., 344, 358
Russell, R. K., 333, 338
Russell, R. L., 15, 21
Ryle, A., 123, 142, 256, 268, 270, 271, 383, 383, 388

S

Sachs, J. S., 266, 271
Safran, J. D., 187, 188, 192, 193, 194, 195, 201, 202, 206, 207, 208, 209, 210, 213, 214, 251, 253, 257, 271

Salmi, S. W., 333, 338
Salovey, P., 122, 128, 141, 143
Sampson, H., 107, 108, 111, 116, 118, 129, 130, 141, 153, 163
Samstag, L. W., 8, 21, 113, 118, 188, 192, 198, 201, 202, 208, 209, 210, 211, 213, 214
Sanavio, E., 51, 67
Sanderson, S., 115, 117
Sandler, J., 70, 100
Sanislow, C. A., 5, 11, 14, 19, 22, 331, 339
Santoro, S., 355, 359
Sapiera, E. P., 260, 271
Sargent, H. D., 78, 100
Sayward, H. 292, 293, 306
Scarf, M., 348, 358
Schacht, T. E., 8, 20, 126, 130, 131, 141, 142, 189, 192, 202, 212, 213, 252, 270, 334, 340
Schaffer, C. E., 292, 295, 296, 306, 308
Schaffer, N., 127, 142
Schaffler, P., 127, 142
Scheffler, R., 344, 358
Scheft, B. K., 51, 62, 66
Scheier, M. F., 71, 98
Schmidt, K. A., 127, 142
Schmitz, M. F., 344, 358
Schmitz, N., 112, 117
Schmitz, P. J., 192, 213
Schneider, M., 62, 67
Schnierda, U., 112, 117
Schwalm, D., 344, 358
Schwartz, E., 48, 67
Scott, N. A., 344, 358
Segal, P. M., 78, 79, 98, 169, 173, 182
Segal, P. S., 93, 99
Seitz, P. F., 125, 126, 142
Seligman, D. A., 6, 9, 11, 21, 105, 106, 117, 331, 341
Seligman, M. E. P., 3, 4, 22, 278, 288, 311, 317, 319, 322, 346, 358
Semel, V. G., 361, 381
Sentell, T., 344, 358
Shadid, L. G., 253, 269, 272

Shaffer, C., 152, 153, 162, 171, 172, 174, 189, 183
Shapiro, D. A., 4, 12, 15, 22, 39, 49, 105, 106, 112, 113, 116, 117, 118, 148, 163, 257, 269, 271, 346, 358
Shapiro, T., 121, 142
Shappell, S., 148, 152, 153, 162, 171, 172, 174, 189, 183
Shaughnessy, P., 253, 271
Shea, T., 28, 45
Shear, M. K., 121, 142
Shearin, E. N., 253, 271
Sherin, E. N., 26, 45
Shmidt, H., 52, 63, 65
Shoemaker, W. E., 344, 358
Sifneos, P. E., 6, 21, 24, 25, 26, 29, 45, 51, 63, 67, 113, 118, 166, 184
Silberschatz, G., 107, 110, 116, 118, 123, 126, 129, 130, 133, 140, 141, 142, 143, 153, 163
Simmens, S., 11, 22
Singer, B. A., 240, 241, 250
Singer, J. L., 128, 129, 141
Sisenwein, F., 10, 22
Sjaastad, M. C., 319, 321
Skovholt, T. M., 326, 327, 328, 340, 341
Slade, A., 202, 214
Sloane, R. B., 56, 67
Smart, D. W., 31, 34, 43, 313, 322
Smelson, D., 48, 67
Smith, M. L., 10, 11, 12, 22, 281, 288, 310, 322
Snyder, C. R., 8, 22
Somberg, D. R., 351, 358
Somberg, E., 51, 53, 67
Sonksen, P. H., 383, 388
Sorbye, O., 170, 180, 183, 319, 321
Sorlie, O., 113, 117
Sorlie, T., 170, 180, 183
Sotsky, S. M., 11, 22
Spanier, C., 267, 270
Spence, D. P., 16, 22, 123, 124, 143
Spiegel, S. B., 147, 151, 162
Spielberger, C. D., 319, 322
Spillman, A., 111, 118, 130, 142

Spruce, D., 242, 250
Spruill, J., 348, 358
Staats, H., 128, 140
Staples, F. R., 56, 67
Startup, M., 105, 106, 112, 118, 346, 358
Steer, R. A., 115, 116
Stein, D. M., 8, 10, 11, 12, 22
Steinberg, P. I., 18, 22, 178, 180, 184, 266, 271
Stern, D. N., 291, 308
Stevens, C., 188, 210, 214
Stich, F., 330, 341
Stiles, T. C., 104, 118, 310, 322
Stiles, W. B., 4, 12, 15, 22, 106, 112, 113, 116, 117, 147, 148, 163, 269, 271
Stinson, C., 129, 141
Stolorow, R., 188, 214, 289, 290, 291, 306
Stoltenberg, C. D., 328, 341
Stone, G. L., 351, 358
Stone, M. H., 252, 271
Stone, M., 51, 53, 67
Stotsky, S., 28, 45
Strachey, J., 166, 184
Strack, M., 128, 140
Strapp, H. H., 14, 19
Street, L. L., 4, 21
Streeter, M. J., 9, 19
Strupp, H. H., 3, 6, 7, 8, 9, 12, 13, 14, 18, 20, 21, 22, 25, 28, 29, 30, 36, 37, 38, 39, 42, 43, 45, 56, 57, 67, 112, 118, 126, 130, 131, 141, 142, 143, 146, 163, 187, 189, 190, 192, 193, 194, 202, 212, 213, 214, 234, 248, 252, 253, 270, 271, 334, 340
Styrsky, E., 276, 281, 283, 288
Sue, D. W., 329, 338, 341
Sue, D., 329, 341
Sue, S., 347, 358
Sullivan, B., 349, 358
Sullivan, H. H., 17, 22, 50, 51, 62, 67, 192, 214, 239, 250, 285, 286, 288
Sullivan, J. M., 166, 183

Summers, F., 290, 308
Svartberg, M., 104, 118, 310, 322
Swatz, L., 334, 340
Symonds, B. D., 187, 213, 290, 307
Szkrumelak, N., 27, 28, 29, 30, 44, 78, 100

T

Talley, P. F., 3, 22
Tallman, K., 3, 22
Tan, J. A., 337, 341
Tang, T. Z., 31, 45
Tarragona, M., 290, 295, 307
Tasman, A., 15, 22
Taylor, G. J., 71, 100
Taylor, L., 353, 354, 358
Taylor, S., 26, 44
Teyber, E., 281, 282, 286, 287, 288
Thelen, M. H., 348, 357
Thompson, B. J., 195, 214
Tichenor, V., 147, 151, 162
Tishby, O., 111, 118, 130, 142
Tolor, A., 71, 76, 100
Tolpin, M., 6, 21
Tomenson, B., 115, 117
Tomita, S. K., 355, 358
Trabin, T., 35, 45
Tress, W., 112, 117
Truax, C. B., 365, 381
Truax, P., 256, 271, 314, 316, 321
Trudeau, L. S., 344, 358
Trujillo, M., 26, 45
Tryon, G., 49, 51, 57, 67
Turk, D. C., 122, 143
Turner, S. M., 51, 66
Turpin, C., 115, 117
Turvey, C., 128, 141
Tyson, R. L., 70, 100

U

Umphress, V., 26, 31, 43, 313, 315, 322
Unger, H. T., 71, 99
Ursano, R. J., 25, 45

V

Vaillant, G. E., 72, 100
VanderBos, G., 351, 356
van der Viuten, P., 52, 63, 65
Van Hasselt, V., 53, 66
Van Ravenswaay, P., 149, 163
VandeCreek, L., 348, 358
VanWagoner, S. L., 238, 250
Vayo, M., 49, 67
Vermeersch, D. A., 31, 34, 43, 313, 322
Visser, P. S., 354, 358
Vorus, N., 311, 317, 321
Voth, H., 71, 99
Vygotsky, L. S., 291, 308

W

Wachtel, P. L., 189, 202, 214
Wagner, L., 350, 358
Waldinger, R. J., 253, 272
Walker, J. A., 336, 337, 340
Wallerstein, R. S., 16, 22, 78, 100
Walter, M. I., 350, 358
Waltz, J., 253, 269, 272
Wampold, B. E., 5, 22, 105, 118, 326, 328, 330, 331, 332, 337, 338, 340, 341, 364, 381
Ward, C. H., 40, 42, 319, 321
Warner, K. K., 10, 22
Warren, C. S., 17, 21, 104, 112, 118, 374, 376, 381
Waskow, I. E., 37, 45
Watkins, J. T., 28, 45
Watkins, L. M., 202, 213
Webster, J. D., 379, 381
Wechsler, D., 34, 45
Wein, S., 292, 295, 306
Weiss, D., 27, 29, 32, 43, 95, 99, 108, 117
Weiss, J., 107, 108, 111, 116, 118, 129, 130, 141, 153, 163

Weissman, M. M., 51, 66, 332, 340
Welfel, E. R., 350, 351, 354, 355, 357, 359
Wells, M. G., 315, 321
Whipple, J. L., 31, 34, 43, 313, 322
Whipple, K., 56, 67
Wiborg, I. M., 112, 118
Wiens, A. N., 68
Wierzbicki, M., 276, 280, 288
Wild, C., 293, 306
Wilkinson, S. M., 233, 249
Winston, A., 8, 21, 25, 44, 45, 51, 67, 113, 118, 167, 168, 180, 184, 198, 202, 208, 209, 210, 213, 214
Wiseman, H., 292, 306
Wiser, S., 266, 270
Wittenberg, I., 275, 278, 279, 282, 285, 288
Wolfe, B., 253, 268, 270
Wolgast, B., 333, 335, 336, 340
Wolleat, P. L., 328, 340
Woodhouse, S. S., 275, 279, 282, 288
Woody, G., 6, 9, 11, 21, 252, 271, 331, 340, 341
Worthen, V., 336, 337, 341
Worthington, R. L., 337, 341
Wright, W. R., 344, 359
Wzontek, N., 294, 298, 299, 302, 303, 308

Y

Yorkston, N. J., 56, 67
Young, K., 347, 358

Z

Zane, N., 347, 358
Zetzel, E., 190, 214
Zevon, M. A., 331, 341
Zuroff, D. C., 5, 11, 14, 19, 22, 331, 339
Zweig, R., 373, 381

Subject Index

A

Academic psychotherapists
  qualities of, 8
Age
  see Supervision
Alexithymia
  see Psychological mindedness
Alliance ruptures
  resolution of transference related, 264
  see Rupture episodes
Alliance threatening interactions
  see Therapeutic alliance,
Anxiety
  and brief therapy, 105, 106
Attachment (maternal), 72

B

Bipolar disorder, 25
Borderline personality disorder, 25, 26, 73
Boundaries
  and self-representation, 293
Brief psychodynamic therapy (BPT)
  adherence to formulated focus, 103
  dose-effect relationship, 103
  effectiveness of, 103
  factors related to progress, 103
  importance of focus, 106-111
  meta-analysis, 103
  outcome factors, 106-116
  patient suitability, 103
  therapist interpretation, 107, 110
Brief psychodynamic therapy (BPT) and other therapies
  cognitive analytic therapy (CAT), 252-267
  cognitive-behavioral therapy, 105, 106
  importance of focus, 106-111
  outcome factors, 106-116
  plan formulation method, 107, 108
  psychodynamic-interpersonal therapy, 105, 106
  supportive therapy, 105, 106
  therapist interpretation, 107, 110
Brief vs. long-term therapy, 25-33, 103, 105

C

Case formulation
  aspects of content and process, 121-123
  defined, 120
  descriptive information, 121
  four goals of, 122
  history of, 124, 125
  methods, 126-140
  narrative communication, 123, 134
  personal-meaning information, 121, 122
  prototypical formulations, 121
  psychodynamic contributions to, 125, 126
Case formulation methods, 126-140
  cognitive analytic therapy (CAT), 251-267
  configural analysis (CA) 126, 128-130, 133-139

core conflictual relationship
theme (CCRT), and, 126-128,
137, 138
Plan Compatibility Intervention
Scale, 108
plan formulation method (PFM),
107, 108, 110
Case study
see June, a case study
Cyclical Maladaptive Patterns,
(CMP), 126, 130, 131, 138
Idiographic Conflict Formulation
Method (ICF), 126, 131-133, 139
Plan Formulation Method
(PFM), 126, 129, 138
CCRT
see core conflictual relationship
theme method
Child Abuse Potential Inventory
as a predicative measure, 34
Child abuse, 80
Clinical trials, 310
Cognitive analytic therapy (CAT)
alliance threatening enactments,
252-264
applications/implications, 267-
269
defined, 252, 254-256
model for enactment resolution,
258-263
psychotherapy outcome, 252
research strategy, 253
task resolution and processes,
257-260
testing the model, 265-267
transference-related ruptures,
252, 254
Cognitive deficits, 25
Communicative-adaptive
approach, 215-217
clinical illustration, 224-228
development of, 217, 218
deviations, 220
existential death anxiety, 221, 222
features of, 216
ground rules, 218-223

predatory/predator death
anxiety, 220-223
Conflictual impulses, 72
Constructing interpretations
accuracy of interpretation, 153,
154
accuracy of transference
interpretation, 154, 155
frequency of interpretation, 150,
151
patient narratives, 148-150
therapist utterances, 147, 148
training exercises, 156-162
transference interpretation, 146,
151-153
see also core conflictual relationship theme, 146; Cognitive
analytic therapy (CAT)
Control, 85-88
Core batteries for outcome
measurement, 33-40
Core Conflictual Relationship
Theme Method (CCRT), 17, 18
episode themes, 17
negative/positive themes, 17
patient narratives, 107
patient transference, 17, 18
rupture episodes, 196, 197, 209
see Case formulation methods
Countertransference
acute vs. chronic, 236
brief relational psychotherapy
and, 242-248
cause-effect-and prevalence of,
240, 242
complementary view, 234
conceptions of, 232
expression vs. emotional
reaction, 237
internal state vs. overt
expression, 236, 237
management of, 237-239, 242
relational conception, 234, 235
totalist view of, 232, 233
Cultural differences, 48
see Multicultural counseling

D

Death anxiety, 220-223
  and the older patient, 368, 378-380
Defense mechanisms, 72, 73
Dependent personality, 26
Depression, 5
  brief psychotherapy and other therapies compared, 105, 106
  and older patients, 366
  and diagnostic criteria, 112, 113
Diagnostic criteria
  and bulimia, 112
  and depression, 112
  and dose-effect, 112, 113
  and outcome, 111-116
  and panic disorder, 112
  and personality disorder, 113
  and psychsomatic disorder, 112, 113
Dose-effect relationship (number of sessions), 102, 112, 113
  and outcome studies, 112-114, 313
  and therapeutic change, 313
Drive theory, 72

E

Effect size
  see meta-analysis
Effectiveness research
  patient-focused approach, 4, 5
  variability in outcome, 10, 11
Effectiveness training, 11-14
Efficacy research, 3-5, 311
Efficacy-for-disorder research, 4
Ego strength, and outcome, 28, 29
Ending therapy
  see Termination phase
Ethical challenges
  adequate informed consent, 350-352
  maintaining confidentiality, 347-350
  reimbursement guidelines, 344, 345, 348
  responsible termination of therapy, 352, 353
  selecting appropriate clients, 343-347
  with minors or older adults, 353-355

F

First-interview tasks, 47, 48
  anatomy of, 51
  limitations of, 48, 49
  patient contributions, 61, 62
  phases of first interview, 62-64
  requirements of, 49
  therapeutic clusters (6 tasks) 55-64
  therapist attitudes, 50, 51
  therapist qualities, 50
  therapist tasks, 51-53
Focal adherence
  and outcome, 107, 108, 110, 111
  and therapy progress, 110, 111
Focality
  see Focus, Focal adherence
Focus
  importance of, 106-111

G

Gender bias
  in patient-client relations, 347
  see Supervision
Gender differences
  internalization of therapy, 297
Geriatric psychotherapy
  see Older adults

H

Health Sickness Rating Scale, 171
Hearing impaired, 48

SUBJECT INDEX

I

Identity, 88
Intelligence
   see Psychological mindedness (PM)
Internalization, 289-293
   as indicator of therapeutic change, 292, 293
   assessment of, 292, 293
   Freud and, 291
   gender differences, 297
   object-representation, 291
   self-representation, 291, 292
Internalization assessment
   Intersession Experience Questionnaire, 295-297
   Therapist Embodiment Scale (TES), 295-297
   Therapist Involvement Scale (TIS), 296-298
   Therapist Representation Inventory (TRI), 295-297
Internalization of therapy, 289-293
Interpretations, 145, 146
   rating accuracy of, 161, 162
   see Constructing interpretations, Transference interpretations
Interventions
   see Rupture episodes, Supervision, Training interventions

J

June, a case study, 383-388
   addendum, 96-98
   case formulation methods, 133-140
   confidentiality, 335, 336
   countertransference, 243-247
   financial responsibility, 335, 336
   informed consent, 335, 336
   transcript, 338-399

L

Loneliness, 73

M

Managed Care
   and outcome measurement, 35, 36
Manuals, 14
Mature-immature defenses, 72, 73
Medicare, see Older adults
Meta-analysis, 103-105, 310, 311
   study flaws, 104, 105
Multicultural counseling, 329, 333, 334
   see also Supervision

N

Narcissistic disorders, 73
Narratives, 107
   constructing interpretations, 148-150
   grand rules, 218-220
   in case formulation, 123, 124
   narrative communication, 123, 124, 148, 149
   see Communicative adaptive approach

O

Object constancy, 88
Object relations, 77, 78
   transference and, 167
Obsessive-compulsive behavior, 26
Older adult curative factors
   collateral impressions of adult children, 373
   consistency of personality, 373, 374
   counterintuitive dynamics, 377, 378
   death anxiety, 368, 378-380
   dependency needs, 377, 378
   depression, 366, 373
   developmental readiness, 374-377
   exploring early experiences, 368-371

in nursing homes, 363, 364, 373
inductive vs. deductive posture, 364, 365
interpretation and insight, 371, 372
Medicare, 361
periodic vs. sustained therapy, 362-364
personality problems, 372
psychodynamic process, 364
reminiscence and life review, 378, 379
transference and, 365-368
Organic brain damage, 25
Outcome measurement
    assessing outcome, 33, 34
    content dimension, 39
    Core Battery Conference (Vanderbilt University), 37-39
    evaluative measures, 34, 35
    feedback systems, 33, 34
    five-dimensional scheme for, 39, 40
    instruments for, 36
    managed care, 35, 36
    multidimensional nature of, 37
    Outcome Measures Project (OMP), 37-39
    predictive measures, 34
    scheme for organizing/conceptualizing outcome measurement, 39, 40
    social level dimension, 39
    source dimension, 40
    task of, 34
    technology dimension, 40
    tests for, 34
    time orientation dimension, 40
Outcome research
    clinical trials, 310
    dose-response relationship, 313
    duration of treatment, 311, 312
    Effectiveness Questionnaire, 311
    efficacy research, 311
    internalization of therapy, 290
    manner of termination, 300-303
    measuring change, 309
    meta-analysis, 310, 311
    patient-focused research, 312-318
    recommendations, 318-321
    self-report, 8, 9
    statistical significance, 314
    see also Constructing interpretations, Focal adherence, Predictors of Outcome, Supervision, Termination phase, Transference interpretations

P

Panic disorder, 112
Passive aggressive personality, 26
Patient dropout, 10
    see Termination phase
Patient narratives, 148-150
    decoding, 218
    see Training exercises
Peer ratings, 6
    effectiveness qualities, 7, 8
    empirical studies, 7
    telephone surveys, 6, 7
PM
    see Psychological mindedness
PMAP
    see Psychological mindedness assessment procedure
Predictive validity, 93, 94
Predictors of outcome
    candidates for short-term therapy, 24, 25
    capacity to relate, 28, 31
    early response to therapy, 30-32
    ego strength, 28, 29, 31, 32
    focality of problem, 30
    motivation to change, 30, 31
    Outcome Questionnaire, 26, 31
    psychological mindedness (PM), 29
    response to trial therapy, 30
    severity of disturbance, 25, 26, 31

Progress
  patient working involvement and, 110
Psychic determinism, 72
Psychodynamic psychotherapy
  drive structural model, 17
  empiricism and research, 15, 16
  process research, 17
  relational model, 17
Psychological mindedness (PM)
  ability to understand and apply interventions, 69-71
  importance of, 75, 76
  measurement approaches, 71, 75-77
  measurement scale, 73
  videotaped interactions, 73
Psychological mindedness assessment procedure (PMAP), 71
  nine levels of PM, 73-76, 95
  predictive validity, 77
  psychometric properties of, 76, 77
Psychosomatic complaints, 25
Psychotherapy
  defined 14
  theory-based, 15, 18
Psychotic vs. nonpsychotic patients
  therapy and, 25
Public Health Model, 4

Q

Quality of object relations (QOR), 77, 92-95
  affect regulation, 79
  assessment, 78, 79, 95
  behavioral manifestations, 79
  collaborative relationship with therapist, 69
  construct validity, 92, 93
  defined, 169
  formation, 84-86, 89
  high vs. low, 177, 178
  historical antecedents, 80
  importance of in STDP, 92-95
  levels in childhood, adolescence, adulthood, 80-83
  narrative formulation, 89-92
  predictive validity, 93-95
  relational meaning of the therapy event, 86-88
  scale development, 79-82
  scoring, 82
  self-esteem regulation, 79
Quality management systems, 23
  optimizing outcome, 23, 24
  psychometric measurement, 24, 36, 39

R

Rupture episodes
  facilitative interventions, 206-212
  misunderstanding events, 195-197
  rupture marker behaviors, 198-206, 209
  withdrawal and control ruptures, 200-202
Rupture Resolution Scale, 211
Rutgers Psychotherapy Progress Scale, 111

S

Self-awareness
  see Psychological mindedness
Session transcripts, 107, appendix
Short-term dynamic psychotherapy (STDP), 92-95
  and intake interview, 70, 71
  capacity for successful engagement in, 69
  importance of, 75, 76
  interventions, 84
Substance abuse, 112
  dependence, 25
Suicide, 25
Supervision
  Association for Counselor Education and Supervision, 336, 337

case conceptualization, 337
client characteristics and treatment plan, 330, 331
factors in 336
focus, 334-336
forming a therapeutic relationship, 330
goals and intentions, 326, 327
multicultural counseling, 329
nature of expertise, 327-329
nontraditional settings (nursing homes), 363, 364
reflectivity, 327-329
supervisory relationship, 333, 334
therapist competence, 331, 332
working alliance, 330, 332, 333

T

Termination, 289, 290
follow up, 290, 291
see Ethical challenges
Termination phase, 275, 276
case study processes, 283-287
conceptualizing the experience, 276, 277
endings by default, 280, 281
forced endings, 281-283
manner of termination, 298-300
negotiated endings, 277, 278, 291
planned endings, 278-280
see Ethical challenges
Therapeutic alliance, 54, 60
alliance threatening interactions, 252
alliance threatening transference reenactments, 252, 253
and cognitive analytic therapy (CAT), 252, 254, 258
applications/implications of the model, 267-269
early parental relationships and, 190
impasses, 191-193
markers of alliance-threatening enactments, 257

model of enactment resolution, 256
process factors and psychotherapy outcome, 252
refined model of RRP enactment resolution, 260-263
research strategy, 253
resolution of alliance ruptures, 264
resolving alliance threats in CAT, 253, 254
rupture in, 188-194
rupture-repair cycles, 194, 195
task analysis, 257
testing the model, 265-267
the empirical analysis, 260
the rational analysis, 258-260
Therapy Experience Questionnaire (TEQ), 253
Type 1 alliance, 190, 191
vs. transference, 189-191
working alliance, 190, 191
see Rupture episodes
Therapist Involvement Scale (TIS)
factors in, 296, 297
Therapist representation
enduring qualities, 300, 301
representational change, 304, 305
Therapist Representation Inventory (TRI), 295, 296
Therapy allegiance, 5, 18, 19
Training exercises,
and CCRT, 156-162
and constructing interventions, 160
and formulating narratives, 157-159
appropriate use of, 168-182
frequency of 151-153
rating accuracy of interpretations, 161, 162
Transference interpretations
see Constructing interpretations
suitability, 170
with high- vs. low-QOR patients, 171-178

with varying patients, 166-182
with the older patient, 365-368
see also Therapeutic alliance
Treatment of Depression
Collaborative Research Program
(TDRCP), 5
Treatment plan
and client characteristics, 330, 331
Triangle of conflict, 107
see Focus
Triangle of person, 107
see Focus

Types of patients
QOR patients, 169, 170
Types of patients
transference and, 167-178

W

Working alliance
supervision and, 330, 332, 333
see also Therapeutic alliance

Lightning Source UK Ltd.
Milton Keynes UK
UKOW06f0903281217
314956UK00007BC/597/P